Present and Future Perspectives of Vascular Interventional Radiology

Present and Future Perspectives of Vascular Interventional Radiology

Editor

Julien Frandon

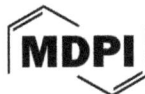

Basel • Beijing • Wuhan • Barcelona • Belgrade • Novi Sad • Cluj • Manchester

Editor
Julien Frandon
Department of Medical
Imaging
Nîmes University Hospital
University of Montpellier
Nimes
France

Editorial Office
MDPI AG
Grosspeteranlage 5
4052 Basel, Switzerland

This is a reprint of articles from the Special Issue published online in the open access journal *Journal of Personalized Medicine* (ISSN 2075-4426) (available at: https://www.mdpi.com/journal/jpm/special_issues/Perspectives_Vascular_Interventional_Radiology).

For citation purposes, cite each article independently as indicated on the article page online and as indicated below:

Lastname, A.A.; Lastname, B.B. Article Title. *Journal Name* **Year**, *Volume Number*, Page Range.

ISBN 978-3-7258-1507-4 (Hbk)
ISBN 978-3-7258-1508-1 (PDF)
doi.org/10.3390/books978-3-7258-1508-1

© 2024 by the authors. Articles in this book are Open Access and distributed under the Creative Commons Attribution (CC BY) license. The book as a whole is distributed by MDPI under the terms and conditions of the Creative Commons Attribution-NonCommercial-NoDerivs (CC BY-NC-ND) license.

Contents

About the Editor vii

Julien Frandon and Jean-Paul Beregi
Special Issue: Present and Future Perspectives of Vascular Interventional Radiology
Reprinted from: *J. Pers. Med.* 2023, 13, 1131, doi:10.3390/jpm13071131 1

Salim A. Si-Mohamed, Alexandra Cierco, Delphine Gamondes, Lauria Marie Restier, Laura Delagrange, Vincent Cottin, et al.
Embolization of Recurrent Pulmonary Arteriovenous Malformations by Ethylene Vinyl Alcohol Copolymer (Onyx®) in Hereditary Hemorrhagic Telangiectasia: Safety and Efficacy
Reprinted from: *J. Pers. Med.* 2022, 12, 1091, doi:10.3390/jpm12071091 4

Gregory Amouyal, Louis Tournier, Constance de Margerie-Mellon, Damien Bouda, Atanas Pachev, Jessica Assouline, et al.
Feasibility of Outpatient Transradial Prostatic Artery Embolization and Safety of a Shortened Deflation Protocol for Hemostasis
Reprinted from: *J. Pers. Med.* 2022, 12, 1138, doi:10.3390/jpm12071138 17

Gregory Amouyal, Louis Tournier, Constance De Margerie-Mellon, Atanas Pachev, Jessica Assouline, Damien Bouda, et al.
Safety Profile of Ambulatory Prostatic Artery Embolization after a Significant Learning Curve: Update on Adverse Events
Reprinted from: *J. Pers. Med.* 2022, 12, 1261, doi:10.3390/jpm12081261 27

Xiang-Ke Niu and Xiao-Feng He
A Nomogram Based on Preoperative Lipiodol Deposition after Sequential Retreatment with Transarterial Chemoembolization to Predict Prognoses for Intermediate-Stage Hepatocellular Carcinoma
Reprinted from: *J. Pers. Med.* 2022, 12, 1375, doi:10.3390/jpm12091375 42

Julien Ghelfi, Ian Soulairol, Olivier Stephanov, Marylène Bacle, Hélène de Forges, Noelia Sanchez-Ballester, et al.
Feasibility of Neovessel Embolization in a Large Animal Model of Tendinopathy: Safety and Efficacy of Various Embolization Agents
Reprinted from: *J. Pers. Med.* 2022, 12, 1530, doi:10.3390/jpm12091530 59

Jean-François Hak, Caroline Arquizan, Federico Cagnazzo, Mehdi Mahmoudi, Francois-Louis Collemiche, Gregory Gascou, et al.
MRI Outcomes Achieved by Simple Flow Blockage Technique in Symptomatic Carotid Artery Stenosis Stenting
Reprinted from: *J. Pers. Med.* 2022, 12, 1564, doi:10.3390/jpm12101564 70

Alexis Coussy, Eva Jambon, Yann Le Bras, Christian Combe, Laurence Chiche, Nicolas Grenier and Clément Marcelin
The Safety and Efficacy of Hepatic Transarterial Embolization Using Microspheres and Microcoils in Patients with Symptomatic Polycystic Liver Disease
Reprinted from: *J. Pers. Med.* 2022, 12, 1624, doi:10.3390/jpm12101624 83

Joël Greffier, Djamel Dabli, Tarek Kammoun, Jean Goupil, Laure Berny, Ghizlane Touimi Benjelloun, et al.
Retrospective Analysis of Doses Delivered during Embolization Procedures over the Last 10 Years
Reprinted from: *J. Pers. Med.* 2022, 12, 1701, doi:10.3390/jpm12101701 95

Chloé Extrat, Sylvain Grange, Alexandre Mayaud, Loïc Villeneuve, Clément Chevalier, Nicolas Williet, et al.
Transarterial Embolization for Active Gastrointestinal Bleeding: Predictors of Early Mortality and Early Rebleeding
Reprinted from: *J. Pers. Med.* 2022, 12, 1856, doi:10.3390/jpm12111856 106

Pierre-Antoine Barral, Mariangela De Masi, Axel Bartoli, Paul Beunon, Arnaud Gallon, Farouk Tradi, et al.
Angio Cone-Beam CT (Angio-CBCT) and 3D Road-Mapping for the Detection of Spinal Cord Vascularization in Patients Requiring Treatment for a Thoracic Aortic Lesion: A Feasibility Study
Reprinted from: *J. Pers. Med.* 2022, 12, 1890, doi:10.3390/jpm12111890 119

Eva Jambon, Yann Le Bras, Gregoire Cazalas, Nicolas Grenier and Clement Marcelin
Pelvic Venous Insufficiency: Input of Short Tau Inversion Recovery Sequence
Reprinted from: *J. Pers. Med.* 2022, 12, 2055, doi:10.3390/jpm12122055 129

Rémi Grange, Lucile Grange, Clément Chevalier, Alexandre Mayaud, Loïc Villeneuve, Claire Boutet and Sylvain Grange
Transarterial Embolization for Spontaneous Soft-Tissue Hematomas: Predictive Factors for Early Death
Reprinted from: *J. Pers. Med.* 2023, 13, 15, doi:10.3390/jpm13010015 138

Arne Estler, Eva Estler, You-Shan Feng, Ferdinand Seith, Maximilian Wießmeier, Rami Archid, et al.
Treatment of Acute Mesenteric Ischemia: Individual Challenges for Interventional Radiologists and Abdominal Surgeons
Reprinted from: *J. Pers. Med.* 2023, 13, 55, doi:10.3390/jpm13010055 151

Jean-François Aita, Thibault Agripnidis, Benoit Testud, Pierre-Antoine Barral, Alexis Jacquier, Anthony Reyre, et al.
Stenting in Brain Hemodynamic Injury of Carotid Origin Caused by Type A Aortic Dissection: Local Experience and Systematic Literature Review
Reprinted from: *J. Pers. Med.* 2023, 13, 58, doi:10.3390/jpm13010058 163

Benjamin Moulin, Massimiliano Di Primio, Olivier Vignaux, Jean Luc Sarrazin, Georgios Angelopoulos and Antoine Hakime
Prostate Artery Embolization: Challenges, Tips, Tricks, and Perspectives
Reprinted from: *J. Pers. Med.* 2023, 13, 87, doi:10.3390/jpm13010087 175

Skander Sammoud, Julien Ghelfi, Sandrine Barbois, Jean-Paul Beregi, Catherine Arvieux and Julien Frandon
Preventive Proximal Splenic Artery Embolization for High-Grade AAST-OIS Adult Spleen Trauma without Vascular Anomaly on the Initial CT Scan: Technical Aspect, Safety, and Efficacy—An Ancillary Study
Reprinted from: *J. Pers. Med.* 2023, 13, 889, doi:10.3390/jpm13060889 186

About the Editor

Julien Frandon

Julien Frandon is a renowned expert in the field of interventional radiology and serves as the Director of the Interventional Radiology Department at Nîmes University Hospital, France. Specializing in interventional oncology and vascular radiology, Pr Frandon has made significant contributions to patient care and medical advancements.

Leading a team in a state-of-the-art facility comprising four dedicated interventional radiology suites, including a cutting-edge 4D spect CT room, Pr Frandon is at the forefront of providing advanced diagnostic and therapeutic interventions. The integration of 4DCT technology allows for real-time dynamic imaging, enhancing precision and accuracy during procedures.

In addition to clinical excellence, Pr Julien Frandon is actively involved in research endeavors, focusing on the development of novel treatments and translating them from laboratory settings to bedside applications. With access to a large animal laboratory, they explore new indications and further refines interventional techniques, pushing the boundaries of medical innovation.

Pr Julien Frandon is not just dedicated to advancing patient care; they are passionate about the education and mentorship of future interventional radiologists. Embracing innovative teaching methodologies, such as gamified learning, they frequently foster an engaging and interactive educational environment. By incorporating game-based approaches that inspire and empower students, Pr Frandon ensures creates a strong foundation of knowledge and skills for anyone they teach.

With an impressive portfolio of accomplishments, Pr Julien Frandon exemplifies leadership, expertise, and a commitment to pushing the frontiers of interventional radiology. Their groundbreaking work in interventional oncology and vascular radiology, state-of-the-art facilities, translational research, and innovative teaching methods make them a respected authority in the field.

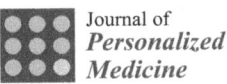

Editorial

Special Issue: Present and Future Perspectives of Vascular Interventional Radiology

Julien Frandon * and Jean-Paul Beregi

Department of Medical Imaging, IPI Plateform, Nîmes University Hospital, University of Montpellier, Medical Imaging Group Nîmes, IMAGINE, 30029 Nîmes, France; jean.paul.beregi@chu-nimes.fr
* Correspondence: julien.frandon@chu-nimes.fr; Tel.: +33-466-683-309

Citation: Frandon, J.; Beregi, J.-P. Special Issue: Present and Future Perspectives of Vascular Interventional Radiology. *J. Pers. Med.* **2023**, *13*, 1131. https://doi.org/10.3390/jpm13071131

Received: 5 July 2023
Accepted: 10 July 2023
Published: 12 July 2023

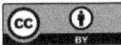

Copyright: © 2023 by the authors. Licensee MDPI, Basel, Switzerland. This article is an open access article distributed under the terms and conditions of the Creative Commons Attribution (CC BY) license (https://creativecommons.org/licenses/by/4.0/).

The field of vascular interventional radiology has witnessed remarkable advancements, transforming the landscape of patient care for both vascular and non-vascular pathologies. Through minimally invasive techniques, we can now offer therapeutic alternatives with reduced complications to patients who are not eligible for conventional treatments. With the emergence of personalized therapies tailored to specific pathologies, disease stages, and patient characteristics, we find ourselves at the forefront of a new era in medicine where treatments are uniquely tailored to each individual.

This Special Issue of the *Journal of Personalized Medicine* features a comprehensive collection of 16 articles, primarily focusing on embolization, a major theme in vascular interventional radiology. Embolization techniques have revolutionized the field, providing effective treatment options for various conditions. Within this issue, we delve into various aspects of embolization, including the embolization of the prostatic artery [1], splenic trauma [2], polycystic liver disease [3], soft tissue hematomas [4], pulmonary arteriovenous malformation [5], gastrointestinal bleeding [6], and even emerging themes such as musculoskeletal embolization [7]. These articles showcase the breadth and depth of research in the field, offering insights into the latest advancements and personalized approaches in embolization therapies.

One prominent focus of this issue revolves around prostatic artery embolization, an increasingly promising technique for treating benign prostatic hyperplasia. The articles within this issue present invaluable insights, offering tips and tricks to enhance the precision of the procedure using real-time navigation [8] devices and showcasing the benefits of radial access in facilitating outpatient management [9]. These techniques not only bolster the safety and efficiency of the procedure but also lead to reduced patient recovery times.

While embolization techniques have effectively addressed vascular pathologies, interventional radiology goes beyond vessel occlusion to include vessel recanalization. In cases of mesenteric ischemia, for instance, revascularization procedures have offered new avenues for treatment, restoring blood flow to ischemic organs and improving patient outcomes [10]. Furthermore, interventional radiologists have played a crucial role in enhancing vascularization by deploying stents in carotid arteries to improve blood supply to the brain [11,12]. Hence, interventional radiology not only occludes vessels but also serves as a powerful tool to reestablish perfusion, ultimately enhancing the overall management of various medical conditions.

In addition to its therapeutic applications, vascular interventional radiology is crucial in the diagnostic realm. By integrating the latest guidance technologies, such as cone beam CT, interventional radiologists can obtain detailed preoperative mapping for complex aortic surgeries [13]. New game-changing technologies such as 4DCT are helping to optimise patient exposure to X-rays for increasingly complex treatments [14]. In the same vein, this issue shows the contribution of MRI in diagnosing pelvic congestion syndrome, a condition often misdiagnosed or misunderstood, causing chronic pain and significant health challenges [15]. The synergy between advanced imaging techniques and interventional radiology empowers clinicians to make informed decisions, resulting in safer and more effective patient treatments.

Beyond vascular pathologies, several articles shed light on the application of vascular interventional radiology in treating non-vascular pathologies, including tendon pathology [7] and hepatocellular cancer [16]. These contributions underscore the importance of comprehending the underlying pathophysiology of these conditions and developing personalized therapeutic approaches.

Collectively, the articles published in this Special Issue of the *Journal of Personalized Medicine* underscore the pivotal role of vascular interventional radiology in contemporary clinical practice. These advances provide patients with innovative, minimally invasive treatment alternatives that reduce complications and enhance their overall quality of life. As personalized medicine continues to evolve, vascular interventional radiology is poised to play an increasingly significant role in delivering tailored treatments that cater to the specific requirements of individual patients.

In conclusion, we extend our gratitude to the authors for their valuable contributions to this Special Issue. Their research and insights hold immense potential to shape the future of vascular interventional radiology, driving the paradigm of personalized medicine. We encourage readers to delve into the articles and embrace the transformative power of innovative interventions in their pursuit of enhanced patient care.

Author Contributions: Conceptualization, J.F. and J.-P.B.; methodology, J.F.; validation, J.F. and J.-P.B.; formal analysis, J.F.; investigation, J.F.; resources, J.F.; data curation, J.F.; writing—original draft preparation, J.F.; writing—review and editing, J.F. and J.-P.B.; visualization, J.-P.B.; supervision, J.-P.B. All authors have read and agreed to the published version of the manuscript.

Funding: This research received no external funding.

Conflicts of Interest: The authors declare no conflict of interest.

References

1. Amouyal, G.; Tournier, L.; De Margerie-Mellon, C.; Pachev, A.; Assouline, J.; Bouda, D.; De Bazelaire, C.; Marques, F.; Le Strat, S.; Desgrandchamps, F.; et al. Safety Profile of Ambulatory Prostatic Artery Embolization after a Significant Learning Curve: Update on Adverse Events. *J. Pers. Med.* **2022**, *12*, 1261. [CrossRef] [PubMed]
2. Sammoud, S.; Ghelfi, J.; Barbois, S.; Beregi, J.-P.; Arvieux, C.; Frandon, J. Preventive Proximal Splenic Artery Embolization for High-Grade AAST-OIS Adult Spleen Trauma without Vascular Anomaly on the Initial CT Scan: Technical Aspect, Safety, and Efficacy—An Ancillary Study. *J. Pers. Med.* **2023**, *13*, 889. [CrossRef] [PubMed]
3. Coussy, A.; Jambon, E.; Le Bras, Y.; Combe, C.; Chiche, L.; Grenier, N.; Marcelin, C. The Safety and Efficacy of Hepatic Transarterial Embolization Using Microspheres and Microcoils in Patients with Symptomatic Polycystic Liver Disease. *J. Pers. Med.* **2022**, *12*, 1624. [CrossRef] [PubMed]
4. Grange, R.; Grange, L.; Chevalier, C.; Mayaud, A.; Villeneuve, L.; Boutet, C.; Grange, S. Transarterial Embolization for Spontaneous Soft-Tissue Hematomas: Predictive Factors for Early Death. *J. Pers. Med.* **2022**, *13*, 15. [CrossRef] [PubMed]
5. Si-Mohamed, S.A.; Cierco, A.; Gamondes, D.; Restier, L.M.; Delagrange, L.; Cottin, V.; Dupuis-Girod, S.; Revel, D. Embolization of Recurrent Pulmonary Arteriovenous Malformations by Ethylene Vinyl Alcohol Copolymer (Onyx®) in Hereditary Hemorrhagic Telangiectasia: Safety and Efficacy. *J. Pers. Med.* **2022**, *12*, 1091. [CrossRef] [PubMed]
6. Extrat, C.; Grange, S.; Mayaud, A.; Villeneuve, L.; Chevalier, C.; Williet, N.; Le Roy, B.; Boutet, C.; Grange, R. Transarterial Embolization for Active Gastrointestinal Bleeding: Predictors of Early Mortality and Early Rebleeding. *J. Pers. Med.* **2022**, *12*, 1856. [CrossRef] [PubMed]
7. Ghelfi, J.; Soulairol, I.; Stephanov, O.; Bacle, M.; de Forges, H.; Sanchez-Ballester, N.; Ferretti, G.; Beregi, J.-P.; Frandon, J. Feasibility of Neovessel Embolization in a Large Animal Model of Tendinopathy: Safety and Efficacy of Various Embolization Agents. *J. Pers. Med.* **2022**, *12*, 1530. [CrossRef] [PubMed]
8. Moulin, B.; Di Primio, M.; Vignaux, O.; Sarrazin, J.L.; Angelopoulos, G.; Hakime, A. Prostate Artery Embolization: Challenges, Tips, Tricks, and Perspectives. *J. Pers. Med.* **2022**, *13*, 87. [CrossRef] [PubMed]
9. Amouyal, G.; Tournier, L.; de Margerie-Mellon, C.; Bouda, D.; Pachev, A.; Assouline, J.; de Bazelaire, C.; Marques, F.; Le Strat, S.; Desgrandchamps, F.; et al. Feasibility of Outpatient Transradial Prostatic Artery Embolization and Safety of a Shortened Deflation Protocol for Hemostasis. *J. Pers. Med.* **2022**, *12*, 1138. [CrossRef] [PubMed]
10. Estler, A.; Estler, E.; Feng, Y.-S.; Seith, F.; Wießmeier, M.; Archid, R.; Nikolaou, K.; Grözinger, G.; Artzner, C. Treatment of Acute Mesenteric Ischemia: Individual Challenges for Interventional Radiologists and Abdominal Surgeons. *J. Pers. Med.* **2022**, *13*, 55. [CrossRef] [PubMed]

11. Aita, J.-F.; Agripnidis, T.; Testud, B.; Barral, P.-A.; Jacquier, A.; Reyre, A.; Alnuaimi, A.; Girard, N.; Tradi, F.; Habert, P.; et al. Stenting in Brain Hemodynamic Injury of Carotid Origin Caused by Type A Aortic Dissection: Local Experience and Systematic Literature Review. *J. Pers. Med.* **2022**, *13*, 58. [CrossRef] [PubMed]
12. Hak, J.-F.; Arquizan, C.; Cagnazzo, F.; Mahmoudi, M.; Collemiche, F.-L.; Gascou, G.; Lefevre, P.-H.; Derraz, I.; Labreuche, J.; Mourand, I.; et al. MRI Outcomes Achieved by Simple Flow Blockage Technique in Symptomatic Carotid Artery Stenosis Stenting. *J. Pers. Med.* **2022**, *12*, 1564. [CrossRef] [PubMed]
13. Barral, P.-A.; De Masi, M.; Bartoli, A.; Beunon, P.; Gallon, A.; Tradi, F.; Hak, J.-F.; Gaudry, M.; Jacquier, A. Angio Cone-Beam CT (Angio-CBCT) and 3D Road-Mapping for the Detection of Spinal Cord Vascularization in Patients Requiring Treatment for a Thoracic Aortic Lesion: A Feasibility Study. *J. Pers. Med.* **2022**, *12*, 1890. [CrossRef] [PubMed]
14. Greffier, J.; Dabli, D.; Kammoun, T.; Goupil, J.; Berny, L.; Benjelloun, G.T.; Beregi, J.-P.; Frandon, J. Retrospective Analysis of Doses Delivered during Embolization Procedures over the Last 10 Years. *J. Pers. Med.* **2022**, *12*, 1701. [CrossRef] [PubMed]
15. Jambon, E.; Le Bras, Y.; Cazalas, G.; Grenier, N.; Marcelin, C. Pelvic Venous Insufficiency: Input of Short Tau Inversion Recovery Sequence. *J. Pers. Med.* **2022**, *12*, 2055. [CrossRef] [PubMed]
16. Niu, X.-K.; He, X.-F. A Nomogram Based on Preoperative Lipiodol Deposition after Sequential Retreatment with Transarterial Chemoembolization to Predict Prognoses for Intermediate-Stage Hepatocellular Carcinoma. *J. Pers. Med.* **2022**, *12*, 1375. [CrossRef] [PubMed]

Disclaimer/Publisher's Note: The statements, opinions and data contained in all publications are solely those of the individual author(s) and contributor(s) and not of MDPI and/or the editor(s). MDPI and/or the editor(s) disclaim responsibility for any injury to people or property resulting from any ideas, methods, instructions or products referred to in the content.

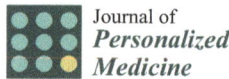 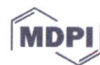

Article

Embolization of Recurrent Pulmonary Arteriovenous Malformations by Ethylene Vinyl Alcohol Copolymer (Onyx®) in Hereditary Hemorrhagic Telangiectasia: Safety and Efficacy

Salim A. Si-Mohamed [1,2,*], Alexandra Cierco [1], Delphine Gamondes [1], Lauria Marie Restier [3], Laura Delagrange [4,5], Vincent Cottin [6], Sophie Dupuis-Girod [4,5] and Didier Revel [1,2]

1. Department of Cardiovascular and Thoracic Radiology, Louis Pradel Hospital, Hospices Civils de Lyon, 59 Boulevard Pinel, 69500 Bron, France; alexandracierco@gmail.com (A.C.); delphine.gamondes@chu-lyon.fr (D.G.); didier.revel@chu-lyon.fr (D.R.)
2. CREATIS, UMR 5220, Univ Lyon, INSA Lyon, Claude Bernard University Lyon 1, 69100 Lyon, France
3. Rockfeller Faculty of Medicine, Lyon Est, Claude Bernard University Lyon 1, 69003 Lyon, France; lauria.restier@etu.univ-lyon1.fr
4. Department of Genetics, Hôpital Femme-Mère-Enfants, Hospices Civils de Lyon, 69677 Bron, France; laura.delagrange@chu-lyon.fr (L.D.); sophie.dupuis-girod@chu-lyon.fr (S.D.-G.)
5. Centre National de Référence Pour la Maladie de Rendu-Osler, 69677 Bron, France
6. National Reference Center for Rare Pulmonary Diseases, Louis Pradel Hospital, Hospices Civils de Lyon, UMR 754, INRAE, Claude Bernard University Lyon 1, Member of ERN-LUNG, 69500 Bron, France; vincent.cottin@chu-lyon.fr
* Correspondence: salim.si-mohamed@chu-lyon.fr; Tel.: +33-4-26-10-94-99; Fax: +33-4-72-07-18-86

Abstract: Objectives: To evaluate short- and long-term safety and efficacy of embolization with Onyx® for recurrent pulmonary arteriovenous malformations (PAVMs) in hereditary hemorrhagic telangiectasia (HHT). Methods: In total, 45 consecutive patients (51% women, mean (SD) age 53 (18) years) with HHT referred to a reference center for treatment of recurrent PAVM were retrospectively included from April 2014 to July 2021. Inclusion criteria included evidence of PAVM recurrence on CT or angiography, embolization using Onyx® and a minimal 1-year-follow-up CT or angiography. Success was defined based on the standard of reference criteria on unenhanced CT or pulmonary angiography if a recurrence was suspected. PAVMs were analyzed in consensus by two radiologists. The absence of safety distance, as defined by a too-short distance for coil/plug deployment, i.e., between 0.5 and 1 cm, between the proximal extremity of the primary embolic material used and a healthy upstream artery branch, was reported. Results: In total, 70 PAVM were analyzed. Mean (SD) follow-up was 3 (1.3) years. Safety distance criteria were missing in 33 (47%) PAVMs. All procedures were technically successful, with a short-term occlusion rate of 100% using a mean (SD) of 0.6 (0.5) mL of Onyx®. The long-term occlusion rate was 60%. No immediate complication directly related to embolization was reported, nor was any severe long-term complication such as strokes or cerebral abscesses. Conclusions: In HHT, treatment of recurrent PAVM with Onyx® showed satisfactory safety and efficacy, with an immediate occlusion rate of 100% and a long-term rate of 60%.

Keywords: hereditary hemorrhagic telangiectasia; Rendu-Osler-Weber disease; thorax; arteriovenous malformations; embolization

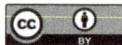

1. Introduction

Arteriovenous malformations are defined as abnormal connections between an artery and a vein and are a common symptom of a rare autosomal dominant orphan disease, the hereditary hemorrhagic telangiectasia (HHT) [1]. Pulmonary arteriovenous malformations (PAVMs) are reported in 30–50% of HHT patients [2]. Because of their abnormal connection, PAVMs bypass the filter of the capillary bed, causing a right-to-left shunt with a high risk of embolic strokes and cerebral abscesses for the patients [3–6].

Embolization is the standard of care for PAVM treatment [7–9]. However, up to 25% of successful embolizations require second treatment due to PAVM recurrence [9,10]. The embolization agents used in the treatment of recurrent PAVMs are solid embolic materials such as coils or plugs. Embolization may be performed according to two different techniques: embolization upstream of the previous embolic materials, more common and technically easier, or embolization downstream of the previous embolic materials, technically difficult but more effective [11]. However, in some cases, retreatment may not be possible because of a too-short afferent artery in case of failure of repeated embolizations (use of numerous coils) or difficult access through the pre-implanted materials [12]. In these cases, the last resort is then surgery.

An ethylene vinyl alcohol copolymer (Onyx®), a liquid embolic agent with physico-chemical properties allowing safe and distal embolization, was recently validated in the treatment of cerebral arteriovenous malformations [13]. It was shown to be non-adherent, to have a progressive solidification, a good cohesion, a high vascular penetration and a very weak inflammatory effect on the endothelium [14]. In the lungs, its use for the treatment of naïve treated PAVM is deemed at too high a risk because of its specific architecture showing high flow in the shunt. However, in the case of recurrent PAVM with a lower flow because of the pre-implanted materials, its use may be an appropriate alternative to solid embolic materials and may allow overcoming inaccessible PAVM embolization.

The objectives of this study were to evaluate in the short- and long-term the safety and efficacy of embolization with Onyx® for recurrent pulmonary arteriovenous malformations in HHT.

2. Materials and Methods

2.1. Study Design

This was a monocentric retrospective study in a reference center. It was approved by the local institutional review board; written consent was waived in accordance with the retrospective character of the study. Clinical, biological and imaging data for all the patients included were extracted from the HHT National Reference Centre database (CIROCO).

2.2. Study Population

In total, 62 consecutive patients were retrospectively reviewed from April 2014 to July 2021; 45 patients were eligible for the study, consisting of 70 embolization procedures (flow chart). Inclusion criteria were the following: HHT diagnosis based on the Curaçao criteria [1], evidence of PAVM recurrence on CT and/or angiography, embolization using Onyx® and a 1-year follow-up CT or angiography examination.

2.3. Clinical and Biological Data

The standard clinical follow-up consisted of an annual consultation with an HHT specialist at our center, with a pneumologist or with organ specialists when necessary (e.g., hepatologist, cardiologist or neurologist). Clinical and biological parameters were recorded during hospitalization and during follow-up to evaluate the embolization safety and efficacy.

2.4. Follow-Up Imaging Protocol

Standard imaging follow-up consisted of unenhanced chest CT one year after embolization. Recurrence was diagnosed based on the standard of reference criteria [8]: efferent vein longer than 2.5 mm and/or increased diameter of the efferent vein or aneurysmal sac. A pulmonary CT angiography or a pulmonary angiography was then performed to conclude the presence of recurrence. This allows defining two groups, i.e., a long-term occlusion (LTO) group for patients with persistent occlusion at follow-up and a short-term occlusion (STO) group for patients with occlusion immediately after embolization but with recurrence at follow-up.

2.5. Pulmonary Arteriovenous Malformation Imaging

Two radiologists (with 1 and 6 years of experience) reviewed in consensus, in a random order, all imaging data, i.e., CT before embolization, follow-up CT, pulmonary angiography during embolization and recurrence follow-up pulmonary angiography. In case of difficulty in reaching a consensus, a third radiologist with 15 years of experience was consulted. The radiologists were blinded to patient, PAVMs status and patient's clinical history for all evaluations. Among the multiple PAVM characteristics collected on CT images, the radiologists recorded the absence of safety distance defined as a too-short distance for coil/plug deployment, i.e., between 0.5 and 1 cm, between the proximal extremity of the primary embolic material used and a healthy upstream artery branch. Recurrence was defined on pre-embolization pulmonary angiogram as recanalization (on the axis perfused by flow through a previously placed coil nest), reperfusion (embolized feeder occluded but presence of small feeders from adjacent normal pulmonary arteries) or both.

Further methods details are provided in Appendix A.

2.6. Embolization

Embolization was performed using the routine procedures of our institution, via a common femoral venous access, under local anesthesia. Catheterization was performed using a 5 French catheter through the pulmonary artery and then with a microcatheter to reach a point as distal as possible within the feeding artery so as to deposit the embolic material (Onyx® 18 or coils).

Concerning the embolic material, a dimethyl sulfoxide compatible microcatheter was required to perform supra-selective catheterization of the feeding artery. Onyx® embolization needed flushing of the microcatheter with a saline solution and then with dimethyl sulfoxide to fill the microcatheter's "dead space". Onyx® was injected slowly into the feeding artery. It was stopped if a leakage in the upstream arterial branches or in the aneurysmal sac downstream of the embolic materials* was identified on non-subtracted angiography. Immediately after embolization, the efficiency of the treatment was evaluated on a selective non-subtracted angiography to confirm the correct deployment of the embolic material (within, downstream or upstream of the previous embolic material) and on angiography to confirm the complete occlusion (absence of vein opacification) and the pulmonary vascularization in the non-involved arterial territory.

2.7. Statistical Analysis

Statistical analyses were performed using the Prism software package (version 8, GraphPad) and the SPSS software (IBM_SPSS Statistics 21; 2020).

All p-values < 0.05 were considered significant. Data are expressed as means ± standard deviations (SD) for normally distributed variables and as medians and interquartile ranges (IQR). Categorical variables are described as frequencies and percentages. Differences in diameter for the efferent vein and the aneurysmal sac between pre-embolization and follow-up CT were calculated. Ordinal qualitative variables were compared between the two groups using a non-parametric Mann–Whitney test, and continuous variables using a two-paired Student t-test or a Wilcoxon rank-sum test, and as function of the normality of the variables using the d'Agostino–Pearson test.

3. Results

3.1. Study Population

In total, 45 consecutive patients (51% women, mean (SD) age 53 (18) years) were retrospectively included from April 2014 to July 2021; 70 embolization procedures were analyzed, corresponding to a mean of 1.4 PAVM per patient (Table 1 and Figure 1). Six PAVMs were treated a second time because of an iterative recurrence after a mean (SD) period of 1.9 (0.7) years. The mean (SD) follow-up period was 3 (1.3) years. Seventeen (24%) PAVMs were treated with a combination of coils and Onyx® because of the poor efficacy of the coils and the absence of distance safety after their deployment.

Table 1. Characteristics of patients.

Population		45
Women		23 (51)
Mean age (SD) (years)		53 (18)
Mean BMI (SD)		25.8 (6.2)
Diabetes mellitus		4 (9)
Tobacco		18 (40)
Mean oxygen saturation (range)		96.3 (92–100)
Curacao criteria		
	Family history of HHT symptoms	45
	Epistaxis	43 (96)
	Telangiectasia	41 (91)
	Liver AVM	7 (16)
	Gastro-intestinal AVM	5 (11)
	Brain AVM	3 (7)
HHT severe complications		
	Hemoptysis	3 (7)
	Brain abscess	5 (11)
	Stroke	7 (16)
Mutation		
	HHT1/ENG	36 (80)
	HHT2/ALK1	5 (11)
	SMAD4	0 (0)
	Unknown/unconfirmed	4 (9)
Unique PAVM		18 (40)
Multiple PAVM		27 (60)

PAVM—pulmonary arteriovenous malformation; HHT—hereditary hemorrhagic telangiectasia; ENG—endogline; SD—standard deviation. Unless otherwise indicated, data are numbers of patients, with percentages in parentheses.

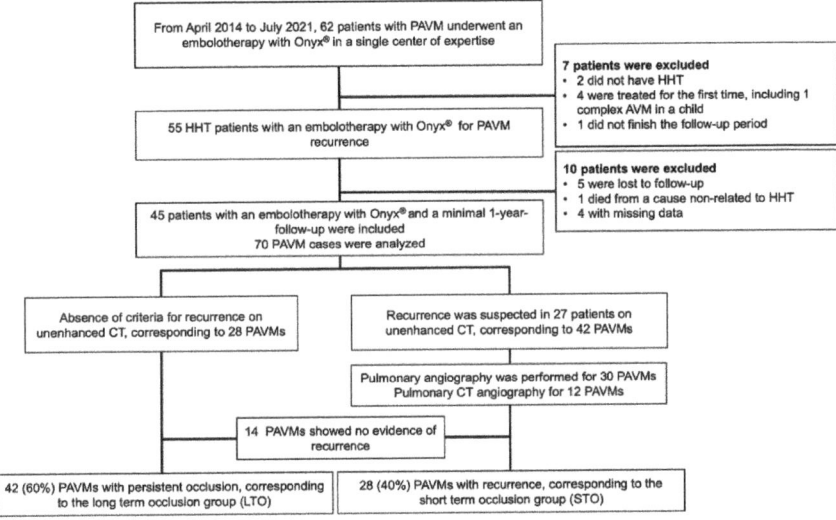

Figure 1. Study flowchart.

3.2. PAVM Characteristics before Embolization

All PAVMs were initially treated with coils. In total, 55 (86%) PAVMs were simple and similarly distributed in the short- and long-term occlusion groups (STO and LTO groups, respectively) (Table 2). The number of embolizations before Onyx® use was significantly higher in the STO group (2.5 ± 1.3 versus 1.8 ± 1.1 in the LTO group, $p = 0.01$). The vein diameter was significantly higher in the STO group, 5.5 ± 5.6 mm versus 3.4 ± 1.0 mm in the LTO group ($p < 0.01$), as well as the aneurysm diameter, 8 ± 6.1 mm versus 3.4 ± 4.1 mm in the LTO group ($p < 0.01$). Recanalization through the embolic materials was found in 98% of the cases in the LTO and 100% in the STO group. On pulmonary angiography, there was no safety distance in 33 (47%) PAVMs, 17 (60%) PAVMs in the LTO group and 16 (43%) PAVMs in the STO group (Table 2).

Table 2. Pulmonary arteriovenous malformation data before embolization in the overall population and in the two groups (short- and long-term occlusion).

Criteria	Total	Long-Term Occlusion	Short-Term Occlusion	p
Previous procedures	70 (100)	42 (60)	28 (40)	NA
PAVMs naive from Onyx®	64 (91)	40 (95)	24 (86)	0.166
PAVMs previously treated with Onyx®	6 (9)	2 (5)	4 (14)	0.166
Simple PAVMs	61 (87)	36 (86)	25 (89)	0.664
Complex PAVMs	9 (14)	6 (15)	3 (13)	0.664
Mean number of embolizations before onyx per PAVM (SD)	2.0 (1.1)	1.8 (1.1)	2.5 (1.3)	0.01
Mean number of recurrence before Onyx® per PAVM	0.9 (1.1)	0.7 (1.0)	1.4 (1.2)	<0.01
PAVMs first treated with coils	70 (100)	42 (100)	28 (100)	1.00
PAVMs first treated with plugs and coils	2 (3)	2 (5)	0	0.245
Length between aneurysm and plug/coil < 10 mm	43 (61)	27 (64)	16 (57)	0.550
Vein diameter (mm)	4.2 (3.7)	3.4 (1.0)	5.5 (5.6)	<0.01
Aneurysm diameter (mm)	5.1 (5.4)	3.4 (4.1)	8 (6.1)	<0.01
Lobar location				
Upper right lobe	13 (19)	9 (21)	4 (14)	0.455
Middle lobe	7 (10)	4 (10)	3 (11)	0.872
Lower right lobe	22 (31)	11 (26)	11 (39)	0.251
Upper left lobe	6 (9)	5 (12)	1 (4)	0.226
Lower left lobe	22 (31)	13 (31)	9 (32)	0.917
Absence of safety distance	33 (47)	17 (60)	16 (43)	0.174
Mechanism of recurrence				
Recanalization	69 (98)	41 (98)	28 (100)	0.414
Reperfusion	10 (14)	7 (17)	3 (11)	0.489
Both	9 (13)	6 (67)	3 (23)	0.664
Incomplete primary treatment	0	0	0	1.000
Territory potentially at risk				
Lobar	2 (3)	1 (2)	1 (4)	0.771
Segmental	18 (26)	9 (21)	9 (32)	0.318
Sub-segmental	50 (71)	32 (76)	18 (64)	0.284

PAVM—pulmonary arteriovenous malformation. Unless otherwise indicated, data are numbers of initially treated PAVMs with percentages in parentheses.

3.3. Safety

No immediate complication related to the injection of dimethyl sulfoxide and Onyx® was reported. A mild anaphylactic reaction was reported during the pulmonary angiography, which did not require the arrest of the procedure.

No downstream leak in the aneurysmal sac or in the efferent vein or upstream leak in the healthy lobar arteries was reported (Table 3). Upstream leaks in the sub-segmental arteries were reported in 39 (56%) PAVMs and in the segmental arteries in 4 (6%) PAVMs.

Table 3. Onyx® embolization data and immediate complications in all PAVMs and in the two groups, short- and long-term occlusion.

Immediate Embolization Characteristics	Total	Long-Term Occlusion	Short-Term Occlusion	p
Per-embolization occlusion	70 (100)	42 (60)	28 (40)	1.00
Treatment type				
Onyx® only	53 (76)	31 (74)	22 (79)	0.65
Onyx® + coils	17 (24)	11 (26)	6 (21)	0.65
Onyx® volume, mL (SD)	0.6 (0.5)	0.5 (0.3)	0.7 (0.6)	0.23
Onyx® distribution **				
Upstream	48 (69)	30 (71)	18 (64)	0.53
Inside coiling	51 (73)	28 (67)	23 (82)	0.16
Downstream	13 (19)	7 (17)	6 (21)	0.62
Upstream + inside	29 (41)	16 (38)	13 (46)	0.49
Downstream + inside	13 (19)	7 (17)	6 (21)	0.62
Upstream + inside + downstream	5 (7)	2 (5)	3 (11)	0.35
Upstream leak outside the target				
At a lobar level	0	0	0	1.00
At a segmental level	4 (6)	2 (5)	2 (7)	1.00
At a sub-segmental level	39 (56)	25 (60)	14 (50)	0.68

Table 3. Cont.

Immediate Embolization Characteristics	Total	Long-Term Occlusion	Short-Term Occlusion	p
Perfusion defect in healthy territory				
Lobar territory	0	0	0	1.00
Segmental territory	0	0	0	1.00
Sub-segmental territory	20 (29)	13 (31)	7 (25)	0.59
Downstream leak in draining vein or aneurysmal sac	0	0	0	1.00
Downstream leak in systemic circulation	0	0	0	1.00
Procedure time, min (SD)	105 (34)	110 (33)	99 (35)	0.15
Volume of contrast agent, mL (SD)	110 (49)	116 (50)	102 (47)	0.19
Adverse events during hospitalization time	5 (7.1)	2 (2.8)	3 (4.3)	0.35
Allergy	1 (20)	0	1 (33.3)	0.22
Chest pain	1 (20)	0	1 (33.3)	0.22
Pleural effusion	0	0	0	1.00
Lung distal infarction	3 (60)	2 (100)	1 (33.3)	0.81
Lung infection	0	0	0	1.00
Brain abscess	0	0	0	1.00
Stroke	0	0	0	1.00
Access site complication	0	0	0	1.00

** Onyx distribution was characterized according to its presence within the pre-implanted embolic materials and/or downstream and/or upstream of it. Unless otherwise indicated, data are numbers of pulmonary arteriovenous malformations, with percentages in parentheses.

No pulmonary perfusion defect was reported in the lobar and segmental lung territories, and 20 (29%) defects were reported in sub-segmental territories. Lung infarctions were reported in three (7%) patients. They resolved spontaneously without requiring longer hospitalization or level 3 analgesics except for one patient for whom it was symptomatic with a 3-day hospitalization. All patients experienced a garlic smell following the dimethyl sulfoxide injection for a couple of days, with no other side effects.

No long-term migration of the Onyx® in the thoracic region was reported, neither brain abscess nor strokes. Hemoptysis due to systemic recruitment of the bronchial arteries from the PAVM was reported in two cases, 3.5 years after retreatment by Onyx® in the first case, related to the systemic reperfusion of a PAVM treated with coils only for the second case. Both were treated by embolization using coils in the bronchial territories.

3.4. Short-Term Efficacy

All procedures were technically successful with complete occlusion of the feeding artery. Procedure times were comparable between the LTO and STO groups (110 ± 33 min versus 99 ± 35 min, $p = 0.15$), as well as the volume of Onyx® delivered (0.5 ± 0.3 in the STO versus 0.7 ± 0.6 mL in the LTO group, $p = 0.23$) (Table 3). Onyx® filled the inside of the previously delivered coils in 73% of cases and the upstream artery in 69% of cases. Case examples are provided in Figures 2–6.

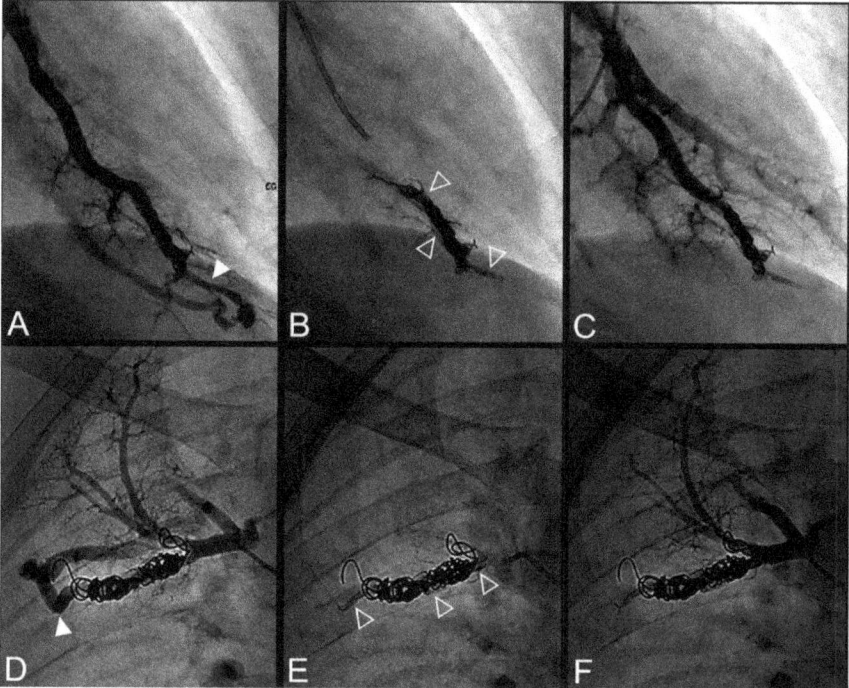

Figure 2. Case examples of a 68-year-old man (**A–C**) and 48-year-old man (**D–F**) treated for a simple recurrent pulmonary arteriovenous malformation. In both cases, digital subtraction angiography unsubtracted images showed a distance >10 mm between the first coil and the aneurysmal sac, which is considered a risk factor for recanalization. (**A–C**). Embolization was performed using Onyx® (0.3 mL) to fill the afferent artery in and downstream of the pre-implanted coils and resulted in an immediate complete occlusion, maintained after 23 months follow-up. No leak in the aneurysm or in the vein was reported. (**A**). Opacification of the afferent artery showed a recanalization through the pre-implanted coils (full arrowhead). (**B**). Opacity within, downstream and upstream of the coils (empty arrowheads) showed the distribution of Onyx® without any evidence of a leak in the aneurysmal sac. (**C**). Opacification of the afferent artery showed the absence of opacification of the aneurysmal sac and the efferent vein in favor of immediate occlusion. The opacification of the healthy arterial branch did not reveal any perfusion defect. (**D–F**). Embolization was performed using Onyx® (0.4 mL) to fill the afferent artery in and downstream of the pre-implanted coils and resulted in an immediate complete occlusion, with a recurrence 36 months after the procedure. No leak in the aneurysm or in the vein was reported. (**D**). Opacification of the afferent artery showed a recanalization through the pre-implanted coils (full arrowhead). (**E**). Opacity within, downstream and upstream of the coils (empty arrowheads) showed the distribution of Onyx® without any evidence of a leak in the aneurysmal sac. (**F**). Opacification of the afferent artery showed the absence of opacification of the aneurysmal sac and the efferent vein in favor of immediate occlusion.

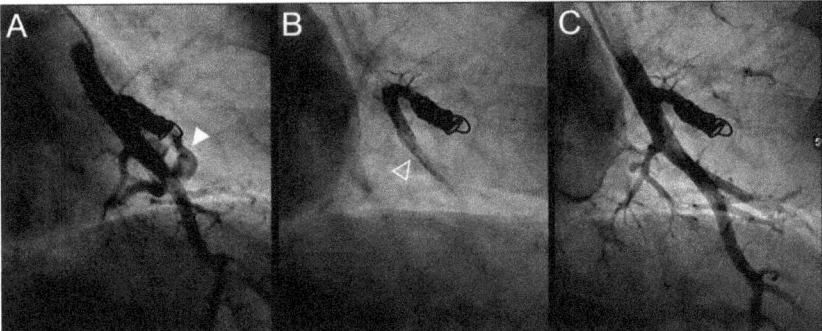

Figure 3. Case example of a 57-year-old woman treated for a simple recurrent pulmonary arteriovenous malformation (PAVM) in the lower left lobe. Digital subtraction angiography unsubtracted images showed a distance between the last coil and a healthy arterial branch too short to add additional coils. Embolization was thus performed using Onyx® (0.4 mL) to fill the afferent artery within the pre-implanted coils and resulted in an immediate complete occlusion, maintained after 13 months follow-up. No leak in the aneurysm or in the vein was reported. A leak upstream the coils in the segmental artery was reported without any consequence on lung perfusion (empty arrowhead). (**A**). Opacification of the afferent artery of a PAVM showed a recanalization through the pre-implanted coils (arrowhead). (**B**). Opacity in the coils and afferent artery showed the distribution of Onyx®, with an upstream leak in a segmental arterial branch (empty arrowhead). (**C**). Opacification of the afferent artery showed the absence of opacification of the aneurysmal sac and the efferent vein in favor of immediate occlusion. The opacification of the healthy arterial branch did not reveal any perfusion defect.

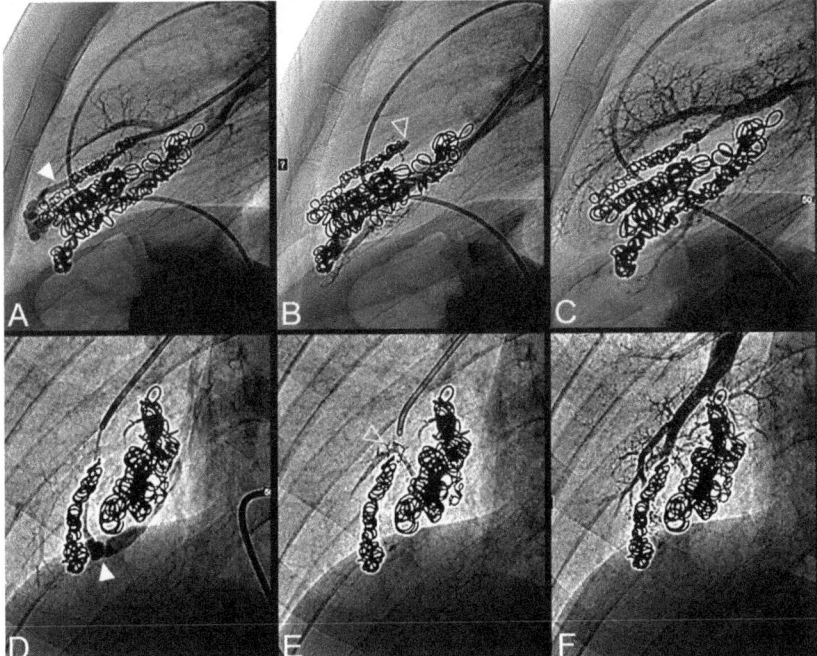

Figure 4. Case example of an 18-year-old man treated for a complex recurrent pulmonary arteriovenous malformation in the middle lobe. Digital subtraction angiography unsubtracted images showed a recanalization in two different segmental feeder arteries (**A–F**). Embolization was performed using Onyx®

(0.5 mL in each artery) to fill the afferent artery upstream and within the pre-implanted coiling and resulted in an immediate complete occlusion, maintained after 43 months follow-up. No leak in the aneurysm or in the vein was reported. (**A**). Opacification of an afferent artery (full head arrow) showed a recanalization through the pre-implanted coils. (**B**). Opacity upstream and in the last coil (empty arrowhead) showed the distribution of Onyx® without any evidence of a leak in the aneurysmal sac or proximal arterial branch. (**C**). Opacification of the afferent artery showed the absence of opacification of the aneurysmal sac and the efferent vein in favor of immediate occlusion. The opacification of the healthy arterial branch did not reveal any perfusion defect. (**D**). Opacification of a second afferent (full head arrow) artery showed a recanalization through the pre-implanted coils. (**E**). Opacity upstream of the coils showed a leak of Onyx® (empty arrowhead) without evidence of any leak in the aneurysmal sac. (**F**). Opacification of the afferent artery showed the absence of opacification of the aneurysmal sac and the efferent vein in favor of immediate occlusion. The opacification of the healthy arterial branch did not reveal any lung perfusion defect.

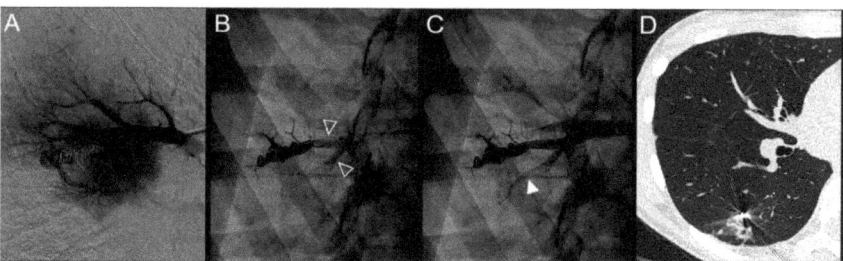

Figure 5. Case example of a 37-year-old woman treated for a simple recurrent pulmonary arteriovenous malformation in the lower right lobe. Embolization was performed using Onyx® (0.5 mL) to fill the afferent artery within the pre-implanted coils and resulted in an immediate complete occlusion, maintained at 34 months follow-up. No leak in the aneurysm or in the vein was reported, but a leak in the upstream sub-segmental arteries was identified. (**A**). Opacification of the afferent artery showed a recanalization through existing coiling. (**B**). Opacity within and upstream of the pre-implanted coils (empty arrowheads) showed the distribution of Onyx®, with a leak in a proximal arterial branch. (**C**). Opacification of the afferent artery showed the absence of opacification of the aneurysmal sac and the efferent vein in favor of immediate occlusion. An altered opacification in the upstream branch (full arrowhead) was identified due to the leak of Onyx®. (**D**). The one-year follow-up chest CT showed a distal lung infarction related to embolization. Of note, the patient did not suffer from chest pain or pleural effusion after the embolization procedure.

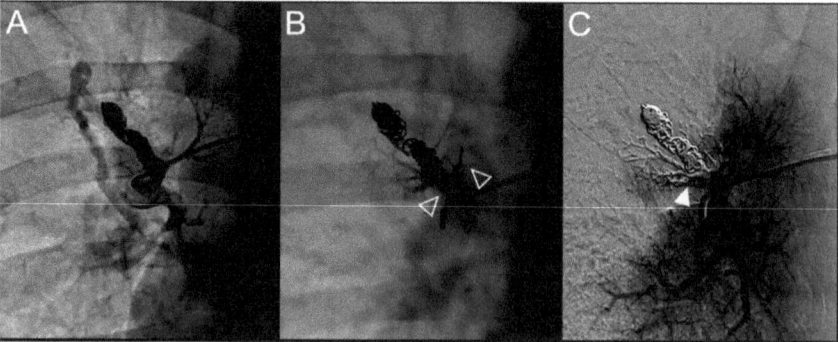

Figure 6. Case example of a 35-year-old man treated for a recurrent simple pulmonary arteriovenous malformation in the right lower lobe. The pulmonary angiograph showed a distance between the last coil and a healthy arterial branch too short to add additional coils. Embolization was thus performed using

Onyx® (0.4 mL) to fill the afferent artery upstream and in the pre-implanted coils, without any leak neither in the aneurysm nor in the vein. It resulted in an immediate complete occlusion until 46 months after the procedure when a recurrence was reported. (**A**). Opacification of the afferent artery of a PAVM in the lower right lobe showing a recanalization through the pre-implanted coils. (**B**). Opacity in and upstream (empty arrowheads) the coils showing the distribution of the Onyx®, without any evidence of a leak in the aneurysmal sac, but with a leak in the small arterial branches. (**C**). Opacification of the afferent artery showing the absence of opacification of the aneurysmal sac and the efferent vein in favor of immediate occlusion. A perfusion defect was identified in a sub-segmental territory (full head arrow), not related to a symptomatic lung infarction.

3.5. Long-Term Efficacy

Recurrence was suspected on CT in 27 patients (60%), a total of 42 PAVMs. Recurrence was further evaluated with pulmonary angiography for 30 PAVMs (25 examinations, 71%), among which 13 (43%) did not show evidence of recurrence, or with pulmonary CT angiography for 12 PAVMs (29%), among which one (8%) did not report recurrence evidence. Overall, 14 (47%) PAVMs showed no evidence of recurrence despite a non-reduction of the vein or aneurysm diameter (Table 4).

Table 4. PAVM follow-up data in the overall population and in the two groups, short- or long-term occlusion.

Long Time Follow-Up		Total	Long-Term Occlusion	Short-Term Occlusion	p
Number of PAVMs		70 (100)	42 (60)	28 (40)	
Follow-up time, months (SD)		34.8 (15.3)	25.2 (13.0)	34.1 (16.7)	0.5
Tobacco consumption		28 (40)	14 (33.3)	14 (50)	0.111
Pack-year of tobacco (SD)		9.3 (17.3)	8.8 (2.8)	11.8 (3.1)	0.133
PAVM characteristics	Aneurysm diameter, mm (SD)	3.9 (4.7)	2.1 (3.2)	7.0 (5.1)	<0.001
	Vein diameter, mm (SD)	2.9 (1.2)	2.4 (0.9)	3.8 (1.0)	<0.001
	Difference in aneurysm diameter, mm (SD) *	22.9 (37.2)	40.5 (39.1)	4.4 (24.4)	<0.01
	Difference in vein diameter, mm (SD) *	18.7 (21.7)	29.9 (18.2)	0.04 (12.1)	<0.001
Complications	Brain abscess	0	0	0	
	Stroke	0	0	0	
	Hemoptysis	2	0	2	
	Hemothorax	0	0	0	

PAVM—pulmonary arteriovenous malformation; SD—standard deviation. Unless otherwise indicated, data are numbers of patients, with percentages in parentheses. * Difference in size was calculated as a proportion of size reduction between baseline and follow-up CT.

A persistent occlusion with a mean reduction between before and after embolization of the aneurysm and vein diameter of 40% and 30% were reported in 42 (60%) PAVMs. On CT follow-up, the vein was significantly larger in the LTO group (3.8 ± 1.0 mm diameter versus 2.4 ± 0.9 mm in the STO group, $p < 0.001$) as well as the aneurysm (7.0 ± 5.1 mm versus 2.1 ± 3.2 mm, respectively, $p < 0.001$). To note, the after rate of success was 56.2% in PAVM treated only once with Onyx®.

4. Discussion

In this retrospective study conducted in an expert center, the safety and efficacy of the Onyx® liquid embolic agent were demonstrated for the embolization of recurrent pulmonary arteriovenous malformation in a hereditary hemorrhagic telangiectasia population. This technique allowed distal endovascular embolization, particularly for PAVMs not eligible for additional coils or plug embolization because of a high risk of occlusion of the collateral branch. All procedures were technically successful, with an immediate occlusion rate of 100%. In the long term, a 60% occlusion rate was reported, with no complications related to the embolization procedure.

Treatment of recurrent PAVM is a challenge. The success rates found in the literature vary from 0 to 80% [11,12,15,16]. In the present study, the long-term occlusion rate was 60%, with a specific 58% rate for recanalized PAVMs and 67% for both recanalized and reperfused PAVMs, in accordance with previous studies. Woodward et al. showed a 66% occlusion rate in 38 PAVMs and 83% for recanalized PAVMs [10]. Another team, Milic et al., showed a 42% occlusion rate in 33 PAVMs (19 patients) [12]. Additionally, embolization failed in 20% of the cases due to the absence of distance safety.

Some baseline variables were significantly different in the success and failure groups and may be determinant factors to consider before embolization. Recurrent PAVMs of the failure group presented the highest number of embolotherapy before retreatment with Onyx®, which may indicate a complicated and refractory type of PAVMs. They also presented large veins and aneurysms, which was not found in a previous study that showed that smaller PAVMs were associated with a higher rate of reperfusion [17]. The presence of a large feeding artery was shown to be a factor of recurrence [12] but was not evaluated in this study because of the pre-implanted embolic materials. Last, the proportion of PAVMs with coils deployed at more than 10 mm from the aneurysm, considered a factor of recurrence [12], was slightly higher in the STO group. Altogether, in our study, the recurrent PAVMs treated with Onyx® were comparable to those treated with standard embolic materials in previous studies.

This study reports, to our knowledge, for the first time, results of embolization of recurrent PAVMs using Onyx®. The choice of this embolic material was supported by the need to fill the pre-implanted materials, as shown in more than 70% of cases in which Onyx® filled the coils packing. Contrary to the glue, Onyx® does not present adhesive properties when in contact with the arterial walls but has "filling" properties which may have facilitated its use for slow and controlled distribution around the pre-implanted materials. It was supported by the lack of a safety distance between the pre-implanted materials and healthy collateral, as reported in 47% of the PAVMs treated. The criteria for embolization arrest were defined before the study started in consensus by our team, based on previous data of Onyx® embolization in other locations and on our experience in limiting the risk of a leak in the systemic circulation and in healthy pulmonary territories. Despite the evidence for treating the nidus in addition to the feeding artery in PAVM naïve of embolization [18,19], we avoided downstream leakages by stopping the procedure when Onyx® would go past the materials, which occurred in 19% of cases. However, no further leak was reported neither in the aneurysm nor in the efferent vein or in the systemic circulation, as confirmed during angiography or follow-up chest CT. The procedure was also stopped when Onyx® would go upstream of the pre-implanted embolic material in a healthy arterial branch. Nevertheless, in 69% of cases, an upstream leak in a non-involved arterial branch was reported, which opens to injection techniques under flow control [20]. Despite this high proportion, only 29% of these cases presented a perfusion defect on pulmonary angiography, from which only 4% of the patients reported a distal lung infarction, which was quasi-asymptomatic and resolved spontaneously. This low rate of perfusion defect, compared to the number of leaks in collaterals, may be explained by the non-obstructive deposition of Onyx® within the healthy artery, hardly differentiable from an obstructive deposition due to the opacity of this material on pulmonary angiogram. In addition, the low rate of lung infarctions, compared to the number of perfusion defects, may be explained either by the presence of asymptomatic infarctions or secondary recurrences of the embolized territory. Nevertheless, this complication is well-known and frequently reported in the endovascular treatment of PAVM [7] and would probably have been more frequent using coils or plugs because of the absence of a significant safety distance [21]. Finally, follow-up of some PAVMs showed no reduction in vein diameter or aneurysm size despite persistent occlusion, which raises the question of the expected reduction in PAVM size [8]. In our practice, we hypothesized this by a loss in vascular compliance after iterative embolization, opening to furthermore investigations.

According to our experience, the success of the procedure was defined according to the standard of reference, i.e., the absence of vein opacification during pulmonary angiography [8]. All procedures resulted in a complete occlusion immediately after Onyx® injection. The mean injected volume was 0.6 mL, low compared to that injected for cutaneous or cerebral arteriovenous malformations [13]. This may be explained by the specific angioarchitecture of PAVMs with a limited volume spare of a recanalized feeding artery and the absence of a nidus. That may explain that contrary to certain techniques of embolization with Onyx® that require a waiting time for polymerization before a second injection, we injected Onyx® continuously until the endpoint was reached.

This study has some limitations, mainly its retrospective and monocentric character. Additionally, the lack of a reference method for the diagnosis of persistent occlusion, i.e., pulmonary angiography, is a limitation. This choice was based on both the current practice in our expert center and on previous results showing sensitivity for recurrence of 98.4% for PAVMs with a vein diameter larger than 2.5 mm (10). Nevertheless, in case of a vein diameter higher than 2.5 mm and/or a recurrent diameter of the aneurysm sac and vein, we performed an injected examination in order to confirm the recurrence.

5. Conclusions

Embolization with Onyx® of recurrent pulmonary arteriovenous malformations allowed a short-term occlusion rate of 100% and a long-term rate of 60%, offering an additional option for the treatment of challenging recurrent pulmonary arteriovenous malformations in HHT.

Author Contributions: Conceptualization, S.A.S.-M., D.R. and D.G.; methodology, S.A.S.-M. and S.D.-G.; software, D.R.; validation, D.R. and S.D.-G.; formal analysis, S.A.S.-M. and A.C.; investigation, A.C., S.A.S.-M., L.M.R., L.D., D.R. and D.G.; resources, D.R. and D.G.; data curation, S.A.S.-M., D.R. and D.G.; writing—original draft preparation, S.A.S.-M. and A.C.; writing—review and editing, A.C., D.R., D.G., S.D.-G., L.D., L.M.R. and V.C.; visualization S.A.S.-M. and D.R.; supervision, D.R.; project administration, L.D. All authors have read and agreed to the published version of the manuscript.

Funding: This research received no external funding.

Institutional Review Board Statement: The study was conducted in accordance with the Declaration of Helsinki and approved by the Institutional Review Board of Hospices Civils de Lyon.

Informed Consent Statement: Patient consent was waived due to the retrospective character of the study.

Acknowledgments: We are deeply grateful to Hélène De Forges for her help in editing the manuscript.

Conflicts of Interest: The authors declare no conflict of interest.

Appendix A

The images were displayed on the PACS workstation in a core lab and were analyzed using the native images, the maximum intensity projection mode and multiplanar reconstructions (MPRs). For CT, analysis was first performed in parenchymal window (WW: 1600 Hounsfield units (HU), WL: −600 HU); the reader was then free to adjust the window width and the level values.

Before embolization, the following variables were collected on CT images lobar location and morphology (simple or complex), length between aneurysm and first embolic material, efferent vein diameter, largest aneurysm diameter, absence of safety distance (too short distance for coil/plug deployment between the proximal extremity of the primary embolic material used and a healthy upstream artery branch). The mechanism of recurrence (recanalization, reperfusion or both) was collected on the pre-embolization pulmonary angiogram. The following criteria were collected on the post-embolization pulmonary angiogram: leak outside the target and perfusion defect in healthy zone at a lobar, segmental or sub-segmental level and leak downstream in the draining vein and/or in the systemic circulation. On the follow-up, CT and pulmonary angiogram were collected for the following variables, the largest diameter of the aneurysmal sac and of efferent vein.

References

1. Shovlin, C.L.; Guttmacher, A.E.; Buscarini, E.; Faughnan, M.E.; Hyland, R.H.; Westermann, C.J.; Kjeldsen, A.D.; Plauchu, H. Diagnostic criteria for hereditary hemorrhagic telangiectasia (Ren-du-Osler-Weber syndrome). *Am. J. Med. Genet.* **2000**, *91*, 66–67. [CrossRef]
2. Berg, J.N.; Guttmacher, A.E.; Marchuk, D.A.; Porteous, M.E. Clinical heterogeneity in hereditary haemorrhagic telangiectasia: Are pulmonary arteriovenous malformations more common in families linked to endoglin? *J. Med. Genet.* **1996**, *33*, 256–257. [CrossRef] [PubMed]
3. Etievant, J.; Si-Mohamed, S.; Vinurel, N.; Dupuis-Girod, S.; Decullier, E.; Gamondes, D.; Khouatra, C.; Cottin, V.; Revel, D. Pulmonary arteriovenous malformations in hereditary haemorrhagic telangiectasia: Correlations between computed tomography findings and cerebral complications. *Eur. Radiol.* **2018**, *28*, 1338–1344. [CrossRef] [PubMed]
4. Shovlin, C.L.; Jackson, J.E.; Bamford, K.B.; Jenkins, I.H.; Benjamin, A.R.; Ramadan, H.; Kulinskaya, E. Primary determinants of ischaemic stroke/brain abscess risks are independent of severity of pulmonary arteriovenous malformations in hereditary haemorrhagic telangiectasia. *Thorax* **2008**, *63*, 259–266. [CrossRef]
5. Cottin, V.; Chinet, T.; Lavolé, A.; Corre, R.; Marchand, E.; Reynaud-Gaubert, M.; Plauchu, H.; Cordier, J.-F. Pulmonary Arteriovenous Malformations in Hereditary Hemorrhagic Telangiectasia: A series of 126 patients. *Medicine* **2007**, *86*, 1–17. [CrossRef]
6. Dupuis-Girod, S.; Cottin, V.; Shovlin, C. The Lung in Hereditary Hemorrhagic Telangiectasia. *Respiration* **2017**, *94*, 315–330. [CrossRef]
7. Shovlin, C.; Condliffe, R.; Donaldson, J.W.; Kiely, D.G.; Wort, S.J. British Thoracic Society Clinical Statement on Pulmonary Arteriovenous Malformations. *Thorax* **2017**, *72*, 1154–1163. [CrossRef]
8. Gamondès, D.; Si-Mohamed, S.; Cottin, V.; Gonidec, S.; Boussel, L.; Douek, P.; Revel, D. Vein Diameter on Unenhanced Multidetector CT Predicts Reperfusion of Pulmonary Arteriovenous Malformation after Embolotherapy. *Eur. Radiol.* **2016**, *26*, 2723–2729. [CrossRef]
9. Remy-Jardin, M.; Dumont, P.; Brillet, P.-Y.; Dupuis, P.; Duhamel, A.; Remy, J. Pulmonary Arteriovenous Malformations Treated with Embolotherapy: Helical CT Evaluation of Long-term Effectiveness after 2–21-Year Follow-up 1. *Radiology* **2006**, *239*, 576–585. [CrossRef]
10. Woodward, C.S.; Pyeritz, R.E.; Chittams, J.L.; Trerotola, S.O. Treated Pulmonary Arteriovenous Malformations: Patterns of Persistence and Associated Retreatment Success. *Vasc. Interv. Radiol.* **2013**, *269*, 8. [CrossRef]
11. Cusumano, L.R. Treatment of Recurrent Pulmonary Arteriovenous Malformations: Comparison of Proximal Versus Distal Embolization Technique. *Cardiovasc. Interv. Radiol.* **2020**, *43*, 29–36. [CrossRef] [PubMed]
12. Milic, A.; Chan, R.P.; Cohen, J.H.; Faughnan, M.E. Reperfusion of Pulmonary Arteriovenous Malformations after Embolotherapy. *J. Vasc. Interv. Radiol.* **2005**, *16*, 1675–1683. [CrossRef] [PubMed]
13. Szajner, M.; Roman, T.; Markowicz, J.; Szczerbo-Trojanowska, M. Onyx® in endovascular treatment of cerebral arteriovenous malformations—A review. *Pol. J. Radiol.* **2013**, *78*, 35–41. [CrossRef] [PubMed]
14. Kilani, M.S.; Izaaryene, J.; Cohen, F.; Varoquaux, A.; Gaubert, J.; Louis, G.; Jacquier, A.; Bartoli, J.; Moulin, G.; Vidal, V. Ethylene vinyl alcohol copolymer (Onyx®) in peripheral interventional radiology: Indications, advantages and limitations. *Diagn. Interv. Imaging* **2015**, *96*, 319–326. [CrossRef]
15. Pollak, J.S.; Saluja, S.; Thabet, A.; Henderson, K.J.; Denbow, N.; White, R.I. Clinical and anatomic outcomes after embolotherapy of pulmonary arteriovenous malformations. *J. Vasc. Interv. Radiol.* **2006**, *17*, 35–45. [CrossRef]
16. White, R.I. Pulmonary arteriovenous malformations: How do we diagnose them and why is it important to do so? *Radiology* **1992**, *182*, 633–635. [CrossRef]
17. Stein, E.J.; Chittams, J.L.; Miller, M.; Trerotola, S.O. Persistence in Coil-Embolized Pulmonary Arteriovenous Malformations with Feeding Artery Diameters of 3 mm or Less: A Retrospective Single-Center Observational Study. *J. Vasc. Interv. Radiol.* **2017**, *28*, 442–449. [CrossRef]
18. Shimohira, M.; Kiyosue, H.; Osuga, K.; Gobara, H.; Kondo, H.; Nakazawa, T.; Matsui, Y.; Hamamoto, K.; Ishiguro, T.; Maruno, M.; et al. Location of embolization affects patency after coil embolization for pulmonary arteriovenous malformations: Importance of time-resolved magnetic resonance angiography for diagnosis of patency. *Eur. Radiol.* **2021**, *31*, 5409–5420. [CrossRef]
19. Brill, R.M.; Guntau, M.; Wildgruber, M.; Brill, E.; Stangl, F.; Taute, B.-M.; Ukkat, J.; Goldann, C.; Wohlgemuth, W.A. Safety and Effectiveness of Ethylene Vinyl Alcohol Copolymer Embolization of Peripheral High-Flow Arteriovenous Malformations: Results of a Prospective Study. *J. Vasc. Interv. Radiol.* **2021**, *32*, 1644–1653.e1. [CrossRef]
20. Shi, Z.-S.; Loh, Y.; Gonzalez, N.; Tateshima, S.; Feng, L.; Jahan, R.; Duckwiler, G.; Viñuela, F. Flow control techniques for Onyx embolization of intracranial dural arteriovenous fistulae. *J. NeuroInterventional Surg.* **2013**, *5*, 311–316. [CrossRef]
21. Brillet, P.-Y.; Dumont, P.; Bouaziz, N.; Duhamel, A.; Laurent, F.; Remy, J.; Remy-Jardin, M. Pulmonary arteriovenous malformation treated with embolotherapy: Systemic collateral supply at multidetector ct angiography after 2–20-year follow-up. *Radiology* **2007**, *242*, 267–276. [CrossRef] [PubMed]

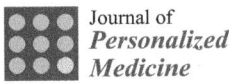

Article

Feasibility of Outpatient Transradial Prostatic Artery Embolization and Safety of a Shortened Deflation Protocol for Hemostasis

Gregory Amouyal [1,2,*], Louis Tournier [2,3], Constance de Margerie-Mellon [2,3], Damien Bouda [2,3], Atanas Pachev [2,3], Jessica Assouline [2,3], Cédric de Bazelaire [2,3], Florent Marques [1], Solenne Le Strat [1], François Desgrandchamps [3,4,5] and Eric De Kerviler [2,3]

[1] Hôpital Privé Geoffroy Saint-Hilaire—Ramsay Santé, 75005 Paris, France; florent.marques@gmail.com (F.M.); docteurlestrat@gmail.com (S.L.S.)
[2] Radiology Department, Hôpital Saint-Louis, 75010 Paris, France; ltourn22@gmail.com (L.T.); constance.de-margerie@aphp.fr (C.d.M.-M.); damien.bouda@aphp.fr (D.B.); atanas.pachev@aphp.fr (A.P.); jessica.assouline@aphp.fr (J.A.); cedric.de-bazelaire@aphp.fr (C.d.B.); eric.de-kerviler@aphp.fr (E.D.K.)
[3] Faculté de Médecine, Université Paris cité, 75006 Paris, France; francois.desgrandchamps@aphp.fr
[4] Urology Department, Hôpital Saint-Louis, 75010 Paris France
[5] SRHI/CEA—Institut de Recherche Clinique Saint-Louis, Hôpital Saint-Louis, 75010 Paris, France
* Correspondence: gregory.amouyal@aphp.fr; Tel.: +33-670132138

Abstract: Background: to evaluate the safety and feasibility of a shorter time to hemostasis applied to outpatient transradial (TR) Prostatic Artery Embolization (PAE). Methods: a retrospective bi-institutional study was conducted between July 2018 and April 2022 on 300 patients treated by outpatient TR PAE. Indications included lower urinary tract symptoms, acute urinary retention, and hematuria. Mean patient height was 176 ± 6.3 (158–192) cm. The primary endpoint was safety of a 45 min deflation protocol for hemostasis. The secondary endpoint was the feasibility of PAE using TR access. Results: technical success was 98.7% (296/300). There was one failure due to patient height. Mean DAP/fluoroscopy times were 16,225 ± 12,126.3 (2959–81,608) $\mu Gy \cdot m^2 / 35 \pm 14.7$ (11–97) min, and mean time to discharge was 80 ± 6 (75–90) min. All access site and embolization-related adverse events were minor. Mild hematoma occurred in 10% (30/300), radial artery occlusion (RAO) in 10/300 (3.3%) cases, and history of smoking was a predictor for RAO. There was no major event. Conclusion: the safety of TR PAE using a 45 min time to hemostasis was confirmed, and TR PAE is feasible in most cases. Radial artery occlusion was still observed and may be favored by smoking.

Keywords: prostatic hyperplasia; embolization; therapeutic; endovascular procedure; radiology; interventional; prostate

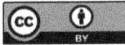

1. Introduction

Prostatic Artery Embolization (PAE) has been proposed for several years as an alternative treatment to surgery for symptomatic Benign Prostatic Hyperplasia (BPH) [1,2]. This endovascular intervention performed by interventional radiologists (IR) has shown safety, efficacy, and comparable outcomes to surgical results [3–6].

PAE was routinely performed during a short hospital stay using transfemoral access (TFA). However, ambulatory PAE is spreading in most IR institutions, as immediate post-operative symptoms are mild and well tolerated. A few reports on the use of transradial access (TRA) in IR procedures showed safety and multiple benefits for the patient [7,8], such as gains in per- and post-procedural comfort (less discomfort during local anesthesia delivery; possibility for elevation of the legs during the procedure, to relieve back pain; possibility for immediate resumption of standing position and ambulation) [9], decreased rate of hemorrhagic adverse events compared to TFA [10], possibility to maintain antiaggregant or anticoagulant medication, shorter time to hemostasis, and faster discharge during ambulatory stays [8].

TRA for PAE has been described with promising initial experiences in terms of feasibility and safety [9,11]. Hemostasis is obtained using a compressive band, with a step-by-step deflation protocol, the duration of which is not yet standardized in IR procedures. As the main challenge is avoiding subsequent post-compression radial artery occlusion (RAO), reflections have been raised on how to reduce the incidence of this complication, among them being the duration of compression.

In this study, an assessment of the feasibility and safety was conducted on a cohort of patients who benefited from outpatient Transradial (TR) PAE, using a shortened deflation protocol, with the objectives to lower the incidence of RAO and to shorten the patients' hospital stay.

2. Materials and Methods

This retrospective, bi-institutional study was conducted on 300 male patients, mean age 68 ± 9.7 (47–102) years, who underwent TR PAE between July 2018 and April 2022. This TRA cohort belonged to a population of 311 consecutive patients treated with PAE, using either TRA or Transfemoral access (TFA), all performed as an outpatient procedure.

Indications for PAE included symptomatic BPH with moderate-to-severe lower urinary tract symptoms and failure of medical treatment, acute urinary retention or macroscopic hematuria due to BPH, and were validated in clinic by a urologist and an IR. Pre-procedural patient assessment was performed as previously described [12].

Ambulatory PAE was performed under local anesthesia (center 1) or anesthesia and neurolept analgesia (center 2) using a subcutaneous peri arterial 4 mL injection of licodaïne mixed with 1 mg of isosorbide dinitrate.

All patients were treated with the intent to use TRA to increase patient comfort and shorten ambulatory stay. Choice for TFA was made only in cases where TRA faced a risk of failure or morbidity, such as excessive height (>195 cm); mental condition unfit for TRA patient installation, such as agitation or dementia; advanced atherosclerosis (defined by a combination of at least 3 factor risks among diabetes, arterial hypertension, smoking, and dyslipidemia in addition to a history of cardiovascular acute event); or obstacles for catheterization in the thoracic or abdominal arterial territory.

In case of TRA, antiaggregant, Direct Oral Anticoagulant (DOA), or Vitamin K Agonist (VKA) medications were not discontinued. When TFA was used, aspirin was maintained; clopidogrel, ticagrelor, or DOA medications were discontinued at least 5 days prior to embolization; and VKAs were transitorily replaced by heparin.

Oxymetric Barbeau test was performed to rule out contraindication for radial puncture, followed by pre-operative left radial artery Doppler Ultrasound (DUS): caliber of the radial artery at puncture site, radial artery patency (RAP), and presence of radial loop were monitored.

Baseline characteristics of the population are presented in Table 1. At time to procedure, 26/300 patients (8.7%) were under anticoagulant medication and 27/300 (9%) under antiaggregant medication. Mean radial artery diameter at puncture site was 2.5 mm ± 0.3 (1.7–3.6), and mean patient height was 176 ± 6.3 (158–192) cm.

TRA was always performed on the left side, as previously described [9,11], using a dedicated 5-Fr sheath for radial puncture (Merit medical, Salt Lake City, UT, USA), composed of a 21-G needle and a 0.018-inch guide wire. In rare situations of a radial artery diameter between 1.7 and 2 mm, a dedicated thinner 5-Fr sheath was used (Terumo Corporation, Tokyo, Japan). Sheath was inserted under ultrasound guidance according to the Seldinger technique.

When patient height was between 175 and 195 cm, "proximal" TRA (pTRA) was performed: radial artery puncture was performed 5 to 10 cm proximally to the usual radial puncture site at an extra-muscular location. When patient height exceeded 195 cm, TFA was chosen.

Table 1. Baseline characteristics of study cohort prior to PAE.

Variable	Study Cohort (n = 300)
Age, years	68 ± 9.7 (47–102)
Height, cm	176 ± 6.3 (158–192)
Radial artery diameter at puncture site, mm	2.5 ± 0.3 (1.7–3.6)
Medication at procedure	53 (17.7)
Aspirin medication	22 (7.3)
Clopidogrel medication	1 (0.3)
Aspirin and clopidogrel medication	2 (0.7)
Aspirin and ticagrelor medication	2 (0.7)
DOA/VKA/Heparin	26 (8.7)
Indication for PAE	
Bothersome LUTS	241 (80.3)
Urinary retention	51 (17)
Macroscopic hematuria	8 (2.7)
IPSS	19 ± 6.9 (4–35)
QOL score	6 ± 1.1 (2–7)
IIEF-15	45 ± 19.3 (4–77)
Prostate volume, mL	92 ± 45.2 (22–280)
Maximum urinary flow, mL/s	8 ± 5 (2.4–31)
Post-voiding residue, mL	98 ± 123 (0–810)
Total PSA, ng/mL	7 ± 5.6 (0.31–28)

Note: values are presented as mean ± SD (range) or as number, n (%). PAE: prostatic artery embolization; DOA: direct oral anticoagulant; VKA: vitamine K ntagonist; LUTS: lower urinary tract symptoms; IPSS: international prostatic symptoms score; QOL: quality of Life; IIEF: international index of erectile function; PSA: prostatic specific antigen.

Following sheath insertion, an antispasmodic and antithrombotic mix of 1 mg of isosorbide dinitrate, 2.5 mg of verapamil, and 3000 IU of heparin was injected in the radial artery through the sheath, after dilution in 20 mL of blood. No additional heparin was injected during the procedure.

TR PAE was performed using a 125 or, when needed, a 135-cm long 5-Fr catheter (Merit medical), a hydrophilic angulated 0.035 guide wire (Terumo Corporation), a 150-cm long microcatheter (Merit medical), a 0.014' micro guide wire (Boston Scientifics, Malborough, MA, USA), and 300–500 μm calibrated trisacryl microparticles (Merit Medical) until complete stasis, as previously described [13]. Coil protection was used in elective cases to prevent extra-prostatic non-target embolization [14,15].

TFA was performed on the right side, using a 5-Fr sheath (Terumo Corporation, Tokyo, Japan, or Cook Medical, Bloomington, IN, USA), a 100-cm long 5-Fr catheter (Terumo Corporation), and a 130-cm long microcatheter (Merit Medical).

Technical success for TRA was defined as completion of the procedure and at least unilateral prostatic artery embolization. Failure was defined as an incapacity for internal iliac or prostatic artery catheterization due to insufficient device length. In case of failure of TRA, the procedure was completed after conversion to TFA.

After complete TR PAE, hemostasis was performed using a hemostatic band (TR Band®, Terumo Corporation, or Prelude Sync®, Merit Medical) as follows: initial inflation of 20 mL of air in the compressive valve was performed to permit a bleeding free sheath retrieval, followed by progressive deflation according to the "patent hemostasis protocol", previously described [16]: when pulsatile reflux of blood was observed through the arteriotomy, 0.5 mL of air was re-inflated to stop the reflux, and palpation of distal radial pulse was reached to confirm artery patency. A first 5 mL deflation was performed at 30 min of compression and a final deflation of the remaining volume at 45 min. In case of bleeding at puncture site during deflation, 2 mL was re-inflated to stop the bleeding, and deflation was reinitiated 15 min later until complete hemostasis. At time to hemostasis, band was retrieved, puncture site cleaned, and a bandage was put on. Prior to this study, the deflation protocol recommended in both institutions for 5-Fr TR embolization procedures was of a 90 min duration, with increments in deflation of 3 mL and the remaining volume at 60, 75, and 90 min.

When patients showed arterial hypertension during hemostasis, no measure was taken to lower blood pressure. Control ultrasound before discharge was performed in selected cases, when radial/distal pulses were not palpated after hemostasis (suspicion of RAO) or when bleeding occurred during/following deflation, in order to rule out pseudo-aneurysm at the puncture site.

Patients were discharged after voiding > 200 mL, 30 to 45 min after hemostasis, and a form was provided to report any adverse event occurring after discharge.

Follow-up consult was performed at 1, 6, and 12 months to assess clinical improvement and monitor adverse events: severity was defined according to the Society of Interventional Radiology Clinical Practice Guidelines [17]. The same documentation as in pre-operative evaluation was obtained, and radial access site DUS monitored RAP and absence of pseudo-aneurysm at one month. Criteria for clinical success were IPSS score decrease of 8 points, QoL score decrease of at least 1 point or value ≤ 3, increase of 2.5 mL/s of Qmax, and successful retrieval of indwelling catheter 15 days after PAE or resolution of hematuria.

Agreement of the Institutional Review board was obtained for this study.

The primary endpoint was safety of a 45 min deflation protocol for hemostasis, described as absence of major adverse events, such as acute hematoma or hand pain requiring hospitalization, and comparable rates of minor adverse events to what was previously described in literature. The secondary endpoint was the feasibility of PAE using TRA, consisting of technical success and no need for conversion to TFA.

Statistical Analysis

Logistic regression was used to determine predictors for access site adverse events. Univariate and multivariate analyses were performed using R software, version 4.1.1. Results are expressed as Odd Ratio (OR) value [95% Confidence Interval, IC] and their p value. A p value < 0.05 was considered significant.

3. Results

Among the cohort of consecutive patients referred for PAE, TFA was chosen over TRA in 11/311 (3.6%) patients: one patient was 197 cm tall, one had a history of kinking of the abdominal aorta, one had a history of occlusion of the left subclavian artery, and the 8 remaining patients had advanced atheroma. Among the TRA cohort, technical success was achieved in 296/300 (98.7%) cases. Bilateral embolization was achieved in 294/296 (99.3%) cases. The four cases of failure of TRA included one case of a painful radial loop preventing completion of the procedure through TRA under local anesthesia, one case showing undocumented occlusion of the left subclavian artery preventing catheterization, one case of combined subclavian artery kinking and aortic aneurysm/tortuosity preventing catheterization of the descendant thoracic aorta, and one case where cannulation of the internal iliac artery was not achieved on one side because of significant iliac tortuosity making the 135-cm long 5-Fr catheter too short for selective angiography (patient's height was 185 cm). Procedural characteristics of the cohort are presented in Table 2.

An angiography review revealed that 48/300 (16%) patient had an accessory prostatic artery originating from a distal branch of the internal pudendal artery ("distal accessory PA") (Figure 1). No lack of microcatheter length was observed, and all but one were successfully catheterized and embolized.

The mean procedure time was 95 ± 26.1 (45–195) min, mean fluoroscopy time and dose-area product (DAP) were 35 ± 14.7 (11–97) min and $16{,}225 \pm 12{,}126.3$ (2959–81,608) µGy·m². Mean time to discharge was 80 ± 6 (75–90) min. Clinical success at one month following TR PAE was 258/300 (86%).

Table 2. Procedure characteristics of the study cohort.

Variable	Study Cohort (n = 300)
Technical success	296 (98.7)
Conversion to TFA	4 (1.3)
Proximal TRA	149 (49.7)
Distal accessory PA	48 (16)
Procedure time, min	95 ± 26.1 (45–195)
Fluoroscopy time, min	35 ± 14.7 (11–97)
DAP, µGy·m^2	16,225 ± 12,126.3 (2959–81,608)
Radiation skin entry, mGy	1557 ± 1098.6 (238–5958)
Closure device	
TR Band	199 (66.3)
Prelude sync	101 (33.7)
Mean time to discharge after completion of procedure, min	80 ± 6 (75–90)

Note: values are presented as mean ± SD (range) or as number, n (%). DAP: dose-area product; min: minute; Gy: Gray; PA: prostatic artery.

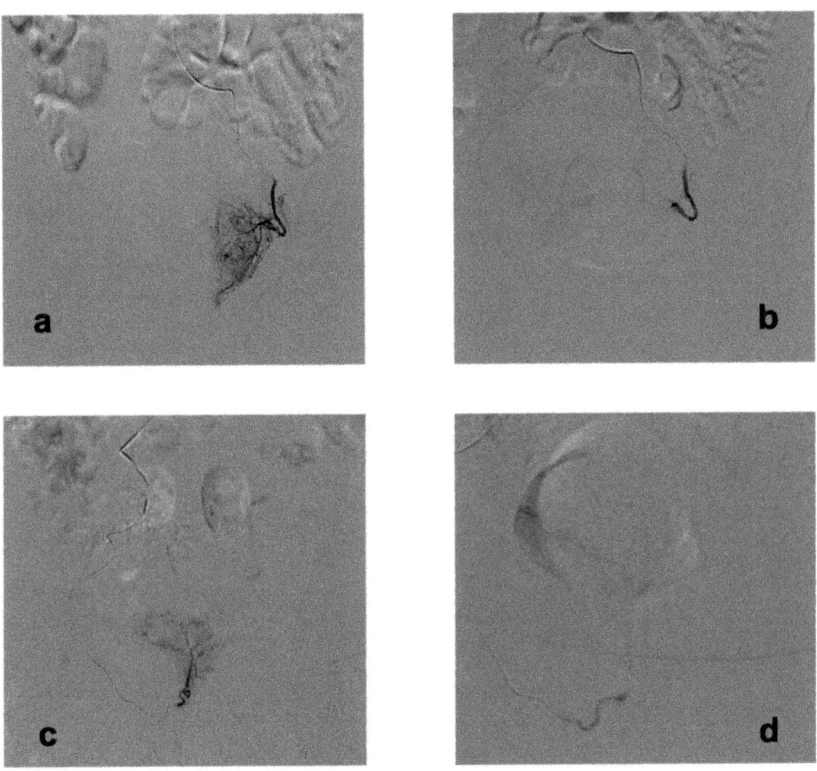

Figure 1. Selective prostatic artery angiograms during transradial prostatic artery embolization. All angiograms are performed on anteroposterior view. (**a**) Selective digital subtraction angiography of the left prostatic artery, showing a full uptake of the left hemi-prostate. (**b**) Selective digital subtraction angiography of the left prostatic artery following embolization, confirming complete stasis in the artery and disappearance of the uptake. (**c**) Selective digital subtraction angiography of an accessory right prostatic artery, arising from the distal part of the internal pudendal artery, and feeding both sides of the prostate. (**d**) Post-embolization selective digital subtraction angiography of the right accessory prostatic artery, confirming complete stasis and absence of uptake.

Adverse Events

There was no major adverse event. There was no case of stroke or any neurological event, including acute pain in the left hand.

All radial pulses were palpated at time to hemostasis. DUS was performed in 2/300 patients prior to discharge because of bleeding during deflation. Mild hematoma at the puncture site was observed in 30 (10/%) cases, and all appeared the next day after discharge. Among them, 4/30 patients were under an anticoagulant and 3/30 patients were under aspirine; none were under clopidogrel medication. Univariate or multivariate logistic regression analysis did not find any significant predictor among age, height, radial artery diameter, pTRA, history of diabetes, arterial hypertension, smoking, dyslipidemia, anticoagulant, or antiaggregant medication for occurrence of hematoma.

There were 2/300 (0.7%) cases of asymptomatic thrombosed pseudo-aneurysm (P-A) of the anterior wall of the radial artery at the puncture site, both diagnosed by DUS: one was observed at day 2 in a patient under VKA medication, who presented in clinic because of a mild hematoma occurring the day before. This P-A had disappeared at control DUS at one month. The second P-A was observed at one-month follow-up DUS in a patient who was under DOA medication.

There were three cases (1%) of arteritis of the left radial artery, manifested by mild swelling and pain in the left arm and wrist along the artery pathway. All three cases occurred after discharge, between day 3 and day 5 following PAE, and one was associated with RAO, which was diagnosed by DUS at the clinic at day 5. After infection was ruled out, they were treated by oral non-steroidal anti-inflammatory drugs, antibiotics, and painkillers and subcutaneous heparinotherapy for the case of associated thrombosis. All evolved favorably under medical treatment within 10 days, but RAO resolved only subcompletely because the patient decided to stop heparinotherapy at day 15.

There were 10/300 (3.3%) cases of radial artery occlusion: nine were asymptomatic and monitored at one month by DUS, and the last one was the one associated with arteritis and diagnosed at day 5 by DUS. No medication was given at one month to treat the asymptomatic occlusions because the diagnosis was considered too late for initiating anticoagulant treatment and because occlusions were asymptomatic. Two RAOs persisted at the 6-month control DUS, one persisted at one-year, the seven other patients were lost to follow-up. Among them, the radial artery diameters varied between 1.85 and 3 mm. Univariate logistic regression analysis found that history of smoking, radial artery diameter < 2 mm (compared to diameter between 2 and 3 mm or <3 mm), and occurrence of hematoma were significant predictive factors for the occurrence of occlusion (OR = 5.63 CI [1.56; 22.62], $p = 0.009$; OR = 4.51 CI [0.92; 17.75], $p = 0.04$ and OR = 4.17 CI [0.86; 16], $p = 0.046$). Multivariate logistic regression found smoking to be a significant predictive factor for the occurrence of RAO (OR = 6.52 CI [1.49; 31.15], $p = 0.013$).

Access site and overall embolization-related adverse events are shown in Tables 3 and 4. Post-embolization syndrome, including mild fever, fatigue, pelvic/anal pain, urethral burning, pollakiuria, and constipation occurring during the first 10 days were not considered adverse events.

Table 3. Access site adverse events.

Variable	Cohort ($n = 300$)
Stroke	0
Hand pain	0
Hematoma after discharge	30 (10)
Thrombosed pseudo-aneurism at puncture site	2 (0.7)
Arteritis	3 (1)
Radial artery occlusion	10 (3.3)

Note: values are represented as mean ± SD (range) or as number, n (%).

Table 4. Embolization-related adverse events.

Variable	Cohort (n = 300)
Acute urinary retention	0
Urinary tract infection	2 (0.7)
Hematuria	5 (1.7)
Bladder ischemia	0
Rectorrhagia	0
Rectal ischemia	0
Balanitis	2 (0.7)
Penile glans necrotic ulcer	0
Erectile dysfunction	0
Hematospermia	6 (2)
Anejaculation	0

Note: values are presented as mean ± SD (range) or as number, n (%).

4. Discussion

4.1. Transradial Access

This study confirmed feasibility and safety of TRA during PAE. There was a low rate of technical failure leading to the conversion to TFA (1.3%). Over the two studies available in the literature on TRA during PAE, Isaacson et al. [9] and Bhatia et al. [11] reported no conversion to TFA in 19 and 32 patients, respectively, but their cohorts were smaller. Still, Bhatia reported 2/32 (6%) conversions to transulnar access.

The results in this study are similar to those of two recent studies on TRA during IR procedures, reporting a 1/91 (1%) [18] and 4/749 (0.5%) [8] rate of conversion to TFA. In the present study, patients in whom TRA failed were 64, 76, 81, and 91 years old. This might suggest that risk for failure may increase with advanced age, but it needs to be confirmed by additional studies. A 1.3% rate of failure in TRA may be of debate, but it is to be balanced with the many benefits of this approach: in addition to those previously described [8], significantly lower DAP and faster ambulatory discharge may be observed compared to TFA [11].

Procedure characteristics were not compared to those of the 11 patients treated using TFA because this TFA cohort was too small for a comparison.

4.2. Adverse Events

This study showed that access site and overall adverse events following a 45 min time to hemostasis in TRA were all minor. To our knowledge, there is no recommended time to hemostasis for 5-Fr TRA in IR procedures. Even though the basic deflation protocol that was locally recommended for previous 5-Fr TR embolization procedures was of a 90 min duration, all TR PAE procedures were performed in both institutions of this study using this 45 min deflation protocol, and the results could therefore not be compared to those of PAE procedures using a 90 min deflation protocol. Isaacson et al. described a deflation protocol, but the total duration was not detailed [9]. Nakhaei et al. described in 91 TRA for uterine fibroid embolization (UFE) a 40 min deflation protocol, with deflation increments at 30, 35, and 40 min and with safe results [18], which supports our results.

Hematoma occurred in 10% of patients in this study. Isaacson et al. reported 11%, and Bhatia et al. 9.4% (TRA) and 12.5% (TFA) [9,11].

In patients manifesting hematoma, anticoagulant, aspirine, or clopidogrel medication were not predictive factors. Still, patients under DOA or VKA medications may be at increased risk of peudoaneurysm at the puncture site. These findings need to be confirmed in further studies.

To our knowledge, there is no report describing pTRA in the literature. pTRA is of benefit when the patient's height is at least 175 cm, as it may prevent the lack of catheter length for cannulation of the IIA or distal accessory PA. Findings in this study suggest that the safety of this puncture seems acceptable. Further studies are needed on this topic.

There was a 3.3% rate of RAO. Isaacson et al. and Bhatia et al. reported none, but their cohorts were smaller ($n = 19$ and $n = 32$) [9,11]. Thakor et al. reported a 0.3% of RAO ($n = 749$) [8], using "patent hemostasis" [16] during TR embolization procedures. These previous results on RAP following TRA were based on post-procedural or follow-up clinical examination, which may underestimate the incidence of RAO compared to DUS, as collateral supply via the superficial palmar arcade may provide retrograde arterial flow in the radial artery at palpation site, distally to the occlusion and maintain distal pulse. This hypothesis may explain why all patients in this study, including those who encountered RAO, had a pulse palpated at time to discharge. Immediate RAO may not be excluded, and control DUS prior to discharge may be of interest to unmask this event. RAO could then be treated early by anticoagulants with a high chance of resorption of the thrombosis. The results in this study may suggest that part of RAO persist in time, when diagnosed "too late" at one month. Some studies in the literature reported the opposite: most cases spontaneously resolved between discharge, 24 h, 1-, and 3-months control DUS [18,19].

This finding on RAO indicates the need for adapted deflation protocols for TR PAE: shorter time to first increment in deflation and/or overall time of compression may be considered.

Alternative maneuvers to reduce RAO were previously described in 5–6F cardiology procedures in randomized studies, such as subcutaneous preprocedural injection at puncture site ($n = 188$) [20] or intra-arterial pre-hemostasis injection ($n = 1706$) [21] of 500 µg of nitroglycerin, ipsilateral ulnar artery compression adding to patent artery compression ($n = 3000$) [19], with significant reduced incidence of RAO (5.4 vs. 14.4%, 8.3 vs. 11.7%, and 0.9% vs. 3%). Heparin sheath injection may play a role [22] (5000 IU in most cardiology procedures vs. 3000 in our study). At last, additional IV injections of 1000 units of heparin every 30 to 60 min during the procedure, to reduced risk of clotting, may be considered.

History of smoking, small caliber artery, and occurrence of hematoma were found to be predictors for RAO. Elective control DUS prior to discharge or within the first days following the procedure for patients in these situations may be of interest in order to early diagnose asymptomatic RAO and start anticoagulant treatment to recover artery patency.

This study reported short-term clinical improvement of 86%. These results are comparable to data in the literature [4,5,9,11].

This study has its limitations, starting with its retrospective nature, its non-randomized nature, the limited follow-up period, and its patients lost to follow-up. This study lacked control groups: this cohort was not compared to another cohort of patients benefiting TRA using a 90 min deflation protocol or TFA. RAP was not monitored at one year in all patients encountering occlusion, which may overestimate the RAO.

5. Conclusions

The safety of transradial access during outpatient PAE using a 45 min time to hemostasis was confirmed and may help to shorten the time to discharge. When purposely chosen, TRA is feasible in most cases of PAE. A low incidence of radial artery occlusion was still observed and may be favored by smoking patients, small caliber arteries, and the occurrence of hematoma. These findings need confirmation by additional studies, and there is a need for comparison between techniques for hemostasis in randomized designs.

Author Contributions: Conceptualization, G.A.; methodology, G.A.; software, L.T.; validation, E.D.K.; formal analysis, L.T.; investigation, G.A.; resources and data curation, C.d.M.-M., D.B., A.P., J.A., C.d.B., F.M., S.L.S. and F.D.; writing—original draft preparation, G.A.; writing—review and editing, E.D.K.; visualization, E.D.K.; supervision, E.D.K. All authors have read and agreed to the published version of the manuscript.

Funding: This research received no external funding.

Institutional Review Board Statement: The study was conducted according to the guidelines of the Declaration of Helsinki and approved by the Institutional Review Board IRB00010835 of HOSPITAL PRIVE GEOFFROY SAINT-HILAIRE, Ramsay Santé Recherche & Enseignement (protocol code COS-RGDS-2020-05-015-AMOUYAL-G, date of approval 18 May 2020).

Informed Consent Statement: Informed consent was obtained from all subjects involved in the study.

Data Availability Statement: Data containing patient characteristics prior and after the intervention, in addition to procedure characteristics, are available and can be found in the PACS and RIS of Hospital privé Geoffroy Saint-Hilaire and Hospital Saint-Louis, where the interventions occurred.

Conflicts of Interest: Gregory Amouyal received financial support from Merit Medical (Salt Lake City, UT, USA) for educational programs. Eric De Kerviler received financial support from Canon Medical (Otawara, Japan) and from Boston Scientific (Malborough, MA, USA) for attending/speaking at symposia/congresses and for educational programs. Other authors have nothing to disclose.

Abbreviations

BPH	Benign Prostatic Hyperplasia
PA	Prostatic Artery
PAE	Prostatic Artery Embolization
LUTS	Lower Urinary Tract Symptoms
AUR	Acute Urinary Retention
IR	Interventional Radiologist
IRB	Institutional Review Board
DSA	Digital Subtracted Angiography
AP view	Antero-posterior view
CBCT	Cone Beam Computed Tomodensitometry
IIA	Internal Iliac Artery
TR	Transradial
TRA	Transradial Access
TFA	Transrfemoral Access
pTRA	Proximal Transradial Access
RAO	Radial Artery Occlusion
DOA	Direct Oral Anticoagulant
VKA	Vitamine K Antagonist
DUS	Doppler Ultrasound
RAP	Radial Artery Patency
APA	Accessory Pudendal Artery
IPA	Internal Pudendal Artery

References

1. Carnevale, F.C.; da Motta-Leal-Filho, J.M.; Antunes, A.A.; Baroni, R.H.; Freire, G.C.; Cerri, L.M.O.; Marcelino, A.S.Z.; Cerri, G.G.; Srougi, M. Midterm Follow-up after prostate embolization in two patients with benign prostatic hyperplasia. *Cardiovasc. Interv. Radiol.* **2011**, *34*, 1330–1333. [CrossRef] [PubMed]
2. Pisco, J.M.; Bilhim, T.; Pinheiro, L.C.; Fernandes, L.; Pereira, J.; Costa, N.V.; Duarte, M.; Oliveira, A.G. Medium- and Long-Term Outcome of Prostate Artery Embolization for Patients with Benign Prostatic Hyperplasia: Results in 630 Patients. *J. Vasc. Interv. Radiol.* **2016**, *27*, 1115–1122. [CrossRef]
3. Cizman, Z.; Isaacson, A.; Burke, C. Short- to Midterm Safety and Efficacy of Prostatic Artery Embolization: A Systematic Review. *J. Vasc. Interv. Radiol.* **2016**, *27*, 1487–1493.e1. [CrossRef] [PubMed]
4. Feng, S.; Tian, Y.; Liu, W.; Li, Z.; Deng, T.; Li, H.; Wang, K. Prostatic Arterial Embolization Treating Moderate-to-Severe Lower Urinary Tract Symptoms Related to Benign Prostate Hyperplasia: A Meta-Analysis. *Cardiovasc. Interv. Radiol.* **2016**, *40*, 22–32. [CrossRef]
5. Malling, B.; Røder, M.A.; Brasso, K.; Forman, J.; Taudorf, M.; Lönn, L. Prostate artery embolisation for benign prostatic hyperplasia: A systematic review and meta-analysis. *Eur. Radiol.* **2018**, *29*, 287–298. [CrossRef] [PubMed]
6. Uflacker, A.; Haskal, Z.J.; Bilhim, T.; Patrie, J.; Huber, T.; Pisco, J.M. Meta-Analysis of Prostatic Artery Embolization for Benign Prostatic Hyperplasia. *J. Vasc. Interv. Radiol.* **2016**, *27*, 1686–1697.e8. [CrossRef] [PubMed]
7. Posham, R.; Biederman, D.M.; Patel, R.S.; Kim, E.; Tabori, N.E.; Nowakowski, F.S.; Lookstein, R.A.; Fischman, A.M. Transradial Approach for Noncoronary Interventions: A Single-Center Review of Safety and Feasibility in the First 1500 Cases. *J. Vasc. Interv. Radiol.* **2015**, *27*, 159–166. [CrossRef]

8. Thakor, A.S.; Alshammari, M.T.; Liu, D.M.; Chung, J.; Ho, S.G.; Legiehn, G.M.; Machan, L.; Fischman, A.M.; Patel, R.S.; Klass, D. Transradial Access for Interventional Radiology: Single-Centre Procedural and Clinical Outcome Analysis. *Can. Assoc. Radiol. J.* **2017**, *68*, 318–327. [CrossRef]
9. Isaacson, A.J.; Fischman, A.M.; Burke, C.T. Technical Feasibility of Prostatic Artery Embolization from a Transradial Approach. *Am. J. Roentgenol.* **2016**, *206*, 442–444. [CrossRef]
10. Kolluri, R.; Fowler, B.; Nandish, S. Vascular access complications: Diagnosis and management. *Curr. Treat. Options Cardiovasc. Med.* **2013**, *15*, 173–187. [CrossRef]
11. Bhatia, S.; Harward, S.H.; Sinha, V.K.; Narayanan, G. Prostate Artery Embolization via Transradial or Transulnar versus Transfemoral Arterial Access: Technical Results. *J. Vasc. Interv. Radiol.* **2017**, *28*, 898–905. [CrossRef] [PubMed]
12. Carnevale, F.C.; Antunes, A.A. Prostatic artery embolization for enlarged prostates due to benign prostatic hyperplasia. How I do it. *Cardiovasc. Interv. Radiol.* **2013**, *36*, 1452–1463. [CrossRef] [PubMed]
13. Picel, A.C.; Hsieh, T.-C.; Shapiro, R.M.; Vezeridis, A.M.; Isaacson, A.J. Prostatic Artery Embolization for Benign Prostatic Hyperplasia: Patient Evaluation, Anatomy, and Technique for Successful Treatment. *RadioGraphics* **2019**, *39*, 1526–1548. [CrossRef] [PubMed]
14. Amouyal, G.; Chague, P.; Pellerin, O.; Pereira, H.; Del Giudice, C.; Dean, C.; Thiounn, N.; Sapoval, M. Safety and Efficacy of Occlusion of Large Extra-Prostatic Anastomoses During Prostatic Artery Embolization for Symptomatic BPH. *Cardiovasc. Interv. Radiol.* **2016**, *39*, 1245–1255. [CrossRef] [PubMed]
15. Bhatia, S.; Sinha, V.; Bordegaray, M.; Kably, I.; Harward, S.; Narayanan, G. Role of Coil Embolization during Prostatic Artery Embolization: Incidence, Indications, and Safety Profile ✩. *J. Vasc. Interv. Radiol.* **2017**, *28*, 656–664.e3. [CrossRef] [PubMed]
16. Pancholy, S.; Coppola, J.; Patel, T.; Roke-Thomas, M. Prevention of radial artery occlusion-Patent hemostasis evaluation trial (PROPHET study): A randomized comparison of traditional versus patency documented hemostasis after transradial catheterization. *Catheter. Cardiovasc. Interv.* **2008**, *72*, 335–340. [CrossRef]
17. Khalilzadeh, O.; Baerlocher, M.O.; Shyn, P.B.; Connolly, B.L.; Devane, A.M.; Morris, C.S.; Cohen, A.M.; Midia, M.; Thornton, R.H.; Gross, K.; et al. Proposal of a New Adverse Event Classification by the Society of Interventional Radiology Standards of Practice Committee. *J. Vasc. Interv. Radiol.* **2017**, *28*, 1432–1437.e3. [CrossRef]
18. Nakhaei, M.; Mojtahedi, A.; Faintuch, S.; Sarwar, A.; Brook, O.R. Transradial and Transfemoral Uterine Fibroid Embolization Comparative Study: Technical and Clinical Outcomes. *J. Vasc. Interv. Radiol.* **2019**, *31*, 123–129. [CrossRef]
19. Pancholy, S.B.; Bernat, I.; Bertrand, O.F.; Patel, T.M. Prevention of Radial Artery Occlusion after Transradial Catheterization: The PROPHET-II Randomized Trial. *JACC Cardiovasc. Interv.* **2016**, *9*, 1992–1999. [CrossRef]
20. Chen, Y.; Ke, Z.; Xiao, J.; Lin, M.; Huang, X.; Yan, C.; Ye, S.; Tan, X. Subcutaneous Injection of Nitroglycerin at the Radial Artery Puncture Site Reduces the Risk of Early Radial Artery Occlusion after Transradial Coronary Catheterization: A Randomized, Placebo-Controlled Clinical Trial. *Circ. Cardiovasc. Interv.* **2018**, *11*, e006571. [CrossRef]
21. Dharma, S.; Kedev, S.; Patel, T.; Kiemeneij, F.; Gilchrist, I.C. A novel approach to reduce radial artery occlusion after transradial catheterization: Postprocedural/prehemostasis intra-arterial nitroglycerin. *Catheter. Cardiovasc. Interv.* **2014**, *85*, 818–825. [CrossRef] [PubMed]
22. Spaulding, C.; Lefèvre, T.; Funck, F.; Thébault, B.; Chauveau, M.; Ben Hamda, K.; Chalet, Y.; Monségu, J.; Tsocanakis, O.; Py, A.; et al. Left radial approach for coronary angiography: Results of a prospective study. *Catheter. Cardiovasc. Diagn.* **1996**, *39*, 365–370. [CrossRef]

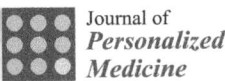

Article

Safety Profile of Ambulatory Prostatic Artery Embolization after a Significant Learning Curve: Update on Adverse Events

Gregory Amouyal [1,2,*], Louis Tournier [2,3], Constance De Margerie-Mellon [2,3], Atanas Pachev [2,3], Jessica Assouline [2,3], Damien Bouda [2,3], Cédric De Bazelaire [2,3], Florent Marques [1], Solenne Le Strat [1], François Desgrandchamps [3,4,5] and Eric De Kerviler [2,3]

1. Ramsay Santé—Hôpital Privé Geoffroy Saint-Hilaire, 75005 Paris, France; florent.marques@gmail.com (F.M.); docteurlestrat@gmail.com (S.L.S.)
2. Radiology Department, Hôpital Saint-Louis, 75010 Paris, France; ltourn22@gmail.com (L.T.); constance.de-margerie@aphp.fr (C.D.M.-M.); atanas.pachev@aphp.fr (A.P.); jessica.assouline@aphp.fr (J.A.); damien.bouda@aphp.fr (D.B.); cedric.de-bazelaire@aphp.fr (C.D.B.); eric.de-kerviler@aphp.fr (E.D.K.)
3. Faculté de Médecine, Université Paris Cité, 75006 Paris, France; francois.desgrandchamps@aphp.fr
4. Urology Department, Hôpital Saint-Louis, 75010 Paris, France
5. SRHI/CEA—Institut de Recherche Clinique Saint-Louis, Hôpital Saint-Louis, 75010 Paris, France
* Correspondence: gregory.amouyal@aphp.fr; Tel.: +33-670132138; Fax: +33-142494126

Abstract: Background: to report the safety of outpatient prostatic artery embolization (PAE) after a significant learning curve. Methods: a retrospective bi-institutional study was conducted between June 2018 and April 2022 on 311 consecutive patients, with a mean age of 69 years ± 9.8 (47–102), treated by outpatient PAE. Indications included lower urinary tract symptoms, acute urinary retention, and hematuria. When needed, 3D-imaging and/or coil protection of extra-prostatic supplies were performed to avoid non-target embolization. Adverse events were monitored at 1-, 6-, and 12-month follow-ups. Results: bilateral PAE was achieved in 305/311 (98.1%). Mean dose area product/fluoroscopy times were 16,408.3 ± 12,078.9 (2959–81,608) µGy.m^2/36.3 ± 1.7 (11–97) minutes. Coil protection was performed on 67/311 (21.5%) patients in 78 vesical, penile, or rectal supplies. Embolization-related adverse events varied between 0 and 2.6%, access-site adverse events between 0 and 18%, and were all minor. There was no major event. Conclusion: outpatient PAE performed after achieving a significant learning curve may lead to a decreased and low rate of adverse events. Experience in arterial anatomy and coil protection may play a role in safety, but the necessity of the latter in some patterns may need confirmation by additional studies in randomized designs.

Keywords: prostatic hyperplasia; embolization; therapeutic; endovascular procedure; radiology; interventional; prostate

1. Introduction

For about ten years, prostatic artery embolization (PAE) has been described as a novel mini-invasive procedure and alternative treatment to surgery for symptomatic benign prostatic hyperplasia (BPH) [1,2]. To date, the literature has shown the efficacy of PAE on lower urinary tract symptoms (LUTSs) close to similar to surgical options, and the majority reports fewer minor events [3–6], its safety profile being mainly based on reports assessing PAE from 2011 to 2016 [7–10].

New evidence has since been published on anatomy [11–13] and technical achievements, such as the coil/gelatin protection of extra-prostatic supplies during PAE [14,15], and the use of different embolic types and sizes [16,17] or new devices, such as a balloon occlusion micro catheter [18–21], all aiming to improve efficacy and decrease non-target embolization. Obviously, in addition to these new tools/technical evolutions, another major asset for safety in performing PAE is the learning curve.

No recent experience of the overall adverse events has been reported since the improvement of knowledge and techniques. In the present study, the results of short-term complications following PAE performed after a significant learning curve are assessed.

2. Materials and Methods

This bi-institutional retrospective study was performed on 311 consecutive male patients between June 2018 and April 2022, with a mean age of 69 years ± 9.8 (47–102). Indications for PAE were patients manifesting symptomatic BPH, described as prostatic volume >35 mL associated with moderate to severe LUTSs, defined as an international prostatic symptoms score (IPSS) > 8 or a quality-of-life score (QoL) > 3/7, and showing failure of optimal medical treatment, or patients with acute urinary retention (AUR) due to BPH and failure of trial without an outer catheter after at least 48 h of alpha-blocker medication, or BPH leading to repeated episodes of bothersome macroscopic hematuria. The exclusion criteria were prostate or bladder cancer, urethral stricture, complicated BPH leading to the dilatation of urinary cavities, and factors preventing the performance of PAE, such as the occlusion of any iliac artery or advanced dementia.

Indications were validated in the clinic by a urologist and interventional radiologist.

Institutional Review Board consent was obtained from each patient for this study. The baseline characteristics of the population are presented in Table 1.

Table 1. Baseline characteristics of the study cohort.

Variable	Study Cohort (n = 311)
Age, yrs	68.7 ± 9.8 (47–102)
Height, cm	176.4 ± 6.5 (158–192)
Radial artery diameter at puncture site, mm	2.5 ± 0.3 (1.7–3.6)
Indication of PAE	
Bothersome LUTSs	246 (79.1)
Urinary retention	56 (18)
Macroscopic hematuria	9 (2.9)
IPSS	18.9 ± 7 (4–35)
QoL score	6 ± 1.1 (2–7)
IIEF-15	44.8 ± 19.5 (4–77)
Prostate volume, mL	91.9 ± 47.3 (22–360)
Maximum urinary flow, mL/s	8.1 ± 5 (2.4–31)
Post-voiding residue, mL	96.6 ± 122.3 (0–810)
Total PSA, ng/mL	6.4 ± 5.6 (0.3–28)

Note: Values are presented as mean ± SD (range) or as number, n (%). PAE: prostatic artery embolization; LUTSs: lower urinary tract symptoms; IPSS: international prostatic symptoms score; QoL: quality of life (range: 1–7); IIEF: international index of erectile function; PSA: prostatic specific antigen.

2.1. PAE Procedure

PAE was performed during ambulatory care for all patients, with the intent to use transradial access (TRA), for comfort issues and in order to shorten their hospital stay. When the left TRA was unfeasible, right transfemoral access (TFA) was used. No Foley catheter was inserted for the performance of the intervention. All patients received per-procedure antibiopropylaxy (intravenous, 1.5 g of cefazoline or 600 mg of clindamycin in case of an allergy to penicillin); no pre- nor post-procedural antibiotherapy was provided. PAE was performed in a 4D CT suite (center 1) or in a c-arm floor-mounted Angio suite equipped with a cone-beam CT (center 2), using 5-Fr TRA or TFA under local anesthesia (center 1) or local anesthesia and intravenous neurolept analgesia (center 2) composed of a mix of intravenous ketamine, midazolam, and fentanyl.

Following selective internal iliac angiography using a 5Fr catheter (Merit Medical, Salt Lake City, UT, USA), the super selective catheterization and angiography of the prostatic artery (PA) was performed on each side using a 2.0-Fr micro catheter (Merit Medical) and 0.014′ micro guide wire (Boston Scientifics, Malborough, MA, USA).

Angio CT or cone-beam CT were performed in selected cases for the detection of the origin of PA, as guidance for selective catheterization, or when angiography alone could not confirm the extra-prostatic supply from the PA.

Extra-prostatic vesical, penile, or rectal supplies were occluded prior to prostatic embolization using coil protection, as previously described [14,15]. PA with penile supplies, previously described as "pattern B PA" [12], were routinely occluded (after angiographic confirmation of at least the unilateral patency of the internal pudendal arteries), except for situations of a reversed flow in the penile arteries oriented toward the apex of the prostate, preventing the anterograde delivery of the embolic agent in the penile arteries during embolization. Rectal supplies from the PA, named "pattern C" [12], were occluded only when selective prostatic catheterization could not prevent early reflux in the rectal artery in pattern C1 and routinely in case of pattern C2 (distal origin of an accessory rectal artery). In cases of an accessory inferior vesical artery (AIVA) or a vesical anastomose originating from the distal part of the PA, coil protection was used only when early reflux was observed during selective prostatic angiography to prevent non-target embolization (Figure 1).

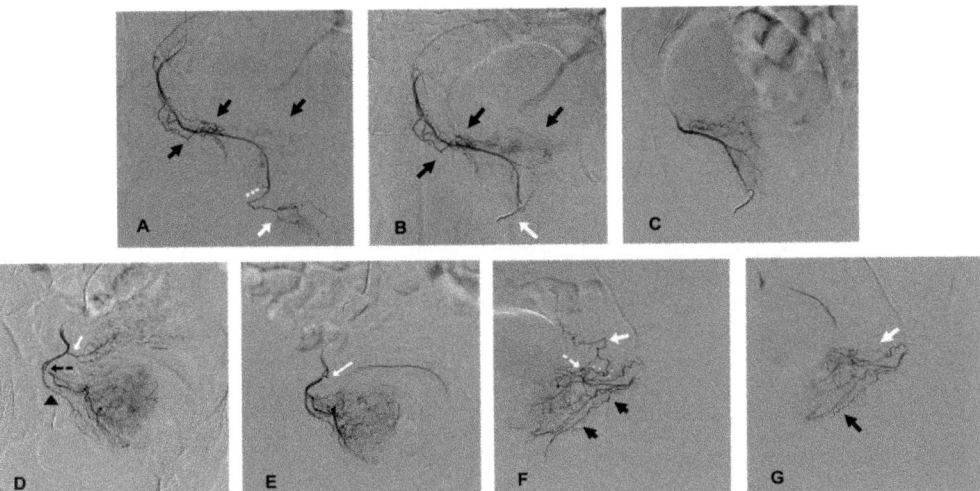

Figure 1. Cases of coil protection of extra-prostatic supplies during PAE and prior to microparticle delivery for safe embolization. (**A–C**) present a case of coil protection of a pattern B prostatic artery (PA). (**A**): selective angiography of the right PA on an ipsilateral oblique view, originating from a right accessory internal pudendal artery (APA). Penile arteries are visible at the end of the APA (white arrow) and distally to the prostatic arterial branches (black arrows); the penile bed should be protected from microparticle non-target prostatic embolization (the elective location of occlusion is marked with white asterisks). (**B**): repeat angiography on ipsilateral oblique view, prior to microparticle delivery, and after a 2 and 3 mm diameter detachable microcoil insertion (white arrow). Penile supply is occluded (penile arteries are no longer opacified) and prostatic vessels are still patent (black arrows). (**C**): repeat angiography on anteroposterior (AP) view prior to prostatic embolization for confirmation of a full uptake of the right hemi prostate. Penile supply is still occluded. (**D,E**) present a case of occlusion of an accessory inferior vesical artery (AIVA). (**D**): selective angiography of the right PA on ipsilateral oblique view. The tip of the microcatheter is inserted in the medial branch of the PA (marked by a black, dotted arrow) and the lateral prostatic branch is marked by a black arrow head. Early reflux is observed in an ipsilateral AIVA (white arrow) originating from the PA, confirming the risk of non-target embolization. (**E**): repeat angiography on AP view prior to PAE and after the insertion of a 2 mm detachable coil in the AIVA (white arrow). The vesical supply is no longer visible and there is a full uptake of the right hemi prostate. (**F,G**) present a case of occlusion of rectal and

vesical supplies. (**F**): selective angiography on ipsilateral oblique view of a left prostatic artery, which carries a common trunk with a rectal artery (black arrows), described as pattern C1. There is an associated anastomosis (arterial loop marked by a white, dotted arrow) between the PA and left inferior vesical artery (IVA, white arrow), which needs to be occluded prior to microparticle delivery (elective location marked by white asterisks). (**G**): repeat angiography on oblique view prior to PAE and after the insertion of 2 mm detachable micro coils in the anastomosis to the IVA (white arrow) and in the rectal artery (black arrow), confirming the occlusion of vesical and rectal supplies.

After ruling out or occluding the extra-prostatic supply from the PA, super selective proximal PAE was performed, using 300–500 µm calibrated trisacryl microparticles, until complete stasis. At a complete bilateral PAE, catheters were retrieved and the access site was closed using a hemostatic band for TRA (TR band®, Terumo Corporation, Tokyo, Japan, or Prelude Sync®, Merit Medical), or a closure device (Exoseal® 5Fr, Cordis, Miami Lakes, FL, USA) in case of TFA. Patients were discharged 75 to 90 min (TRA) or 180 to 240 min (TFA) after the completion of PAE.

Technical success was defined as achieving at least unilateral PAE. Clinical success was defined as an IPPS decrease of at least 8 points, a QoL score decrease of 1 point or score <3, the ability to stop any medication later than 15 days following PAE, the successful retrieval of the Foley catheter at day 15, or the disappearance of hematuria. The removal of the indwelling catheter was delayed by 10 days in case of ongoing urinary tract infection (UTI) after elective oral antibiotic treatment.

Follow-up was performed at 1, 6, and 12 months to assess clinical success using identical documentation as pre-procedural workup. Post-embolization syndrome and minor/major complications following PAE were defined according to the Society of Interventional Radiology classification of complications [22], and were monitored at one month using a standardized questionnaire filled out by the patient. Additional left radial artery Doppler ultrasound simultaneously monitored TRA adverse events. Mid-term adverse events were monitored at a 6-month follow-up, when a short-term adverse event was observed at the 1-month follow-up. Patients were deemed lost to follow-up when the questionnaire regarding adverse events was not filled out at 1 month, or when no documentation regarding an ongoing adverse event or no follow-up exams were obtained at 6- and 12-month visits.

2.2. Statistical Analysis

The differences between the baseline and 1-month data were assessed using Student's paired t-test and R software, version 4.1.1. The results are expressed as mean ± SD (range) and their *p*-values. A *p*-value < 0.05 was considered significant.

2.3. Results

A total of 315 patients were referred by the urologist for PAE (Figure 2). Over the course of the pre-procedural assessment, prostatic MRI revealed two cases of advanced prostatic cancer extending to the bladder neck, one case of a T2a staged prostatic cancer, and one case of advanced bladder cancer extending to the prostate. These four patients did not undergo PAE and were referred back to the urologist, because LUTSs were not caused by BPH but by locally advanced cancer (*n* = 3) or because prostatic cancer required oncological treatment (*n* = 1).

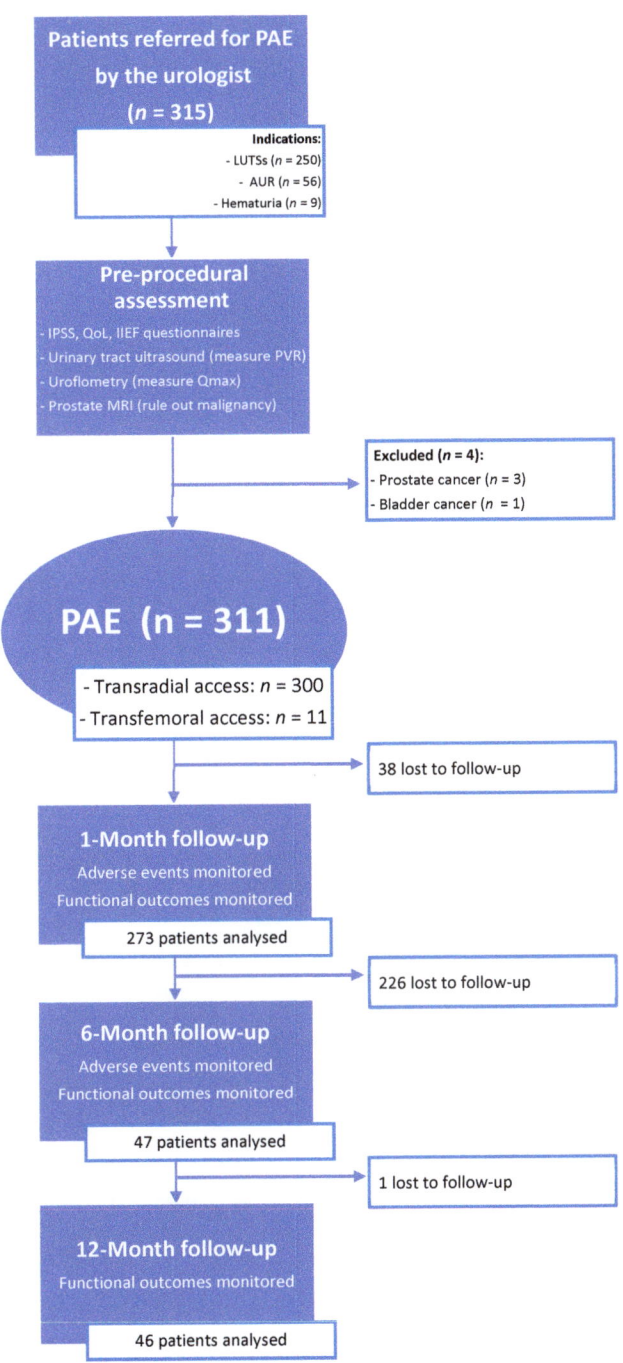

Figure 2. Patient flowchart. PAE: prostatic artery embolization; LUTSs: lower urinary tract symptoms; AUR: acute urinary retention; IPSS: international prostatic symptoms score; QoL: quality of life; IIEF: international index of erectile function; PVR: post-voiding residue; Qmax: maximum urinary flow.

A total of 300/311 (96.4%) patients underwent transradial outpatient PAE and 11/311 (3.6%) transfemoral outpatient PAE. Bilateral embolization was performed in 305/311 (98.1%) cases. Mean DAP/fluoroscopy times were $16{,}408.3 \pm 12{,}078.9$ (2959–81,608) $\mu Gy.m^2/36.3 \pm 15.7$ (11–97) minutes. Angio CT or CBCT was needed for 10/311 (3.2%) patients; 6 mappings of the PA, 4 to rule out extra-prostatic supplies. The procedure characteristics are presented in Table 2 and the distribution of prostatic arterial vasculature in Table 2 and Figures 3 and 4, according to Assis's and Amouyal's classification [11,12].

Table 2. Procedure characteristics of the study cohort.

Variable	Study Cohort (n = 311)
Transfemoral access	11 (3.6)
Transradial access	300 (96.4)
Unilateral embolization	6 (1.9)
Procedure time, min	96.5 ± 27.4 (45–195)
Fluoroscopy time, min	36.3 ± 15.7 (11–97)
DAP, $\mu Gy.m^2$	$16{,}408.3 \pm 12{,}078.9$ (2959–81,608)
Radiation skin entry, mGy	1585.7 ± 1115.7 (238–5958)
Mean time to discharge after completion of procedure, min	80.3 ± 7.1 (75–240)
Angiographic review and 3D-angriographic guidance	
Mapping of PA	6 (1.9)
Rule out extra-prostatic supply	4 (1.3)
Coil protection of extra-prostatic supply from prostatic artery	
Vesical accessory artery	23 (7.4)
Prostato-penile anastomose (pattern B)	30 (9.6)
Middle rectal artery from prostato-rectal artery (pattern C1)	20 (6.4)
Accessory rectal artery from prostato-rectal artery (pattern C2)	5 (1.6)
	Hemi-Pelvis (n = 622)
Solitary prostatic artery per side	493 (79.3)
Multiple prostatic arteries par side	129 (20.7)

Note: Values are presented as mean ± SD (range) or as number, n (%). Min: minute; DAP: dose-area product; Gy: gray; PA: prostatic artery; patterns B, C1, and C2 refer to the classification proposed by Amouyal et al.

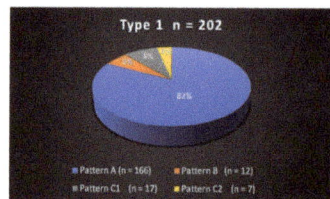
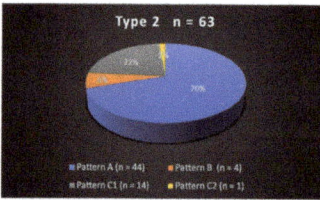
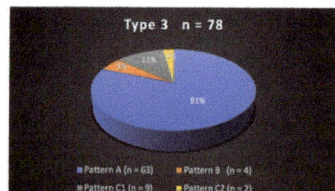
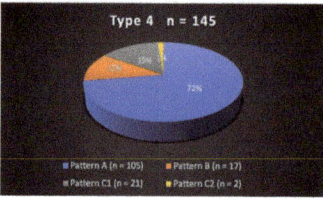
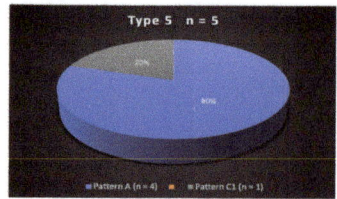

Figure 3. Distribution in study cohort of the origins of the solitary prostatic arteries according to the different patterns. Types 1 to 5 represent the possible origins of the prostatic artery (PA), according to the Assis classification. The values are presented as a number, n. Patterns A, B, and C1 and C2 correspond to the different intra/extra-prostatic supplies of the prostatic artery in case of a solitary PA (one artery per side, n = 493/622 (79.3%) in this study), according to the Amouyal classification. The values are presented as a number (n) and %.

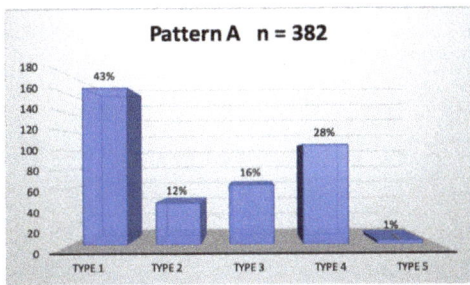
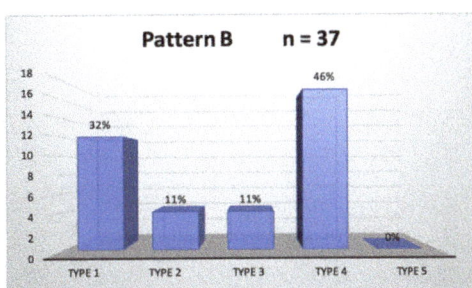
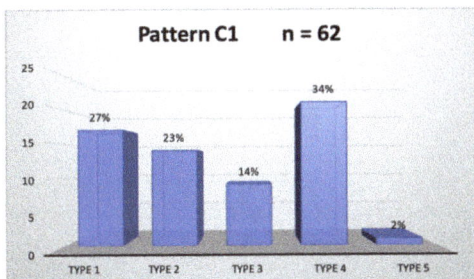
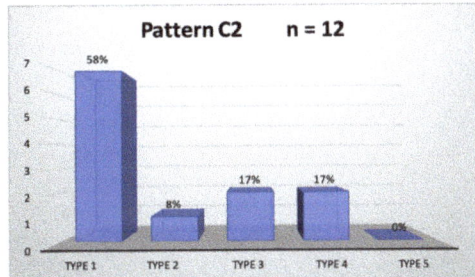

Figure 4. Distribution in study cohort of the patterns of the solitary prostatic arteries according to the different origins. Patterns A, B, and C1 and C2 correspond to the different intra/extra-prostatic supplies of the prostatic artery in the case of a solitary PA (one artery per side, n = 493/622 (79.3%) in this study), according to the Amouyal classification. The values are presented as number, n. Types 1 to 5 represent the possible origins of the PA, according to the Assis classification. The values are presented as a percentage, %.

Coil protection was considered as necessary to prevent non-target embolization in 67/311 (21.5%) patients in 78 extra-prostatic supplies. Among pattern B PAs, 30/37 (81%) benefited from coil protection: 4 did not because of a reversed flow in the penile arteries and 3 because the coil protection of pattern B PA had already been performed on the contralateral side. Among C1 and C2 pattern arteries, 20/62 (32%) middle rectal arteries were protected because of early reflux from the prostatic branch (C1) and 5/12 accessory rectal artery (42%) (C2) when its super selective catheterization was achievable. Among AIVA/vesical anastomoses, 23/58 (40%) required protection.

Mean follow-up was 4.35 months.

Post-embolization syndrome was observed in 264/311 (84.9%) patients, and urethral burning and pollakiuria were the predominant symptoms. The mean duration increased for most symptoms with prostate volume (Table 3); the overall mean durations for urethral burning and pollakiuria were 4 ± 3.9 (0–12) and 4.2 ± 3.4 (0–12) days. There were 8/311 (2.6%) cases of transient hematospermia that spontaneously resolved within 1 to 90 days. For each patient, control MRI did not present a seminal vesicle signal or enhancement abnormality. The overall post-embolization symptoms and their durations according to prostate volume are presented in Table 3.

Table 3. Duration of post-embolization syndrome according to prostate volume.

Variable	Mean Duration, Days					
	PV < 40	PV (40–50)	PV (50–80)	PV (80–100)	PV > 100	Overall PV
Mild fever	0	1.4 ± 3.1 (0–7)	0.1 ± 0.3 (0–1)	0.5 ± 1 (0–2)	0.5 ± 1.5 (0–5)	0.4 ± 1.4 (0–7)
Urethral burning	1 ± 1.4 (0–2)	4.2 ± 5.8 (0–11)	3.7 ± 3.8 (0–10)	3.8 ± 3.3 (0–10)	5.1 ± 4.1 (0–12)	4 ± 3.9 (0–12)
Pollakiuria	0	2 ± 3.9 (0–9)	3.8 ± 3.2 (0–10)	4 ± 2.3 (2–9)	6.2 ± 3.1 (3–12)	4.2 ± 3.4 (0–12)
Constipation	0	1 ± 1.4 (0–3)	0.8 ± 1.1 (0–3)	0.3 ± 2.8 (0–2)	1.2 ± 1.6 (0–3)	0.7 ± 1.2 (0–4)
Pelvic pain	1 ± 1.4 (0–2)	6.4 ± 6.3 (0–15)	2.8 ± 5.3 (0–20)	2.8 ± 3.2 (0–9)	2.6 ± 3.8 (0–12)	3.1 ± 4.5 (0–20)
Anal burning/pain	0	3 ± 6.7 (0–15)	2 ± 4.3 (0–15)	0.04 ± 0.8 (0–2)	1.2 ± 2.8 (0–10)	1.5 ± 3.7 (0–15)
Hematospermia	0	7 ± 12 (0–28)	12.4 ± 25.6 (0–90)	4 ± 6 (0–16)	0	6.5 ± 17.2 (0–90)

Note: Values are represented as mean ± SD (range) or as number, n (%). PV: prostatic volume (mL) represented as range.

2.4. Adverse Events

All adverse events were minor, most occurred in the first 21 days (Tables 4 and 5), and all but one were monitored at the 1-month follow-up control or reported by the patient prior to the visit. There was no major adverse event. Access-site adverse events are presented in Table 5 and are mostly represented by hematoma.

Table 4. Embolization-related adverse events.

Variable	Study Cohort (n = 311)
Acute urinary retention	0
Foley catheter-related urinary tract infection	2 (0.6)
Urinary tract infection (catheter-free)	0
Hematuria	8 (2.6)
Rectorrhagia	2 (0.6)
Balanitis	2 (0.6)
Detachment of prostatic fragment	1 (0.3)
Worsening of erectile dysfunction	1 (0.3)
Transient ejaculate volume decrease	5 (1.7)
Anejaculation	0
Bladder ischemia	0
Rectal ischemia	0
Penile glans necrotic ulcer	0

Note: Values are presented as mean ± SD (range) or as a number, n (%).

Table 5. Access-site adverse events.

Variable	TRA (n = 300)	TFA (n = 11)
Stroke	0	0
Hand pain	0	0
Groin pain	–	2 (18)
Hematoma	30 (10)	1 (9)
Pseudo-aneurysm at puncture site	0	0
Thrombosed pseudo-aneurysm at puncture site	2 (0.7)	0
Arteritis	3 (1)	0
Radial artery occlusion	10 (3.3)	–

Note: Values are represented as mean ± SD (range) or as a number, n (%). TRA: transradial access; TFA: transfemoral access.

Embolization-related complications ranged from 0.6 to 2.6%: there were 2/311 (0.6%) cases of urinary tract infection in patients treated for AUR, for whom an indwelling catheter was still in place, occurring at days 10 and 12, manifested by moderate fever and a positive urinary sample test. Both were successfully treated by oral antibiotics for 15 days. Catheter removal was attempted 10 days after relief of fever: one was successful, the other failed, and so did a second attempt 15 days later.

There were 2/311 (0.6%) cases of transient balanitis appearing at days 2 and 3, manifested by bilateral asymptomatic zones of fibrin on the mucosa of the glans that were successfully treated with local antiseptic and antibiotics and resolved within 15 days with no sequelae.

An angiographic review of these two cases reported the presence for each patient of an accessory PA supplying the gland from the apex ("distal pudendal PA"), originating from the distal portion of the internal pudendal artery (IPA), in close proximity to the penile vessels.

There were 8/311 (2.6%) cases of macroscopic hematuria occurring between days 1 and 20, except for one case associated with fragment detachment at day 90. All were spontaneously resolved within 24 h. A retrospective angiographic review revealed a bilateral type-1 origin of the PA according to De Assis (common origin with the vesical arteries) in two patients and a unilateral type-1 origin in six patients. The coil protection of an AIVA was performed on one patient.

There were 2/311 (0.6%) cases of a single episode of rectorrhagia manifested by traces of blood in the stool occurring at days 1 and 3, in a context of constipation, also resolved in 24 h. An angiographic review reported bilateral pattern A origins for both patients and no coil protection of rectal arteries.

There was one case (1/311, 0.3%) of transient worsening of erectile dysfunction following coil protection of a pattern B PA. In this patient, there was a short and proximal occlusion of the ipsilateral IPA, whereas contralateral IPA was patent. As IPA was patent on one side, the decision was made to use coil protection. The revascularization of the occluded IPA was proposed to the patient at day 21 with the aim to improve erectile function, which he refused, and instead preferred tadalafil oral medication with limited efficacy. LUTS improved within 15 days and erectile dysfunction spontaneously improved to reach pre-embolization status within six months with no further need for tadalafil.

There was one case (0.3%) of detachment of the prostatic fragment occurring at three months. At the 1-month follow-up, patient symptoms had improved: IPSS/QoL scores and the prostatic volume changed from 26, 7, and 120 mL to 4, 1, and 80. Approximately three months following PAE, the patient suddenly presented an episode of hematuria associated with a recurrence of dysuria and pelvic pain during urination. He described the spontaneous expulsion of several small fragments of prostatic tissue and a clot during micturition, for 48 h. As the symptoms persisted, the patient visited the urology department and a cystoscopic examination performed five days later revealed a clot and necrotic scar on the median lobe wall, from which a centimetric fragment was removed with no subsequent bleeding. No MRI was performed in this urgent context. Dysuria/pain disappeared after the fragment removal and there was no anejaculation following this partial resection.

There were 5/311 (1.7%) cases of a transient reduction in ejaculate volume lasting from 15 days to 4 months. There were no cases of anejaculation.

There was no case of acute urinary retention, glans, rectal or vesical partial ischemia, or radiodermitis.

Apart from radial artery occlusion at the puncture site, no persistent adverse event was observed at 6- and 12-month follow-up controls.

2.5. Clinical Success

The successful removal of the Foley catheter on day 15 for patients treated for AUR was observed in 44/56 (78.6%) patients. Overall clinical success was 268/311 (86.2%) at the 1-month follow-up control: mean IPSS and QoL scores decreased from 18.9 ± 7 (4–35) and 6 ± 1.1 (2–7) to 8.7 ± 7.2 (0–35) ($p < 0.001$) and 3 ± 1.7 (1–7) ($p < 0.001$). There was no significant change in mean IIEF score values ($p = 0.83$); mean maximum urinary flow increased from 8.1 ± 5 (2.4–31) mL/s to 13.4 ± 6.1 (3–32) ($p < 0.001$); and mean post-voiding residue, prostate volume, and total PSA decreased significantly ($p < 0.001$) (Table 6).

Table 6. Baseline and follow-up characteristics in study cohort.

Variable	Baseline	1 Month
IPSS	18.9 ± 7 (4–35)	8.7 ± 7.2 (0–35) ($p < 0.001$)
QoL score	6 ± 1.1 (2–7)	3 ± 1.7 (1–7) ($p < 0.001$)
IIEF-15	44.8 ± 19.5 (4–77)	47.6 ± 19.1 (5–72) ($p = 0.83$)
Prostate volume, mL	91.9 ± 47.3 (22–360)	69.4 ± 32 (20–190) ($p < 0.001$)
Maximum urinary flow, mL/s	8.1 ± 5 (2.4–31)	13.4 ± 6.1 (3–32) ($p < 0.001$)
Post-voiding residue, mL	96.6 ± 122.3 (0–810)	39.3 ± 59 (0–270) ($p < 0.001$)
Total PSA, ng/mL	6.4 ± 5.6 (0.3–28)	4 ± 3.1 (0.4–15) ($p < 0.001$)

Note: Values are presented as mean ± SD (range) (p-value). Comparison of the data is conducted from its baseline value. p-values were obtained using Student's paired t-test. A p-value < 0.05 represents a significant difference. IPSS: international prostatic symptoms score; QoL: quality of life (range: 1–7); IIEF: international index of erectile function; PSA: prostatic specific antigen; mL: milliliter; mL/s: milliliter/second.

3. Discussion

The present study of ambulatory PAE reported low rates (0.6 to 2.6%) of embolization-related minor adverse events and no major adverse event. Major adverse events remain rare and each one is estimated to occur in 0.08% to 0.24% of cases [7–10].

3.1. Embolization-Related Adverse Events

As most major and minor complications follow non-target embolization, a possible explanation for their absence/low rate in this report may be the increased knowledge concerning the management of extra-prostatic communications during PAE [14,15] and prostatic arterial anatomy [11–13]. Three-dimensional imaging during selective angiography used as a routine practice may help to rule out extra-prostatic supplies, and its need may decrease over time and eventually be restricted to elective cases once a significant learning curve is achieved.

Early minor events ranged from 0.6 to 2.6%, which were lower than those previously reported [7–10]. Multiple adverse events previously described in the literature and meta-analyses were not observed in this study, which may suggest a significant decrease in non-target embolization and may be explained by the improvement of experience during recent years.

There was no AUR compared to the 4.55, 7, 9 and 7.8% previously described [7–10]. AUR is favored by bladder distension during and after PAE and the increase in urethral stricture and bladder outlet obstruction due to post-embolization intra-prostatic oedema. Foley catheter insertion during PAE was not necessary as less invasive measures, such as urinating moments prior to entering the Angio suite, a urinal at their disposal during the procedure, and immediate voiding after PAE, were efficient to prevent retention. Furthermore, TRA permits urination in a standing position, moments after the procedure, which facilitates micturition.

Hematuria occurred in 2.6%, which was lower compared to the 5.51, 9, 4.45, and 4.38% previously reported [7–10]. As the angiographic review reported the close proximity of the vesical arteries to the PA (at least one type-1 PA per patient), these events may suggest that non-target vesical embolization due to reflux of the embolic agent was possibly the cause of hematuria. Nonetheless, the short duration of this event (24 h in all cases except the one associated with prostatic fragment detachment) may suggest the bleeding of prostate tissue necrosis during its healing process following PAE.

One case of 24 h-lasting hematuria and no micturition symptom followed coil protection of an AIVA or a vesical anastomosis, which suggests the safety of this technique for bladder viability and confirms the findings of a previous report in the literature [15]. On the other hand, the absence of coil protection of a vesical artery or anastomose in proximity to the prostatic artery may lead to bladder ischemia: a previous case report reported focal bladder necrosis following non-target vesical embolization during PAE using 100–300 μm microparticles, that was successfully treated by Foley catheter placement for several weeks [23].

There was a 0.6% rate of rectorrhagia, which was lower than the 4.8, 3.9, 3.02, and 3.02% previously reported [7–10]. The hypothesis for rectal bleeding following PAE is non-target embolization and ischemic ulceration of the rectum. This was previously described in a case report for PAE using 100–300 μm particles, where coil protection was not performed, with the spontaneous resolution of ulcerations within 5 days [24]. In this study, both cases of rectorrhagia did not present arterial anatomy at risk of non-target rectal embolization. As the amount and duration of bleeding were negligible, the traces of blood in stool that were reported by the patients may instead be attributed to hemorrhoid hemorrhage provoked by constipation. Furthermore, there were interestingly 7/12 (58%) cases of pattern C2 PA where the accessory rectal artery could not be coil-protected and was therefore fully embolized with no post-operative complication. This may suggest that the embolization of pattern C2 PAs using 300–500 μm particles does not necessarily require coil protection. This supposition could have been stronger in case of a control group purposely not performing coil protection, but the case report mentioned regarding the above [24] made the safety of such a design questionable.

This hypothesis will need further comparative studies for confirmation, but the safety profile of future study designs must be considered. As the size of the microparticles used may play a role in the occurrence of adverse events [23,24], the choice of particle size of the type of embolic should be carefully made, and choosing to use 300–500 μm particles may be the best option for future randomized trials. In our opinion, the choice of a control group performing the abstention of coil protection may be too risky, and coil protection should be compared to the balloon occlusion micro-catheter technique. Concerning small rectal arteries arising from the PA (pattern C2), the results of this study may suggest another safety profile other than vesical, penile, or large rectal extra-prostatic supplies in case of non-target embolization using 300–500 μm particles.

There was no sign of rectal ischemia following coil protection, which confirmed the results of the previous reports [14,15].

Balanitis was observed in 0.6%, which is comparable to the 0.6, 0.3, and 0.7% reported [8–10]. This event occurred in a particular anatomical pattern previously described. Penile adverse events, secondary to non-target microparticle embolization, are more likely to occur in situations where the PA is close to penile vessels, such as pattern B PA, accessory distal pudendal PA, or type-4 PA, and, despite cautious microparticle delivery, can lead to ischemic balanitis or, in the worst case, necrosis of the glans penis [25]. The findings in this study may suggest cautious particle delivery when embolizing the PA in a situation of distal pudendal PA: reflux during embolization may be at a higher risk of adverse events and should be avoided. Coil protection of pattern B PA, when possible, was safe in this study, as previously reported [14,15]. When coil protection is precluded, a balloon occlusion micro catheter may be of use [21] to prevent reflux.

UTIs were found in 0.6% in this cohort, only in patients with a Foley catheter in place because of an AUR, which was lower compared to the 3.1, 2.7, and 3.32% described in the literature [7,9,10]. No distinction was made in previous reports between patients with a Foley catheter or catheter-free. In several studies assessed in meta-analyses, Foley catheter insertion during PAE was performed to facilitate the procedure [4,26,27], which was not the case for patients from this cohort. The findings in this study suggest that the insertion and/or presence of Foley catheter may increase the risk of UTIs.

There was one case of a transient worsening of erectile dysfunction (ED) following the coil protection of a prostato-penile artery in a situation of ipsilateral IPA occlusion. De novo ED following PAE is rare and has been reported [5], but never occurred after coil protection [14,15,28–30].

We believe that coil protection should be avoided in situations of poor IPA vasculature. IPA revascularization may also be considered [31] to permit safe bilateral PAE in a two-step process.

There was one case of the detachment of prostate fragments three months after PAE. This rare event was reported in three case reports and a retrospective report in a total of 8 patients and occurred at 2 to 10 weeks: spontaneous tissue elimination of fragment(s) ranging from a 10 to 15 mm diameter and up to 60 mm long was reported after PAE using 250 μm (1 case) [32] or 100–300 ± 300–500 μm microparticles (3 cases) [33], and 4 cases of detachment following 250 μm particles PAE [34,35] required cystoscopic removal of multiple fragments. In the latter (3/48 patients, 6.3%), predictors for the detachment of prostatic tissue were proposed, such as indwelling catheter, high central gland index, and inflammation. Detachment seems to be correlated with the use of small size embolics <300 μm. Torres et al. reported in a randomized study no clinical benefit of 100–300 μm compared to 300–500 μm trisacryl microparticles, and more frequent minor adverse events [17].

Hematospermia was observed in 2.6%, compared to the 3.63, 4.09, and 5.2 reported [7–9]. Occurrence may vary from a study to another as its identification relies on sexual activity. Previous reports link its occurrence to the non-target embolization of seminal vesicles [2]. Ischemia of the seminal vesicles following PAE was described [36,37], but as all control MRI in this study did not show morphological/enhancement abnormalities of the SV in patients manifesting hematospermia, bleeding from necrotic prostatic tissue during ejaculation may not be excluded. This is why it was decided in this report to consider hematospermia as a post-embolization symptom rather than an adverse event.

No case of anejaculation was reported. There is, to our knowledge, no report of anejaculation following PAE using 300–500 μm trisacryl microparticles. Anejaculation following PAE ranges in the radiologic literature from 0 to 2.3% [7–10]. The reasons are unclear. A recent urological report of PAE using 250–400 μm polyzene microparticles [38] reported an unexpected 4/25 (16%) rate of anejaculation and 40% of decreased ejaculation volume assessed by a 4-item sexual questionnaire 3 months after PAE. Among patients facing anejaculation, 3/4 had undergone endoscopic enucleation of the prostate following symptomatic detachment of prostatic tissue after PAE. Furthermore, longer follow-up (>3 months) on ejaculation was not available.

3.2. Access-Site Adverse Events

Complications concerning TRA during PAE in this study were comparable to the previous reports on TRA during PAE: there [14,15] were 10% and 3.3% rates of hematoma and radial artery occlusion. Bhatia et al. [39] and Isaacson et al. [40] described 9 and 11% of hematoma and no radial artery occlusion; the number of patients (32 and 19) was lower.

3.3. Clinical Success

There was 86.2% of clinical success following PAE, and baseline characteristics evolved favorably within one month with results comparable to what was previously described in the literature [7–10]. As efficacy was not the topic of this study, and as clinical success was previously shown to be similar between patients undergoing PAE using coil/gelatin protection and the basic technique [14], clinical success was not compared in the population of this study benefiting from coil protection with a control group.

3.4. Follow-Up

There was a 12.2% (38/311) rate of loss to follow-up at one month, and 84.9% and 85.2% (264/311 and 265/311) at 6 and 12 months. The amount of missing data after the one-month follow-up needs to be considered. Still, as all but one adverse events were monitored at one month because they occurred during the first days following PAE and had, except for a few rare events, resolved within the first month prior to the one-month follow-up visit, the loss of follow-up may not have a significant impact on estimating the overall occurrence of adverse events and only limits the results on mid-term functional outcomes and clinical success. Furthermore, patients manifesting adverse events lasting longer than one month or occurring between months 1 and 6, such as transient decreased ejaculate volume, prostate fragment detachment, or radial artery occlusion, were all observed in the clinic at 6- and 12-month visits.

This report has some limitations, including its retrospective nature, the limited number of studied patients, the loss of follow-up at mid-term visits, and the short period of follow-up time. Additionally, this study lacks control groups, especially concerning measures used for the protection of extra-prostatic arterial supplies. Most adverse events were retrospectively monitored and based on patient testimony only, and were not confirmed by clinical examination or assessed by urinary/blood tests or imaging at the time of occurrence. This may have led to the over- or underestimation of their occurrence.

4. Conclusions

This study showed that outpatient PAE using 300–500 µm calibrated microparticles with improved anatomical knowledge and techniques can lead to fewer and lower rates of minor embolization-related adverse events than previously reported. These findings demand confirmation by complementary studies. The extensive use of coil protection may be questioned, and its comparison to the balloon occlusion microcatheter or other innovative techniques in randomized designs is necessary to assess its utility in different situations of an acknowledged risk of non-target embolization. Furthermore, there is a need to identify predictors for rare adverse events.

Author Contributions: Conceptualization, G.A. Methodology, G.A. Software, G.A. and L.T. Validation, E.D.K. Formal Analysis, G.A. and L.T. Investigation, G.A. Resources and Data Curation, C.D.M.-M., D.B., A.P., J.A., C.D.B., F.M., S.L.S. and F.D. Writing—Original Draft Preparation, G.A. Writing—Review and Editing, E.D.K. Visualization, E.D.K. Supervision, E.D.K. All authors have read and agreed to the published version of the manuscript.

Funding: This research received no external funding.

Institutional Review Board Statement: The study was conducted according to the guidelines of the Declaration of Helsinki and approved by the Institutional Review Board IRB00010835 of HOSPITAL PRIVE GEOFFROY SAINT-HILAIRE, Ramsay Santé Recherche & Enseignement (protocol code: COS-RGDS-2020-05-015-AMOUYAL-G; date of approval: 18 May 2020).

Informed Consent Statement: Informed consent was obtained from all subjects involved in the study.

Data Availability Statement: Data containing patient characteristics prior to and after the intervention, in addition to procedure characteristic, are available and can be found in the PACS and RIS of Hospital privé Geoffroy Saint-Hilaire and Hospital Saint-Louis, where the interventions occurred.

Conflicts of Interest: G.A. received financial support from Merit Medical (Salt Lake City, Utah) for educational programs. L.T., C.d.M.-M., A.P., J.A., D.B., C.d.B., F.M., S.L.S. and F.D. declare no conflicts of interest. E.d.K. received financial support from Canon Medical (Otawara, Japon) and Boston Scientific (Malborough, Massachusetts) for attending/speaking at symposia/congresses and educational programs.

Abbreviations

PAE	Prostatic Artery Embolization
BPH	Benign Prostatic Hyperplasia
LUTSs	Lower Urinary Tract Symptoms
IPSS	International Prostatic Symptoms Score
QoL	Quality-of-Life Score
AUR	Acute Urinary Retention
TRA	Transradial Access
TFA	Tranfemoral Access

PA	Prostatic Artery
AIVA	Accessory Inferior Vesical Artery
UTI	Urinary Tract Infection
AP view	Antero-Posterior View
CBCT	Cone-Beam Computed Tomodensitometry
APA	Accessory Pudendal Artery
IPA	Internal Pudendal Artery

References

1. Carnevale, F.C.; da Motta-Leal-Filho, J.M.; Antunes, A.A.; Baroni, R.H.; Freire, G.C.; Cerri, L.M.O.; Marcelino, A.S.Z.; Cerri, G.G.; Srougi, M. Midterm Follow-Up After Prostate Embolization in Two Patients with Benign Prostatic Hyperplasia. *Cardiovasc. Interv. Radiol.* **2011**, *34*, 1330–1333. [CrossRef] [PubMed]
2. Pisco, J.M.; Bilhim, T.; Pinheiro, L.C.; Fernandes, L.; Pereira, J.; Costa, N.V.; Duarte, M.; Oliveira, A.G. Medium- and Long-Term Outcome of Prostate Artery Embolization for Patients with Benign Prostatic Hyperplasia: Results in 630 Patients. *J. Vasc. Interv. Radiol.* **2016**, *27*, 1115–1122. [CrossRef]
3. Gao, Y.A.; Huang, Y.; Zhang, R.; Yang, Y.D.; Zhang, Q.; Hou, M.; Wang, Y. Benign prostatic hyperplasia: Prostatic arterial embolization versus transurethral resection of the prostate—A prospective, randomized, and controlled clinical trial. *Radiology* **2014**, *270*, 920–928. [CrossRef] [PubMed]
4. Carnevale, F.C.; Iscaife, A.; Yoshinaga, E.M.; Moreira, A.M.; Antunes, A.A.; Srougi, M. Transurethral Resection of the Prostate (TURP) Versus Original and PErFecTED Prostate Artery Embolization (PAE) Due to Benign Prostatic Hyperplasia (BPH): Preliminary Results of a Single Center, Prospective, Urodynamic-Controlled Analysis. *Cardiovasc. Interv. Radiol.* **2016**, *39*, 44–52. [CrossRef]
5. Abt, D.; Hechelhammer, L.; Müllhaupt, G.; Markart, S.; Güsewell, S.; Kessler, T.M.; Schmid, H.-P.; Engeler, D.; Mordasini, L. Comparison of prostatic artery embolisation (PAE) versus transurethral resection of the prostate (TURP) for benign prostatic hyperplasia: Randomised, open label, non-inferiority trial. *BMJ* **2018**, *361*, k2338. [CrossRef]
6. Insausti, I.; de Ocáriz, A.S.; Galbete, A.; Capdevila, F.; Solchaga, S.; Giral, P.; Bilhim, T.; Isaacson, A.; Urtasun, F.; Napal, S. Randomized Comparison of Prostatic Artery Embolization versus Transurethral Resection of the Prostate for Treatment of Benign Prostatic Hyperplasia. *J. Vasc. Interv. Radiol.* **2020**, *31*, 882–890. [CrossRef] [PubMed]
7. Uflacker, A.; Haskal, Z.J.; Bilhim, T.; Patrie, J.; Huber, T.; Pisco, J.M. Meta-Analysis of Prostatic Artery Embolization for Benign Prostatic Hyperplasia. *J. Vasc. Interv. Radiol.* **2016**, *27*, 1686–1697.e8. [CrossRef]
8. Cizman, Z.; Isaacson, A.; Burke, C. Short- to Midterm Safety and Efficacy of Prostatic Artery Embolization: A Systematic Review. *J. Vasc. Interv. Radiol.* **2016**, *27*, 1487–1493.e1. [CrossRef]
9. Feng, S.; Tian, Y.; Liu, W.; Li, Z.; Deng, T.; Li, H.; Wang, K. Prostatic Arterial Embolization Treating Moderate-to-Severe Lower Urinary Tract Symptoms Related to Benign Prostate Hyperplasia: A Meta-Analysis. *Cardiovasc. Interv. Radiol.* **2017**, *40*, 22–32. [CrossRef]
10. Malling, B.; Røder, M.A.; Brasso, K.; Forman, J.; Taudorf, M.; Lönn, L. Prostate artery embolisation for benign prostatic hyperplasia: A systematic review and meta-analysis. *Eur. Radiol.* **2018**, *29*, 287–298. [CrossRef] [PubMed]
11. de Assis, A.M.; Moreira, A.M.; de Paula Rodrigues, V.C.; Harward, S.H.; Antunes, A.A.; Srougi, M.; Carnevale, F.C. Pelvic Arterial Anatomy Relevant to Prostatic Artery Embolisation and Proposal for Angiographic Classification. *Cardiovasc. Interv. Radiol.* **2015**, *38*, 855–861. [CrossRef] [PubMed]
12. Amouyal, G.; Pellerin, O.; Del Giudice, C.; Dean, C.; Thiounn, N.; Sapoval, M. Variants of Patterns of Intra- and Extra-prostatic Arterial Distribution of the Prostatic Artery Applied to Prostatic Artery Embolization: Proposal of a Classification. *Cardiovasc. Interv. Radiol.* **2018**, *41*, 1664–1673. [CrossRef] [PubMed]
13. DeMeritt, J.S.; Wajswol, E.; Wattamwar, A.; Osiason, A.; Chervoni-Knapp, T.; Zamudio, S. Duplicated Prostate Artery Central Gland Blood Supply: A Retrospective Analysis and Classification System. *J. Vasc. Interv. Radiol.* **2018**, *29*, 1595–1600.e9. [CrossRef] [PubMed]
14. Amouyal, G.; Chague, P.; Pellerin, O.; Pereira, H.; Del Giudice, C.; Dean, C.; Thiounn, N.; Sapoval, M. Safety and Efficacy of Occlusion of Large Extra-Prostatic Anastomoses During Prostatic Artery Embolization for Symptomatic, B.P.H. *Cardiovasc. Interv. Radiol.* **2016**, *39*, 1245–1255. [CrossRef]
15. Bhatia, S.; Sinha, V.; Bordegaray, M.; Kably, I.; Harward, S.; Narayanan, G. Role of Coil Embolization during Prostatic Artery Embolization: Incidence, Indications, and Safety Profile. *J. Vasc. Interv. Radiol.* **2017**, *28*, 656–664.e3. [CrossRef] [PubMed]
16. Wang, M.Q.; Zhang, J.L.; Xin, H.N.; Yuan, K.; Yan, J.; Wang, Y.; Zhang, G.D.; Fu, J.X. Comparison of Clinical Outcomes of Prostatic Artery Embolization with 50-mum Plus 100-mum Polyvinyl Alcohol (PVA) Particles versus 100-mum PVA Particles Alone: A Prospective Randomized Trial. *J. Vasc. Interv. Radiol.* **2018**, *29*, 1694–1702. [CrossRef]
17. Torres, D.; Costa, N.V.; Pisco, J.; Pinheiro, L.C.; Oliveira, A.G.; Bilhim, T. Prostatic Artery Embolization for Benign Prostatic Hyperplasia: Prospective Randomized Trial of 100–300 mum versus 300–500 mum versus 100- to 300-mum + 300- to 500-mum Embospheres. *J. Vasc. Interv. Radiol.* **2019**, *30*, 638–644. [CrossRef]
18. Keasler, E.; Isaacson, A.J. Changes in Prostatic Artery Angiography with Balloon Occlusion. *J. Vasc. Interv. Radiol.* **2017**, *28*, 1276–1278. [CrossRef] [PubMed]

19. Isaacson, A.J.; Hartman, T.S.; Bagla, S.; Burke, C.T. Initial Experience with Balloon-Occlusion Prostatic Artery Embolization. *J. Vasc. Interv. Radiol.* **2018**, *29*, 85–89. [CrossRef]
20. Ayyagari, R.; Powell, T.; Staib, L.; Chapiro, J.; Schoenberger, S.; Devito, R.; Pollak, J. Case-Control Comparison of Conventional End-Hole versus Balloon-Occlusion Microcatheter Prostatic Artery Embolization for Treatment of Symptomatic Benign Prostatic Hyperplasia. *J. Vasc. Interv. Radiol.* **2019**, *30*, 1459–1470. [CrossRef] [PubMed]
21. Bilhim, T.; Costa, N.V.; Torres, D.; Pisco, J.; Carmo, S.; Oliveira, A.G. Randomized Clinical Trial of Balloon Occlusion versus Conventional Microcatheter Prostatic Artery Embolization for Benign Prostatic Hyperplasia. *J. Vasc. Interv. Radiol.* **2019**, *30*, 1798–1806. [CrossRef]
22. Khalilzadeh, O.; Baerlocher, M.O.; Shyn, P.B.; Connolly, B.L.; Devane, A.M.; Morris, C.S.; Cohen, A.M.; Midia, M.; Thornton, R.H.; Gross, K.; et al. Proposal of a New Adverse Event Classification by the Society of Interventional Radiology Standards of Practice Committee. *J. Vasc. Interv. Radiol.* **2017**, *28*, 1432–1437.e3. [CrossRef] [PubMed]
23. Moschouris, H.; Stamatiou, K.; Kornezos, I.; Kartsouni, V.; Malagari, K. Favorable Outcome of Conservative Management of Extensive Bladder Ischemia Complicating Prostatic Artery Embolization. *Cardiovasc. Interv. Radiol.* **2018**, *41*, 191–196. [CrossRef] [PubMed]
24. Moreira, A.M.; Marques, C.F.S.; Antunes, A.A.; Nahas, C.S.R.; Nahas, S.C.; Ariza, M.D.G.; Carnevale, F.C. Transient Ischemic Rectitis as a Potential Complication after Prostatic Artery Embolization: Case Report and Review of the Literature. *Cardiovasc. Interv. Radiol.* **2013**, *36*, 1690–1694. [CrossRef] [PubMed]
25. Kisilevzky, N.; Neto, C.L.; Cividanes, A. Ischemia of the Glans Penis following Prostatic Artery Embolization. *J. Vasc. Interv. Radiol.* **2016**, *27*, 1745–1747. [CrossRef]
26. de Assis, A.M.; Moreira, A.M.; de Paula Rodrigues, V.C.; Yoshinaga, E.M.; Antunes, A.A.; Harward, S.H.; Srougi, M.; Carnevale, F.C. Prostatic artery embolization for treatment of benign prostatic hyperplasia in patients with prostates > 90 g: A prospective single-center study. *J. Vasc. Interv. Radiol.* **2015**, *26*, 87–93. [CrossRef] [PubMed]
27. Amouyal, G.; Thiounn, N.; Pellerin, O.; Yen-Ting, L.; Del Giudice, C.; Dean, C.; Pereira, H.; Chatellier, G.; Sapoval, M. Clinical Results After Prostatic Artery Embolization Using the PErFecTED Technique: A Single-Center Study. *Cardiovasc. Interv. Radiol.* **2016**, *39*, 367–375. [CrossRef]
28. Laborda, A.; De Assis, A.M.; Ioakeim, I.; Sánchez-Ballestín, M.; Carnevale, F.C.; De Gregorio, M. Radiodermitis After Prostatic Artery Embolization: Case Report and Review of the Literature. *Cardiovasc. Interv. Radiol.* **2015**, *38*, 755–759. [CrossRef]
29. Bagla, S.; Smirniotopolous, J.B.; Vadlamudi, V. Crossing a Prostatic Artery Chronic Total Occlusion to Perform Prostatic Arterial Embolization. *J. Vasc. Interv. Radiol.* **2016**, *27*, 295–297. [CrossRef]
30. Kably, I.; Dupaix, R. Prostatic Artery Embolization and the Accessory Pudendal Artery. *J. Vasc. Interv. Radiol.* **2016**, *27*, 1266–1268. [CrossRef]
31. Diehm, N.; Marggi, S.; Ueki, Y.; Schumacher, D.; Keo, H.H.; Regli, C.; Do, D.D.; Moeltgen, T.; Grimsehl, P.; Wyler, S.; et al. Endovascular Therapy for Erectile Dysfunction—Who Benefits Most? Insights from a Single-Center Experience. *J. Endovasc. Ther.* **2019**, *26*, 181–190. [CrossRef] [PubMed]
32. Costa, N.V.; Pereira, J.; Fernandes, L.; Bilhim, T.; Pisco, J.M. Prostatic Tissue Expulsion after Prostatic Artery Embolization. *J. Vasc. Interv. Radiol.* **2016**, *27*, 601–603. [CrossRef]
33. Leite, L.C.; Moreira, A.M.; Harward, S.H.; Antunes, A.A.; Carnevale, F.C.; De Assis, A.M. Prostatic Tissue Elimination After Prostatic Artery Embolization (PAE): A Report of Three Cases. *Cardiovasc. Interv. Radiol.* **2017**, *40*, 937–941. [CrossRef] [PubMed]
34. Ghelfi, J.; Poncet, D.; Sengel, C.; Charara, S.; Delouche, A.; Guillaume, B.; Fiard, G.; Long, J.A.; Ferretti, G. Prostatic Fragment Requiring Endoscopic Management After Prostatic Artery Embolization for Indwelling Bladder Catheter. *Cardiovasc. Interv. Radiol.* **2018**, *41*, 1295–1297. [CrossRef] [PubMed]
35. Hechelhammer, L.; Müllhaupt, G.; Mordasini, L.; Markart, S.; Güsewell, S.; Betschart, P.; Schmid, H.-P.; Engeler, D.S.; Abt, D. Predictability and Inducibility of Detachment of Prostatic Central Gland Tissue after Prostatic Artery Embolization: Post Hoc Analysis of a Randomized Controlled Trial. *J. Vasc. Interv. Radiol.* **2019**, *30*, 217–224. [CrossRef] [PubMed]
36. Wang, M.; Zhang, G.; Yuan, K.; Duan, F.; Yan, J.; Wang, Y. Seminal Vesicle Ischemia: An Unusual Complication Occurring after Prostatic Artery Embolization for the Treatment of Benign Prostatic Hyperplasia. *J. Vasc. Interv. Radiol.* **2015**, *26*, 1580–1582. [CrossRef] [PubMed]
37. Zhang, J.L.; Yuan, K.; Wang, M.Q.; Yan, J.Y.; Wang, Y.; Zhang, G.D. Seminal vesicle abnormalities following prostatic artery embolization for the treatment of benign prostatic hyperplasia. *BMC Urol.* **2018**, *18*, 92. [CrossRef] [PubMed]
38. Abt, D.; Müllhaupt, G.; Hechelhammer, L.; Markart, S.; Güsewell, S.; Schmid, H.-P.; Mordasini, L.; Engeler, D.S. Prostatic Artery Embolisation Versus Transurethral Resection of the Prostate for Benign Prostatic Hyperplasia: 2-yr Outcomes of a Randomised, Open-label, Single-centre Trial. *Eur. Urol.* **2021**, *80*, 34–42. [CrossRef] [PubMed]
39. Bhatia, S.; Harward, S.H.; Sinha, V.K.; Narayanan, G. Prostate Artery Embolization via Transradial or Transulnar versus Transfemoral Arterial Access: Technical Results. *J. Vasc. Interv. Radiol.* **2017**, *28*, 898–905. [CrossRef]
40. Isaacson, A.J.; Fischman, A.M.; Burke, C.T. Technical Feasibility of Prostatic Artery Embolization from a Transradial Approach. *Am. J. Roentgenol.* **2016**, *206*, 442–444. [CrossRef]

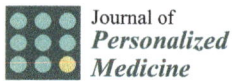

Article

A Nomogram Based on Preoperative Lipiodol Deposition after Sequential Retreatment with Transarterial Chemoembolization to Predict Prognoses for Intermediate-Stage Hepatocellular Carcinoma

Xiang-Ke Niu [1,2] and Xiao-Feng He [2,*]

1. Department of Interventional Radiology, Affiliated Hospital of Chengdu University, Chengdu 610081, China
2. Department of Interventional Radiology, Nanfang Hospital, Southern Medical University, Guangzhou 510515, China
* Correspondence: ozonetherapy@163.com

Abstract: (1) Background: Conventional transarterial chemoembolization (cTACE) is the mainstay treatment for patients with Barcelona Clinic Liver Cancer (BCLC) B-stage hepatocellular carcinoma (HCC). However, BCLC B-stage patients treated with cTACE represent a prognostically heterogeneous population. We aim to develop and validate a lipiodol-deposition-based nomogram for predicting the long-term survival of BCLC B-stage HCC patients after sequential cTACE. (2) Methods: In this retrospective study, 229 intermediate-stage HCC patients from two hospitals were separately allocated to a training cohort (n = 142) and a validation cohort (n = 87); these patients underwent repeated TACE (≥4 TACE sessions) between May 2010 and May 2017. Lipiodol deposition was assessed by semiautomatic volumetric measurement with multidetector computed tomography (MDCT) before cTACE and was characterized by two ordinal levels: ≤50% (low) and >50% (high). A clinical lipiodol deposition nomogram was constructed based on independent risk factors identified by univariate and multivariate Cox regression analyses, and the optimal cutoff points were obtained. Prediction models were assessed by time-dependent receiver-operating characteristic curves, calibration curves, and decision curve analysis. (3) Results: The median number of TACE sessions was five (range, 4–7) in both cohorts. Before the TACE-3 sessions, the newly constructed nomogram based on lipiodol deposition achieved desirable diagnostic performance in the training and validation cohorts with AUCs of 0.72 (95% CI, 0.69–0.74) and 0.71 (95% CI, 0.68–0.73), respectively, and demonstrated higher predictive ability compared with previously published prognostic models (all $p < 0.05$). The prognostic nomogram obtained good clinical usefulness in predicting the patient outcomes after TACE. (4) Conclusions: Based on each pre-TACE lipiodol deposition, two sessions are recommended before abandoning cTACE or combining treatment for patients with intermediate-stage HCC. Furthermore, the nomogram based on pre-TACE-3 lipiodol deposition can be used to predict the prognoses of patients with BCLC B-stage HCC.

Keywords: transarterial chemoembolization; hepatocellular carcinoma; lipiodol; nomogram; overall survival

Citation: Niu, X.-K.; He, X.-F. A Nomogram Based on Preoperative Lipiodol Deposition after Sequential Retreatment with Transarterial Chemoembolization to Predict Prognoses for Intermediate-Stage Hepatocellular Carcinoma. J. Pers. Med. 2022, 12, 1375. https://doi.org/10.3390/jpm12091375

Academic Editors: Julien Frandon and Kenneth P.H. Pritzker

Received: 25 June 2022
Accepted: 24 August 2022
Published: 25 August 2022

Publisher's Note: MDPI stays neutral with regard to jurisdictional claims in published maps and institutional affiliations.

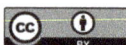

Copyright: © 2022 by the authors. Licensee MDPI, Basel, Switzerland. This article is an open access article distributed under the terms and conditions of the Creative Commons Attribution (CC BY) license (https://creativecommons.org/licenses/by/4.0/).

1. Introduction

Hepatocellular carcinoma (HCC) is the fifth most commonly diagnosed form of cancer and the second leading cause of cancer-related death worldwide [1]. Patients with Barcelona Clinic Liver Cancer (BCLC) stage B disease are considered ineligible for surgical resection, and the median overall survival (OS) is approximately 2 years, even after optimal treatment [2]. Conventional transarterial chemoembolization (cTACE) is one of the most widely performed digital subtraction angiography (DSA)-guided catheter-based therapies for the treatment of BCLC stage B HCC, and a meta-analysis based on randomized controlled trials showed that cTACE has a positive effect on survival in patients in this stage of disease [3]. cTACE generally uses ethiodized oil, or lipiodol, mixed with chemotherapeutic agents. This mixed liquid is superselectively injected into tumor-feeding arteries, followed by bland embolization of the tumor blood supply [4].

However, some questions remain to be addressed. First, resulting from the enormous heterogeneity of BCLC stage B HCC patients, the prediction of outcome is also heterogeneous for patients treated with cTACE [5,6]. Various scoring systems predicting the prognosis of HCC patients receiving cTACE are available, such as albumin-bilirubin (ABLI) grade and up-to-7 criteria [5,7]. Unfortunately, these predictive models need sophisticated calculation and are not fully validated. Second, a previous study by Hiraoka et al. [8] concluded that repeated TACE gradually reduces hepatic reserve function. Moreover, in clinical practice, some patients cannot tolerate TACE treatment, which may manifest as TACE resistance. Thus, an appropriate judgment of the number of TACEs that should be performed has become important to avoid harmful TACE and for less-effective patients switching to multiple systemic therapies in a timely and effective manner.

Lipiodol, an injectable agent, can be visualized with pretreatment multidetector computed tomography (MDCT). Several studies have shown that lipiodol can be detected within a treated tumor for several months after injection [9–11]. Lipiodol deposition on intraprocedural cone-beam computed tomography (CBCT) has been utilized to predict treatment response [12–14]. Unfortunately, CBCT is not widely used, especially in developing countries. In routine clinical practice, MDCT is applied to guide treatment planning before each TACE procedure. In this study, based on a 3D quantification of preoperative lipiodol deposition, we develop and validate a new predictive nomogram for assessing the prognoses of patients with BCLC B-stage HCC after sequential cTACE treatment, which may be used to assess individualized prognosis and can help to select patients suitable for sequential cTACE treatments.

2. Methods

2.1. Patients and Tumor Selection

The diagnosis of HCC was based on pathology or noninvasive imaging features outlined by the American Association for the Study of Liver Disease guidelines [15,16]. Patients treated with TACE at Southern Medical University Nanfang Hospital from May 2010 to May 2017 were included in the training cohort. From May 2010 to May 2017, the independent validation cohort consisted of patients who underwent TACE treatments at the Affiliated Hospital of Chengdu University. The study included patients who were partially reported by our recent research [17]. We used the following inclusion criteria in both cohorts (Figure 1): (a) BCLC B-stage disease with preserved liver function (Child–Pugh class A or B); (b) patients were $\geq$ 18 years old with a performance status (PS) score $\leq$ 2 at the time of the first TACE treatment; (c) preoperative MDCT imaging was performed within 24 h–72 h prior to each TACE treatment; and (d) TACE was performed as monotherapy, and at least four TACE sessions were performed by a single patient. Overall survival (OS) was defined as the interval from the time of each cTACE session to the time of death or last follow-up. This study was censored on 15 March 2020.

The study was approved by the Ethics Committee of the Affiliated Hospital of Chengdu University and the Ethics Committee of the Southern Medical University Nanfang Hospital. The study protocol conformed to the ethical guidelines of the 1975 Declaration of Helsinki. All patients or their relatives provided written informed consent.

2.2. cTACE Protocol

Briefly, we performed superselective catheterization of the tumor-feeding branches with a microcatheter, and an emulsion containing a 50 mg doxorubicin (Adriamycin; Pharmacia & Upjohn, Peapack, NJ, USA) mixture with lipiodol (Lipiodol; Guerbet, Paris, France) was infused with a microcatheter, followed by delivery of a gelfoam slurry (Upjohn, Kalamazoo, MI, USA) or microsphere particles (Embosphere Microspheres; Biosphere Medical, Rockland, MA, USA) until tumor blood flow stagnation was seen on DSA imaging.

cTACE was performed by interventional radiologists with 10 years of experience in hepatic interventions at each institution. The procedure was conducted on demand, and cTACE was discontinued in the case of a complete radiological response. In addition, the presence of Child–Pugh type C cirrhosis, vascular invasion, extensive liver involvement, extrahepatic metastases, or a PS score >2 were considered contraindications to TACE retreatment [18].

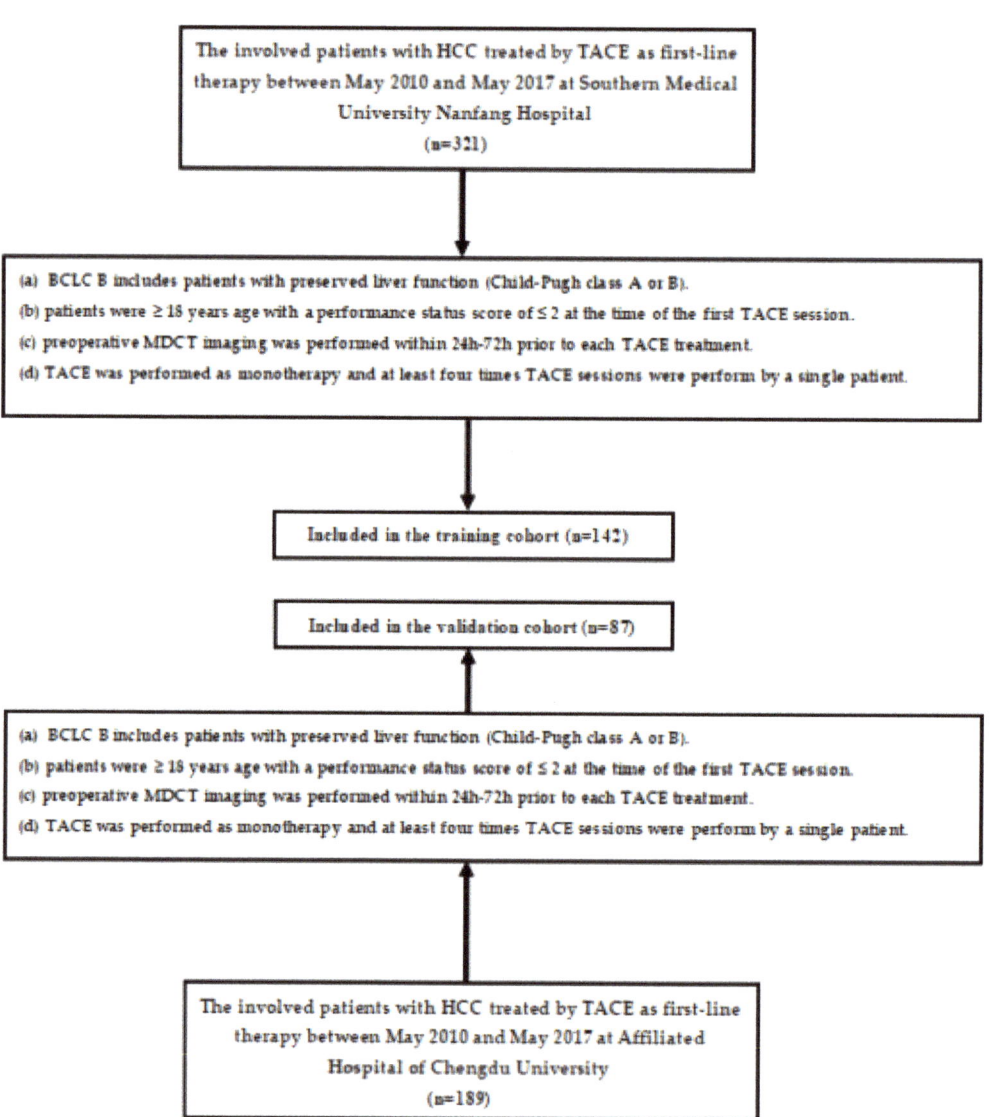

Figure 1. Flowchart for inclusion and exclusion of patients within the training and validation cohorts. TACE: transarterial chemoembolization; BCLC: Barcelona Clinic Liver Cancer; MDCT: multi-detector computed tomography; HCC: hepatocellular carcinoma.

2.3. Quantification of Volumetric Oil Deposition

Unenhanced abdominal CT scans were performed 24 h–72 h before each cTACE procedure with a multislice CT scanner (Discovery CT750 HD (GE Medical System), Sensation 64 CT (Siemens), Somatom Definition (Siemens)). Standard liver scan protocol was used in the present study and can be seen in our recent research [17].

In the training cohort, images were interpreted independently by two radiologists (who had experience interpreting liver images for at least 5 years). In the validation cohort, images were interpreted by a single radiologist (who had experience in interpreting liver images for at least 5 years). Overall tumor volumes, as well as the amount of lipiodol deposition (in cm^3), were measured using semiautomated quantification software (ITK-SNAP software (http://www.itksnap.org/pmwiki/pmwiki.php)). The total tumor volume was measured using pretreatment portal venous phase imaging, while the volume of lipiodol deposition was determined using noncontrast imaging. The lipiodol deposition rate was recorded as the ratio of the oil deposition volume to the total tumor volume. The rate of lipiodol retention before each TACE was classified as follows: (1) high level: >50% tumor volume and categorized as a responder; and (2) low level: ≤50% tumor volume and categorized as a nonresponder (Figure 2). The index lesion method was used to determine the tumor response [19–21]. The related clinical data were extracted from the electronic medical record system at each institution. The characteristics of the tumors, including the largest tumor size, number of lesions (with either three or more tumors, regardless of size) [22], and tumor capsule, were determined by a radiologist with experience in liver imaging.

2.4. Statistical Analysis

The clinical data and imaging characteristics were assessed by Student's t-test, the chi-squared test, or the Mann–Whitney U test, as appropriate. Interobserver reproducibility was assessed using the intraclass correlation coefficient (ICC).

The Kaplan–Meier (KM) method was used for the survival curves and was compared with the results of the log-rank test. Univariate and multivariate Cox regression analyses were conducted to identify the independent predictive factors, and a nomogram was built. For example, nomogram I represented the pre-TACE-2 lipiodol deposition combined with pretreatment valuable predictors, and nomogram II represented the pre-TACE-3 lipiodol deposition combined with pretreatment valuable predictors (Figure 3). The performance of each model was evaluated with the concordance index (C-index). The highest diagnostic nomogram was compared with eight well-recognized models (six-and-twelve, seven-eleven criteria, hepatoma arterial embolization prognostic (HAP) score, modified HAP 3 score, BCLC-B subclassification system, ALBI grade, and assessment for retreatment (ART); as well as the alpha fetoprotein, Barcelona Clinic Liver Cancer, Child–Pugh increase, and tumor response (ABCR) score) by the time-dependent area under receiver-operating characteristic curve (AUROC). The clinical utility of the nomogram in both datasets was evaluated by calibration curve and a decision curve analysis (DCA).

In addition, the training set was divided into two subgroups (high- and low-score groups) based on the best cutoff points obtained from the "surv_cutpoint" function of the "survminer" R package. Patients in the validation sets were also categorized into two subgroups based on the same best cutoff points used in the training set. OS rates at 1, 2, and 3 years were calculated for each group, and KM survival curves were generated. Statistical significance was defined as $p < 0.05$. All statistical analyses were performed using R software (version 3.6.2).

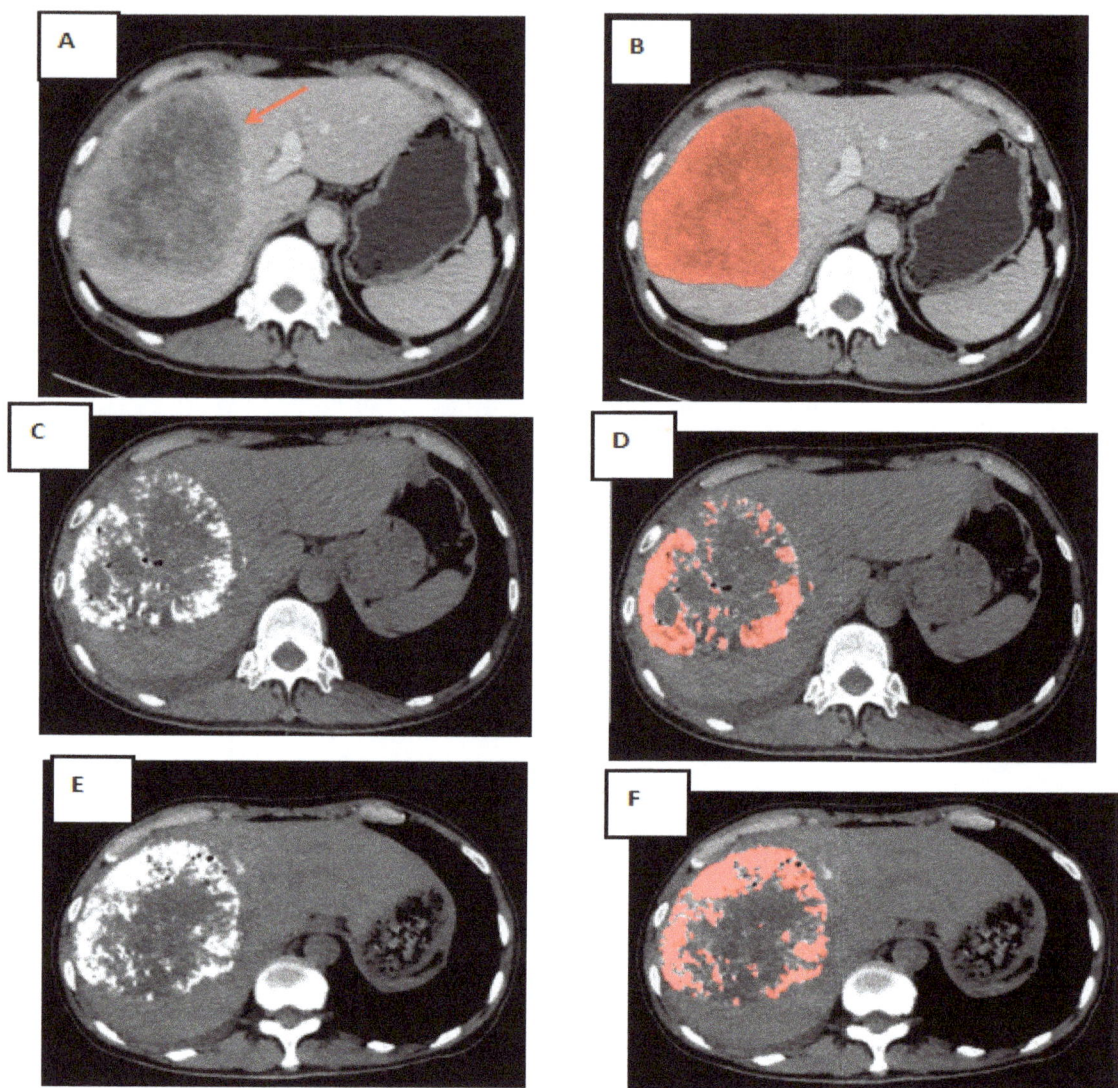

Figure 2. 3D volumetric semi-automatic evaluation of diffuse lipiodol retention from one representative patient. (**A**): A large HCC in right hepatic lobe (red arrow) seen on preprocedural contrast-enhanced CT images as a hypoattenuating tumor in the portal venous phase. (**B**): The red shaded area depicts semi-automated segmentation of the tumor; the tumor volume on the pretreatment MDCT was 512.6 cm^3. (**C**): Lipiodol retention on noncontrast CT imaging in pre-TACE-2. (**D**): The red shaded area depicts the lipiodol volume on noncontrast CT imaging of 121.7 cm^3 in pre-TACE-2. (**E**): Lipiodol retention on noncontrast CT imaging in pre-TACE-3. (**F**): The red shaded area demonstrates the lipiodol volume on noncontrast CT imaging as 174.8 cm^3 in pre-TACE-3. After two cycles of TACEs, the volume of lipiodol was less than 50% of total tumor volume. TACE: transarterial chemoembolization; BCLC: Barcelona Clinic Liver Cancer; MDCT: multi-detector computed tomography; HCC: hepatocellular carcinoma.

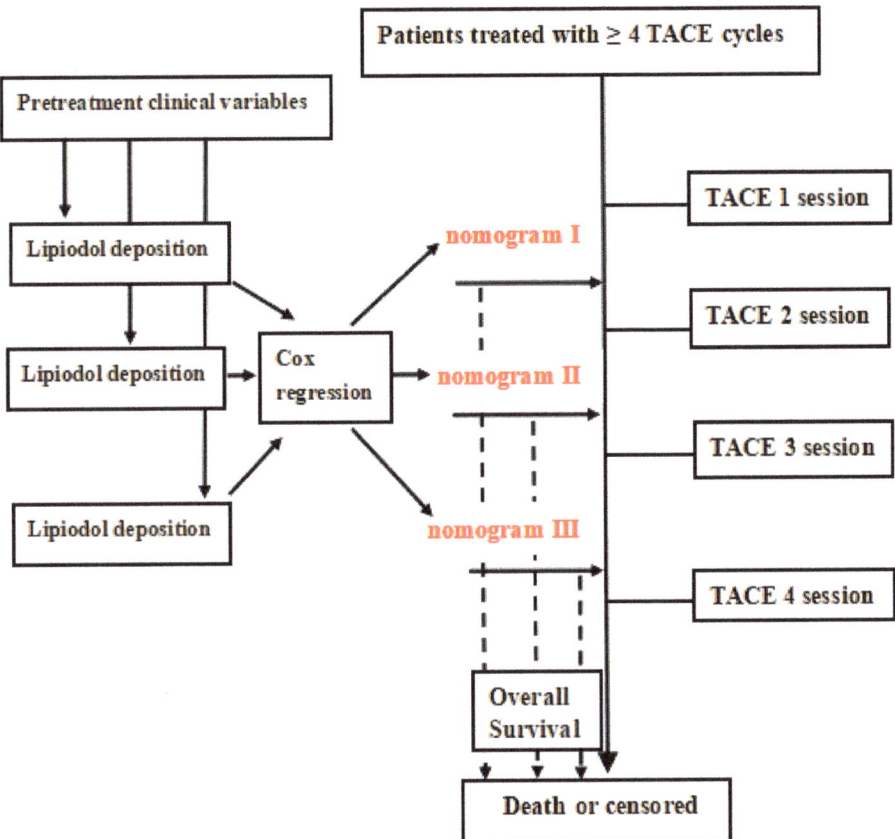

Figure 3. Study design for nomogram construction. Nomograms were built by Cox regression analyses based on each pretreatment lipiodol deposition and clinical variables. TACE: transarterial chemoembolization.

3. Results

3.1. Baseline Characteristics

A total of 510 patients with HCC received TACE as monotherapy between May 2010 and May 2017. A total of 142 patients were included in the training cohort, and 87 were enrolled in the validation cohort. The median follow-up time was 45.9 months (interquartile range, 23.3–58.2 months) for the training cohort and 42.4 months (interquartile range, 27.2–62.2 months) for the validation cohort. The median OS values of the training and validation cohorts were not significantly different (median OS 31.4 [95% CI 23.2–36.2] months vs. 29.6 [95% CI 23.7–37.1] months, $p = 0.212$). The median number of TACE sessions for both cohorts was five (range, 4–7). Table 1 describes the baseline characteristics of patients in these cohorts before the first cTACE treatment.

Table 1. Patient characteristics.

Characteristic	Training Cohort		Validation Cohort		p-Value
	N = 142	%	N = 87	%	
Age (yr)					0.731
<60	90	63	52	60	
≥60	52	37	35	40	
Sex					0.329
Male	95	67	49	56	
Female	47	33	38	44	
HBsAg status					0.941
Positive	112	79	69	80	
Negative	30	21	18	20	
Child–Pugh class					0.881
A	89	62	54	62	
B	53	38	33	38	
Largest tumor size (cm)					0.227
<5					
mean ± SD	96	67	47	54	
≥5	46	33	40	46	
Tumor number					0.258
≤3	91	64	49	56	
>3	51	36	38	44	
AFP ((IU/mL)					0.341
<200	40	28	27	31	
≥200	102	72	60	69	
AST (U/L)					0.319
<40	50	35	37	42	
≥40	92	65	50	58	
ALT(U/L)					0.431
<40	53	37	31	35	
≥40	89	63	56	65	
ALB (g/L)					0.351
<35	41	29	21	24	
≥35	101	71	66	76	
Capsule					0.239
Absent	67	47	32	36	
Present	75	53	55	64	
Up-to-seven criteria					0.651
Within	44	30	22	25	
Beyond	98	70	65	75	

BCLC: Barcelona Clinic Liver Cancer; HBsAg: hepatitis B surface antigen; AST: aspartate aminotransferase; ALT: alanine transaminase; AFP: alpha fetoprotein; ALB: albumin.

3.2. Interobserver Agreement

Lipiodol retention levels were assessed by the ICC test, and excellent interobserver reproducibility was demonstrated (ICC, 0.866; 95% CI, 0.812–0.914).

3.3. Consecutive Oil Deposition

For the training cohort, the response rate to the first cTACE was 76 of 142 (53.5%; 95% CI: 43.7, 67.7). Among patients who did not respond to the first cTACE, the response rate after the second cTACE was 34 of 66 (51.5%; 95% CI: 47.8, 54.6). Among patients who did not respond to second cTACE, the response rate after the third cTACE was 7 of 32 (21.8%; 95% CI: 18.7, 23.7). Subsequently, among patients who did not respond to third cTACE, the corresponding rate after the fourth cTACE was low, at 3 of 25 (12%; 95% CI: 9.1, 15.2) (Table 2).

Table 2. Nonresponders to previous cTACEs after next cTACE sessions in the training cohort.

Parameter	No. of Patients	Responders	Nonresponders
Response after Second Chemoembolization Response after First Chemoembolization Nonresponders	66	34 (51.5) (47.8, 54.6)	32 (48.5) (42.2, 52.3)
Response after Third Chemoembolization Response after Second Chemoembolization Nonresponders	32	7 (21.8) (18.7, 23.7)	25 (78.2) (71.3, 82.4)
Response after Third Chemoembolization Response after Fourth Chemoembolization Nonresponders	25	3 (12.0) (9.1, 15.2)	22 (88.0) (82.9, 91.4)

Data in parentheses are percentages; data in brackets are 95% CIs.

In the training cohort, the overall survival rates at 1, 2, and 3 years were significantly lower for nonresponders to the first cTACE than responders ($p < 0.001$). For patients who did not respond to the first cTACE but who underwent the second cTACE, overall survival rates at 1, 2, and 3 years after a the second cTACE were significantly lower for nonresponders than for responders ($p < 0.001$). For patients who did not respond to the second cTACE but received a third cTACE, long-term survival outcomes were similar for nonresponders and responders ($p = 0.198$). A similar trend was observed in patients who did not respond to the third cTACE but received the fourth cTACE ($p = 0.268$) (Table 3).

Table 3. Survival outcomes for responders and nonresponders in the training cohort.

Parameter	Median OS (mo)	1-Year OS	2-Year OS	3-Year OS	p-Value
Survival outcomes after cTACE-1					$p < 0.001$
Responders	39.2 ± 0.5	91.4 (82.6, 92.9)	56.2 (47.2, 60.4)	33.8 (28.2, 38.2)	
Nonresponders	26.1 ± 1.2	88.4 (81.2, 91.3)	26.1 (21.1, 30.2)	13.4 (10.1, 18.8)	
Survival outcomes for nonresponders to cTACE-1 who underwent cTACE-2					$p < 0.001$
Responders	38.1 ± 0.9	90.2 (85.2, 94.1)	60.1 (56.2, 68.1)	36.2 (32.2, 40.1)	
Nonresponders	24.2 ± 0.8	86.2 (81.3, 90.5)	28.9 (22.1, 31.3)	14.8 (11.2, 18.2)	
Survival outcomes for nonresponders to cTACE-2 who underwent cTACE-3					$p = 0.198$
Responders	31.2 ± 0.7	86.4 (81.2, 91.3)	57.1 (48.1, 62.2)	30.7 (26.4, 35.2)	
Nonresponders	28.4 ± 0.9	85.2 (82.7, 90.2)	54.3 (48.1, 61.2)	26.5 (22.1, 30.4)	
Survival outcomes for nonresponders to cTACE-3 who underwent cTACE-4					$p = 0.268$
Responders	19.1 ± 0.9	61.4 (55.2, 66.3)	14.2 (10.9, 18.4)	8.2 (5.2, 11.7)	
Nonresponders	17.4 ± 1.6	59.2 (54.9, 65.7)	10.8 (6.2, 14.3)	6.1 (2.2, 10.8)	

Note: median data are means ± standard deviation; data in parentheses are 95% CIs. cTACE-1: first conventional transarterial chemoembolization (cTACE) session; cTACE-2: second cTACE session; cTACE-3: third cTACE session; cTACE-4: fourth cTACE session; OS: overall survival.

3.4. Model Building and Evaluation

Based on the results of the Cox proportional hazards model, the largest tumor size (all $p < 0.001$ for nomograms I, II, and III), the tumor number (all $p < 0.001$ for nomograms I, II, and III), and the pretreatment lipiodol deposition ($p = 0.032$ and $p < 0.001$ for nomograms I and II, respectively) were identified as independent predictors of survival for the training cohort. Several prediction models (nomograms I, II, and III) were constructed to predict patient prognosis (Table 4, Tables S1 and S2). Nomogram II had a higher predictive value than nomograms I and III (Table 5) and is shown in Figure 4. In comparison to eight other well-recognized prognostic models, the time-dependent AUROC analysis showed that nomogram II had improved diagnostic performance in the training cohort (Table 6; Figure 5A).

Table 4. Predictors of death for patients with intermediate-stage HCC before second TACE.

Variable	Univariate Analysis			Multivariate Analysis		
Before Second TACE	Hazard Ratio	95% CI	*p*-Value	Hazard Ratio	95% CI	*p*-Value
Age (yr) <60/≥60	0.68	0.32–1.03	0.171			
Sex male/female	0.81	0.42–1.27	0.233			
HBsAg status positive/negative	0.54	0.23–0.76	0.234			
Child–Pugh class A/B	1.32	0.63–1.34	0.338			
Largest tumor size (cm) <5/≥5	1.34	1.17–3.04	0.007	1.56	0.45–2.43	<0.001
Tumor number ≤3/m>3	1.31	1.01–2.98	0.004	1.45	1.07–3.00	<0.001
AFP (IU/mL) <200/≥200	0.62	0.22–1.09	0.018	1.45	1.04–2.01	0.078
AST (U/L) <40/≥40	0.54	0.27–0.94	0.081			
ALT(U/L) <40/≥40	0.53	0.12–0.78	0.079			
ALB (g/L) <35/≥35	1.34	0.82–2.34	0.043	1.45	1.01–1.71	0.073
Capsule absent/present	1.87	1.34–3.97	0.018	1.46	0.09–2.76	0.093
Up-to-seven criteria within/beyond	1.32	1.10–1.87	0.032	1.67	1.00–1.76	0.098
Pre-TACE-2 lipiodol deposition responder/nonreponder	1.89	0.71–2.87	0.038	1.98	0.87–2.89	0.032

BCLC: Barcelona Clinic Liver Cancer; HBsAg: hepatitis B surface antigen; AST: aspartate aminotransferase; ALT: alanine transaminase; AFP: alpha fetoprotein; ALB: albumin.

Table 5. Comparison of the performance and discriminative ability of constructed nomogram models.

Cohort	Models	1-yr AUROC (95% CI)	2-yr AUROC (95% CI)	3-yr AUROC (95% CI)	C-Index (95% CI)	*p*-Value
Training	Nomogram I	0.70 (0.69–0.73)	0.65 (0.63–0.67)	0.61 (0.60–0.63)	0.66 (0.64–0.68)	0.032
	Nomogram II	0.74 (0.71–0.77)	0.71 (0.69–0.73)	0.67 (0.65–0.69)	0.72 (0.69–0.74)	Ref.
	Nomogram III	0.61 (0.59–0.66)	0.59 (0.53–0.63)	0.53 (0.50–0.57)	0.56 (0.52–0.62)	<0.01
Validation	Nomogram I	0.67 (0.65–0.69)	0.64 (0.61–0.67)	0.61 (0.59–0.63)	0.63 (0.60–0.65)	0.028
	Nomogram II	0.72 (0.69–0.74)	0.70 (0.68–0.73)	0.65 (0.63–0.67)	0.71 (0.68–0.73)	Ref.
	Nomogram III	0.59 (0.53–0.63)	0.57 (0.53–0.61)	0.52 (0.50–0.57)	0.53 (0.51–0.57)	<0.01

AUROC: area under receiver-operating characteristic curve; CI: confidence interval; Ref.: reference.

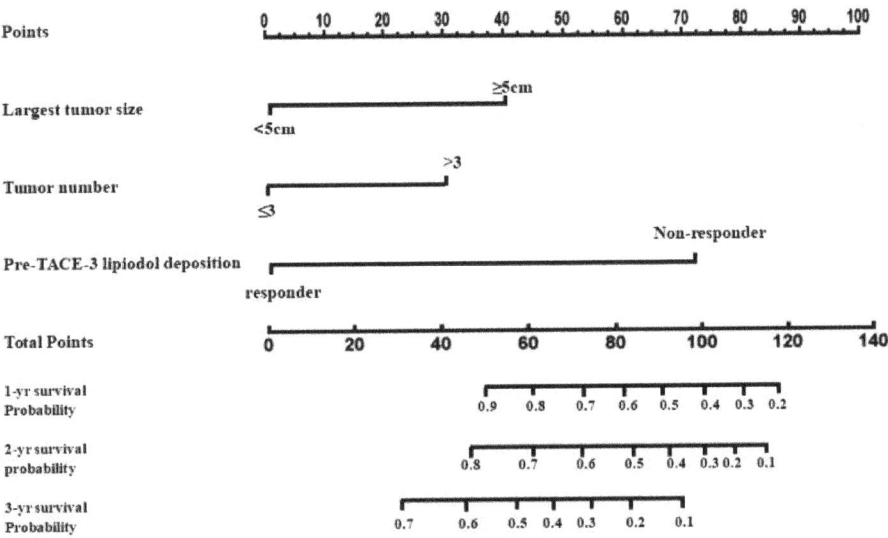

Figure 4. Prognostic nomogram showing the assessment of 1-, 2-, and 3-year survival in patients with intermediate-stage HCC after cTACE. (To use this nomogram in clinical practice, a vertical line is first drawn from the factor axis to the "Points" scale to determine the number of points for each factor ("Largest tumor size," "Tumor number," and "Pre-TACE-3 lipiodol deposition.") Then, these numbers are summed and located on the axis of the total points. Finally, a downward line is drawn from the axis of the total points to the survival axes to calculate the 1-, 2-, and 3-year survival probabilities.) TACE: transarterial chemoembolization.

Table 6. Comparison of the performance and discriminative ability between the current model and other models.

Cohort	Models	1-yr AUROC (95% CI)	2-yr AUROC (95% CI)	3-yr AUROC (95% CI)	C-Index (95% CI)	p-Value
Training	Nomogram II	0.74 (0.71–0.77)	0.71 (0.69–0.73)	0.67 (0.65–0.69)	0.72 (0.69–0.74)	Ref.
	Six-and-Twelve	0.71 (0.69–0.73)	0.66 (0.64–0.68)	0.62 (0.60–0.65)	0.67 (0.65–0.69)	0.032
	Seven-Eleven Criteria	0.69 (0.67–0.71)	0.63 (0.61–0.67)	0.59 (0.55–0.62)	0.63 (0.61–0.65)	0.023
	HAP	0.55 (0.51–0.59)	0.54 (0.52–0.57)	0.53 (0.50–0.55)	0.56 (0.53–0.59)	<0.01
	mHAP 3	0.61 (0.59–0.63)	0.59 (0.54–0.62)	0.52 (0.50–0.55)	0.61 (0.58–0.64)	<0.01
	BCLC-B subclassification	0.58 (0.56–0.63)	0.54 (0.52–0.58)	0.52 (0.50–0.56)	0.57 (0.55–0.61)	<0.01
	ALBI grade	0.66 (0.64–0.69)	0.61 (0.59–0.64)	0.59 (0.55–0.65)	0.63 (0.60–0.69)	0.038
	ART score	0.61 (0.58–0.64)	0.59 (0.56–0.63)	0.57 (0.54–0.60)	0.60 (0.56–0.64)	<0.01
	ABCR score	0.67 (0.63–0.70)	0.65 (0.62–0.68)	0.61 (0.57–0.65)	0.65 (0.62–0.69)	0.036
Validation	Nomogram II	0.72 (0.69–0.74)	0.70 (0.68–0.73)	0.65 (0.63–0.67)	0.71 (0.68–0.73)	Ref.
	Six-and-Twelve	0.70 (0.68–0.73)	0.65 (0.62–0.68)	0.61 (0.58–0.63)	0.66 (0.64–0.69)	0.048
	Seven-Eleven Criteria	0.68 (0.66–0.71)	0.62 (0.59–0.65)	0.57 (0.55–0.61)	0.62 (0.60–0.64)	0.041
	HAP	0.54 (0.51–0.56)	0.52 (0.50–0.55)	0.50 (0.49–0.53)	0.54 (0.52–0.56)	<0.01
	mHAP 3	0.60 (0.57–0.63)	0.56 (0.52–0.61)	0.51 (0.48–0.54)	0.60 (0.58–0.63)	<0.01
	BCLC-B subclassification	0.56 (0.54–0.60)	0.52 (0.50–0.55)	0.50 (0.48–0.53)	0.55 (0.53–0.60)	<0.01
	ALBI grade	0.65 (0.62–0.67)	0.60 (0.58–0.63)	0.56 (0.54–0.60)	0.61 (0.58–0.64)	0.039
	ART score	0.62 (0.57–0.66)	0.56 (0.52–0.60)	0.54 (0.51–0.58)	0.59 (0.56–0.63)	<0.01
	ABCR score	0.68 (0.64–0.71)	0.66 (0.62–0.70)	0.63 (0.59–0.67)	0.66 (0.62–0.70)	0.041

AUROC: area under receiver-operating characteristic curve; CI: confidence interval; HAP: hepatoma arterial embolization prognostic; mHAP: modified HAP; BCLC: Barcelona Clinic Liver Cancer; ALBI: albumin–bilirubin; ART: assessment for retreatment; ABCR: alpha fetoprotein, Barcelona Clinic Liver Cancer, Child–Pugh increase, tumor response; Ref.: reference.

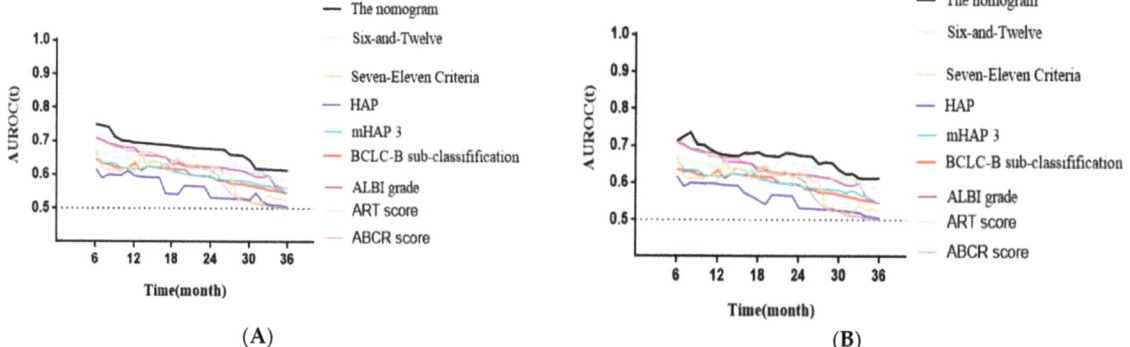

Figure 5. Time-dependent AUROC values of the current model and other available models. (**A**): Time-dependent AUROC values in training set. (**B**): Time-dependent AUROC values in validation set. HAP: hepatoma arterial embolization prognostic; mHAP 3: modified HAP 3; ALBI: albumin-bilirubin; ART: assessment for retreatment; ABCR: alpha fetoprotein, Barcelona Clinic Liver Cancer, Child–Pugh increase, tumor response; AUROC: area under receiver-operating characteristic curve; BCLC: Barcelona Clinic Liver Cancer.

3.5. Validation

After the new prognostic model (nomogram II) was established, its performance was evaluated. In the validation cohort, nomogram II maintained adequate discriminative performance (C-statistic of 0.71; 95% CI, 0.68–0.73). Generally, the time-dependent AUROC values of nomogram II were higher than those of the other models in the validation cohort (Figure 5B). In addition, the calibration curves demonstrated the favorable calibration of nomogram II in both cohorts (Figure 6A,B). The decision curves displayed a good performance of nomogram II in terms of clinical utility (Figure 6C).

3.6. Survival Stratification

To identify the prognostic stratification of patients receiving cTACE, we calculated the optimal cutoff points for nomogram II in the training set using the "surv_cutpoint" function of the "survminer" R package, which was 70 points. Therefore, patients in the training cohort were divided into two subgroups: the low-score group (total score ≤ 70) and the high-score group (total score > 70). The KM survival analysis showed that the OS in the training group was significantly different between the two subgroups (median OS values of the low-score group and the high-score group were 42.1 months (95% CI 37.2–48.2) and 23.4 months (95% CI 17.2–28.2), respectively; log-rank test: $p < 0.05$) (Figure 7A). A similar trend was observed in the validation set (median OS values of the low-score group and high-score group were 43.4 months (95% CI 37.5–49.1) and 21.2 months (95% CI 16.9–26.3), respectively; log-rank test: $p < 0.05$) (Figure 7B).

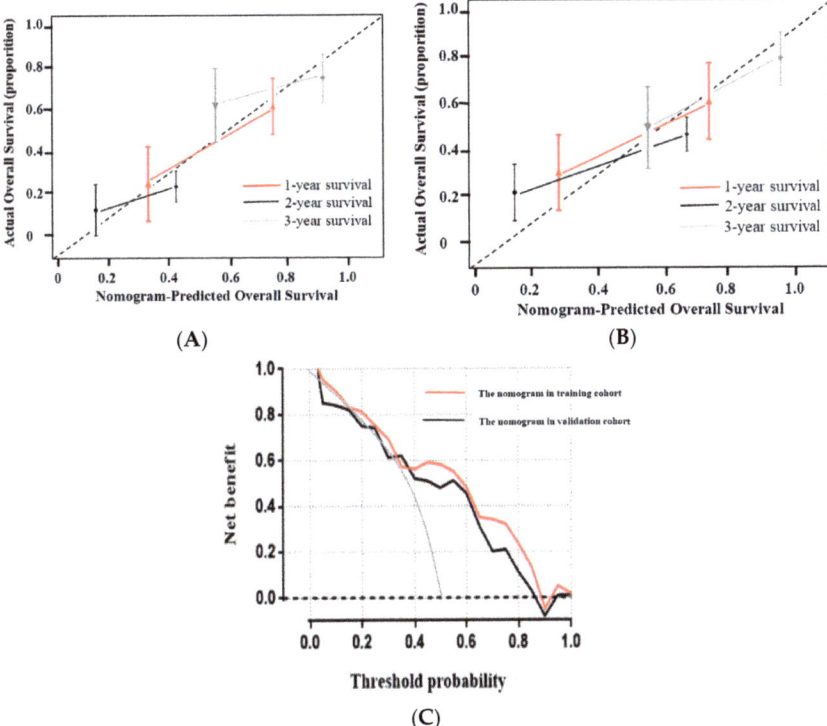

Figure 6. Calibration and decision curve analyses. (**A**): Calibration curves of the nomogram on the training dataset. The Hosmer–Lemeshow test yielded a p-value of 0.121 in the training dataset. (**B**): Calibration curves of the nomogram on the validation dataset. The Hosmer–Lemeshow test yielded a p-value of 0.137 in the validation dataset. (**C**): Decision curve analysis for the newly constructed nomogram (nomogram II) in the training cohort and the validation cohort. The y-axis represents the net benefit, and the x-axis represents the threshold probability. The newly constructed nomogram obtained more benefit than either the treat-all-patients scheme (gray line) or the treat-none scheme (horizontal black dashed line) within certain ranges of threshold probabilities for predicting therapeutic response to sequential cTACE in HCC.

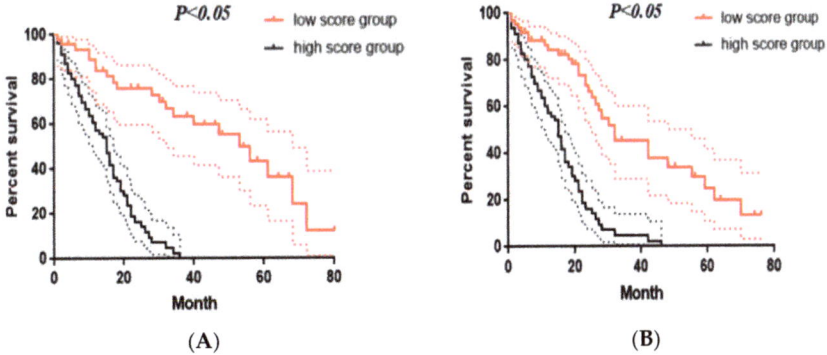

Figure 7. Kaplan–Meier survival curves for overall survival (OS) of patients according to the nomogram-II-based subgroups in the training set (**A**) and validation set (**B**).

4. Discussion

The majority of HCC patients who undergo TACE have varying degrees of cirrhosis, which may limit the potential survival benefit of the procedure. This is further complicated by the fact that HCC patients commonly need multiple TACE sessions to obtain an optimal tumor response [23]. Hiraoka et al. [8] suggested that 9–14% of liver function deteriorates to CP-B after each TACE procedure, and hepatic function is also essential in the tyrosine kinase inhibitor (TKI) and immunotherapy eras. Therefore, evaluation of the benefits of each TACE is critical to decision-making in clinical practice. Our study had two major findings. First, we confirmed that approximately 50% of patients who were nonresponsive to the first cTACE showed a significant response after the second TACE, which is consistent with results by Georgiades et al. [24]. Second, the nomogram constructed by pre-TACE-3 lipiodol deposition combined with clinical variables could be used to predict relatively long-term patient survival, and its diagnostic value was higher than that of other existing clinical predictive models.

Lipiodol deposition has been proved to be strongly associated with OS in patients with BCLC B-stage HCC treated with cTACE [12]. Several studies have shown that lipiodol deposition on intraoperative CBCT can be utilized to predict tumor response [13,25]. However, CBCT has inherent shortcomings. CBCT clarity and real resolution are not equivalent to CT; moreover, motion artifacts, especially from respiration, can affect imaging analysis. As an alternative, magnetic resonance imaging (MRI) can be used to diagnose residual tumors after cTACE in a timely manner, with superior performance compared to CT [26]. However, peritumoral inflammation due to TACE can also lead to a false-positive diagnosis of tumor necrosis [27]. An inaccurate assessment of treatment response may have harmful consequences, especially misleading the interventional radiologist to subsequently choose an inappropriate TACE. Varzaneh et al. [28] reported that post-TACE lipiodol deposition in MDCT could accurately predict tumor necrosis (treatment response) in treated HCC lesions. Therefore, we used CT imaging to evaluate the tumor treatment response and found that the lipiodol deposition level combined with pretreatment clinical data could be used to predict HCC patients who underwent multiple TACEs.

It remains controversial whether treatment should be changed during repeated TACE or whether the effect obtained at a certain time helps to predict patient survival [29]. The optimal number of sessions before abandoning cTACE or requiring combined treatment is also controversial. The Japan Society of Hepatology (JSH) proposed "TACE refractoriness" and recommended that at least two TACE treatments be performed before abandonment [30]. This TACE refractoriness concept has gradually been accepted by various HCC panels [22,31,32]. Notably, in the present study, after the second TACE procedure, approximately 50% of patients with BCLC B-stage HCC who did not respond to the first chemoembolization procedure showed a significant response, while less than 25% of patients who did not respond to the second and third cTACE sessions responded to the third and fourth sessions, respectively. Therefore, two sessions of TACE were sufficient to evaluate the treatment response and, thereafter, patients could consider abandoning cTACE or the need for combined treatment. This result was consistent with the recommendation of the European Association for the Study of the Liver (EASL) guideline that cTACE should be abandoned when a significant tumor treatment response has not been achieved after two cycles of treatment [33]. Regarding survival analyses, the results showed that a largest tumor size greater than 5 cm and a tumor number over 3 were independently associated with inferior OS; these results are consistent with previous studies [34,35].

In recent years, several individualized prediction models have been established to evaluate patient prognosis after cTACE, including tumor burden evaluation models such as the six-and-twelve system and liver reserve evaluation systems such as ALBI grade. Our present study proved that the nomogram based on pre-TACE-3 lipiodol deposition had the highest value for predicting patient outcomes among all the analyzed models. Compared with our constructed nomogram, current commonly used prediction models were built by preprocedure clinical variables. The ALBI grade can provide an objective method for assessing liver function in HCC patients with good prognosis [36]. However, a study by Chi et al. [37] demonstrated that "ALBI-grade migration" was an independent risk factor associated with poor progress-free survival (PFS) and short-term OS. Research by Hiraoka et al. [8] and Lin et al. [38] illustrated that dynamic changes in the ALBI score are a good predictive parameter for prognosis in patients receiving cTACE. Therefore, the application of pretreatment prediction (which cannot independently assess the effect of predictor changes on outcome) and posttreatment prediction models (which cannot independently evaluate the effect of a patient's underlying condition on outcomes) alone may not be sufficient to accurately predict outcome. Recent studies by Adhoute et al. [39] and Wang et al. [40] concluded that pretreatment clinical variables (such as tumor size and tumor number) combined with post-TACE data (presence or absence of radiological response) could have higher values than other pretreatment prediction and posttreatment prediction models. The newly built nomogram combined the best predictive variables in the pretreatment and posttreatment periods to achieve the optimum prediction, which, not surprisingly, was more efficient than other well-known prediction models. The recent 2022 BCLC guidelines were updated, and two novel concepts were introduced: treatment stage migration (TSM) and untreatable progression [41]. Untreatable progression is defined when either treatment failure or progression after the selected treatment approach occur, but patients still fit into their initial BCLC stage, thus warranting the consideration of a therapy corresponding to a more advanced stage. Given the Barcelona Clinic Liver Cancer 2022 update and the successful validation of our newly constructed model (nomogram II), we proposed a novel algorithm for TACE retreatment (Figure 8).

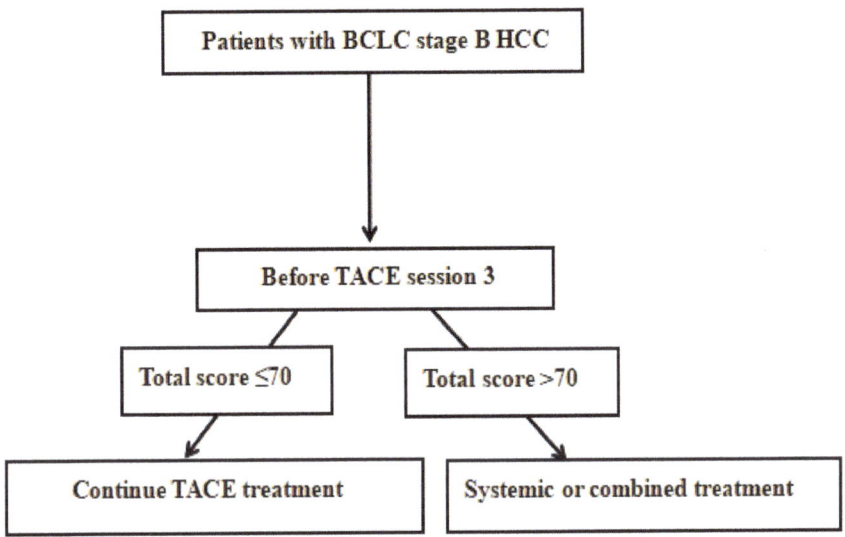

Figure 8. Proposal for nomogram-II-guided retreatment strategy with TACE. TACE: transarterial chemoembolization; BCLC: Barcelona Clinic Liver Cancer; HCC: hepatocellular carcinoma.

To guide the best options for TACE retreatment in HCC patients, Sieghart et al. [42] developed a scoring system called the ART score. Another published scoring system, known as the ABCR score, also aims to select patients who are not capable of benefitting from continued TACE [43]. A time-dependent AUC curve analysis showed that the prognostic value was significantly lower than that of our newly constructed model. There are two major reasons to explain the results: (1) In our study, as well as in research by Georgiades et al. [24], it was demonstrated that, after one TACE session, evaluating the tumor response may not be appropriate. (2) The ART and ABCR scores use the EASL criteria to assess tumor response; however, in tumors with patchy and irregular necrosis, compared to computer-assisted semiautomated measurement, the accurate determination of the tumor border is problematic and susceptible to interobserver variation when using the EASL criteria [10].

The present study has some limitations. First, this retrospective study had potential patient selection bias. Second, the sample size was small; therefore, our results need to be validated with a larger sample size. Finally, the accuracy of semiautomated volume measurement is limited by computer technologies and is dependent on precise contour delineation. Radiomics, a burgeoning technology that could transform potential pathological and physiological information from routine-acquired images into high-dimensional, quantitative, and mineable imaging data, has been demonstrating great potential in the survival predictions of HCC [17,44]. In the future, we aim to build a larger database and use artificial intelligence (AI) for data processing.

5. Conclusions

In summary, based on pre-TACE lipiodol deposition, two sessions were recommended before abandoning cTACE or considering the need for combined treatment for patients with intermediate-stage HCC. Furthermore, we developed and validated a relatively reliable prognostic nomogram to predict the long-term OS in patients with BCLC B-stage HCC after cTACE. Subsequently, the use of this nomogram should be encouraged to improve decision making by providing individualized survival information.

Supplementary Materials: The following are available online at https://www.mdpi.com/article/10.3390/jpm12091375/s1, Table S1: Predictors of death for patients with intermediate-stage HCC before third TACE, Table S2: Predictors of death for patients with intermediate-stage HCC before fourth TACE.

Author Contributions: X.-F.H. conceived the study; X.-K.N. and X.-F.H. oversaw the statistical analysis plan; X.-F.H. conducted the statistical analysis; X.-F.H. contributed to data acquisition; X.-K.N. contributed to data quality assurance and data quality analysis; X.-F.H. contributed to data interpretation; X.-K.N. drafted the initial manuscript, and all the remaining authors critically revised the manuscript. All authors have read and agreed to the published version of the manuscript.

Funding: This research was supported by the Beijing Medical Award Foundation (Project No. YXJL-2020-0972-0420), the Medical Association Project of Sichuan Province (Project Nos. 2021HR04 and Q20050), and the Innovation Team Foundation of the Affiliated Hospital of Chengdu University (Project No. CDFYCX202204).

Institutional Review Board Statement: This study was reviewed and approved by the Ethics Committees of the Affiliated Hospital of Chengdu University and Southern Medical University Nanfang Hospital. All patients or their relatives provided written informed consent.

Informed Consent Statement: Informed consent was obtained from all subjects involved in the study.

Data Availability Statement: The original contributions presented in the study are included in the article and supplementary materials; further inquiries can be directed to the corresponding author.

Acknowledgments: We are grateful to all the patients who participated in this study.

Conflicts of Interest: The authors declare that there is no conflict of interest related to this study.

References

1. Bray, F.; Ferlay, J.; Soerjomataram, I.; Siegel, R.L.; Torre, L.A.; Jemal, A. Global cancer statistics 2018: GLOBOCAN estimates of incidence and mortality worldwide for 36 cancers in 185 countries. *CA Cancer J. Clin.* **2018**, *68*, 394–424. [CrossRef] [PubMed]
2. Cabibbo, G.; Enea, M.; Attanasio, M.; Bruix, J.; Craxi, A.; Cammà, C. A meta-analysis of survival rates of untreated patients in randomized clinical trials of hepatocellular carcinoma. *Hepatology* **2010**, *51*, 1274–1283. [CrossRef] [PubMed]
3. Llovet, J.M.; Bruix, J. Systematic review of randomized trials for unresectable hepatocellular carcinoma: Chemoembolization improves survival. *Hepatology* **2003**, *37*, 429–442. [CrossRef] [PubMed]
4. Salem, R.; Lewandowski, R.J. Chemoembolization and radioembolization for hepatocellular carcinoma. *Clin. Gastroenterol. Hepatol.* **2013**, *11*, 604–611. [CrossRef] [PubMed]

5. Burroughs, A.; Dufour, J.-F.; Galle, P.R.; Mazzaferro, V.; Piscaglia, F.; Raoul, J.L.; Sangro, B.; Bolondi, L. Heterogeneity of patients with intermediate (BCLC B) Hepatocellular Carcinoma: Proposal for a subclassification to facilitate treatment decisions. *Semin. Liver Dis.* **2012**, *32*, 348–359. [CrossRef]
6. Ha, Y.; Shim, J.H.; Kim, S.-O.; Kim, K.M.; Lim, Y.-S.; Lee, H.C. Clinical appraisal of the recently proposed Barcelona Clinic Liver Cancer stage B subclassification by survival analysis. *J. Gastroenterol. Hepatol.* **2014**, *29*, 787–793. [CrossRef]
7. Johnson, P.J.; Berhane, S.; Kagebayashi, C.; Satomura, S.; Teng, M.; Reeves, H.L.; O'Beirne, J.; Fox, R.; Skowronska, A.; Palmer, D.; et al. Assessment of liver function in patients with hepatocellular carcinoma: A new evidence-based approach-the ALBI grade. *J. Clin. Oncol.* **2015**, *33*, 550–558. [CrossRef] [PubMed]
8. Hiraoka, A.; Kumada, T.; Kudo, M.; Hirooka, M.; Koizumi, Y.; Hiasa, Y.; Tajiri, K.; Toyoda, H.; Tada, T.; Ochi, H.; et al. Hepatic Function during Repeated TACE Procedures and Prognosis after Introducing Sorafenib in Patients with Unresectable Hepatocellular Carcinoma: Multicenter Analysis. *Dig. Dis.* **2017**, *35*, 602–610. [CrossRef] [PubMed]
9. Loffroy, R.; Lin, M.; Yenokyan, G.; Rao, P.P.; Bhagat, N.; Noordhoek, N.; Radaelli, A.; Blijd, J.; Liapi, E.; Geschwind, J.-F. Intraprocedural C-arm dual-phase cone-beam CT: Can it be used to predict short-term response to TACE with drug-eluting beads in patients with hepatocellular carcinoma? *Radiology* **2013**, *266*, 636–648. [CrossRef]
10. Monsky, W.L.; Kim, I.; Loh, S.; Li, C.-S.; Greasby, T.A.; Deutsch, L.-S.; Badawi, R.D. Semiautomated segmentation for volumetric analysis of intratumoral ethiodol uptake and subsequent tumor necrosis after chemoembolization. *Am. J. Roentgenol.* **2010**, *195*, 1220–1230. [CrossRef]
11. Suk, O.J.; Jong, C.H.; Gil, C.B.; Giu, L.H. Transarterial chemoembolization with drug-eluting beads in hepatocellular carcinoma: Usefulness of contrast saturation features on cone-beam computed tomography imaging for predicting short-term tumor response. *J. Vasc. Interv. Radiol.* **2013**, *24*, 483–489. [CrossRef] [PubMed]
12. Letzen, B.S.; Malpani, R.; Miszczuk, M.; de Ruiter, Q.M.; Petty, C.W.; Rexha, I.; Nezami, N.; Laage-Gaupp, F.; Lin, M.; Schlachter, T.R.; et al. Lipiodol as an intra-procedural imaging biomarker for liver tumor response to transarterial chemoembolization: Post-hoc analysis of a prospective clinical trial. *Clin. Imaging* **2021**, *78*, 194–200. [CrossRef] [PubMed]
13. Wang, Z.; Chen, R.; Duran, R.; Zhao, Y.; Yenokyan, G.; Chapiro, J.; Schernthaner, R.; Radaelli, A.; Lin, M.; Geschwind, J.F. Intraprocedural 3D Quantification of Lipiodol Deposition on Cone-Beam CT Predicts Tumor Response after Transarterial Chemoembolization in Patients with Hepatocellular Carcinoma. *Cardiovasc. Interv. Radiol.* **2015**, *38*, 1548–1556. [CrossRef] [PubMed]
14. Chen, R.; Geschwind, J.F.; Wang, Z.; Tacher, V.; Lin, M. Quantitative assessment of lipiodol deposition after chemoembolization: Comparison between cone-beam CT and multidetector CT. *J. Vasc. Interv. Radiol.* **2013**, *24*, 1837–1844. [CrossRef]
15. Bruix, J.; Sherman, M.; Llovet, J.M.; Beaugrand, M.; Lencioni, R.; Burroughs, A.K.; Christensen, E.; Pagliaro, L.; Colombo, M.; Rodés, J. Clinical management of hepatocellular carcinoma. Conclusions of the Barcelona-2000 EASL conference. European Association for the Study of the Liver. *J. Hepatol.* **2001**, *35*, 421–430. [CrossRef]
16. Bruix, J.; Sherman, M. American Association for the Study of Liver Diseases. Management of hepatocellular carcinoma: An update. *Hepatology* **2011**, *53*, 1020–1022. [CrossRef]
17. Niu, X.K.; He, X.F. Development of a computed tomography-based radiomics nomogram for prediction of transarterial chemoembolization refractoriness in hepatocellular carcinoma. *World J. Gastroenterol.* **2021**, *27*, 189–207. [CrossRef]
18. Peck-Radosavljevic, M.; Sieghart, W.; Kölblinger, C.; Reiter, M.; Schindl, M.; Ulbrich, G.; Steininger, R.; Müller, C.; Stauber, R.; Schöniger-Hekele, M.; et al. Austrian Joint ÖGGH-ÖGIR-ÖGHO-ASSO position statement on the use of transarterial chemoembolization (TACE) in hepatocellular carcinoma. *Wien. Klin. Wochenschr.* **2012**, *124*, 104–110. [CrossRef]
19. Riaz, A.; Miller, F.H.; Kulik, L.M.; Nikolaidis, P.; Yaghmai, V.; Lewandowski, R.J.; Mulcahy, M.F.; Ryu, R.K.; Sato, K.T.; Gupta, R.; et al. Imaging response in the primary index lesion and clinical outcomes following transarterial locoregional therapy for hepatocellular carcinoma. *JAMA* **2010**, *303*, 1062–1069. [CrossRef]
20. Llovet, J.M.; Di Bisceglie, A.M.; Bruix, J.; Kramer, B.S.; Lencioni, R.; Zhu, A.X.; Sherman, M.; Schwartz, M.; Lotze, M.; Talwalkar, J.; et al. Design and endpoints of clinical trials in hepatocellular carcinoma. *J. Natl. Cancer Inst.* **2008**, *100*, 698–711. [CrossRef]
21. Lencioni, R.; Llovet, J.M. Modified RECIST (mRECIST) assessment for hepatocellular carcinoma. *Semin. Liver Dis.* **2010**, *30*, 52–60. [CrossRef]
22. European Association for the Study of the Liver. EASL Clinical Practice Guidelines: Management of hepatocellular carcinoma. *J. Hepatol.* **2018**, *69*, 182–236. [CrossRef]
23. Terzi, E.; Golfieri, R.; Piscaglia, F.; Galassi, M.; Dazzi, A.; Leoni, S.; Giampalma, E.; Renzulli, M.; Bolondi, L. Response rate and clinical outcome of HCC after first and repeated cTACE performed "on demand". *J. Hepatol.* **2012**, *57*, 1258–1267. [CrossRef]
24. Georgiades, C.; Geschwind, J.-F.; Harrison, N.; Hines-Peralta, A.; Liapi, E.; Hong, K.; Wu, Z.; Kamel, I.; Frangakis, C. Lack of response after initial chemoembolization for hepatocellular carcinoma: Does it predict failure of subsequent treatment? *Radiology* **2012**, *265*, 115–123. [CrossRef] [PubMed]
25. Wang, Z.; Chapiro, J.; Schernthaner, R.; Duran, R.; Chen, R.; Geschwind, J.-F.; Lin, M. Multimodality 3D Tumor Segmentation in HCC Patients Treated with TACE. *Acad. Radiol.* **2015**, *22*, 840–845. [CrossRef]
26. Miyayama, S.; Yamashiro, M.; Nagai, K.; Tohyama, J.; Kawamura, K.; Yoshida, M.; Sakuragawa, N. Evaluation of tumor recurrence after superselective conventional transcatheter arterial chemoembolization for hepatocellular carcinoma: Comparison of computed tomography and gadoxetate disodium-enhanced magnetic resonance imaging. *Hepatol. Res.* **2016**, *46*, 890–898. [CrossRef]

27. Tezuka, M.; Hayashi, K.; Kubota, K.; Sekine, S.; Okada, Y.; Ina, H.; Irie, T. Growth rate of locally recurrent hepatocellular carcinoma after transcatheter arterial chemoembolization: Comparing the growth rate of locally recurrent tumor with that of primary hepatocellular carcinoma. *Dig. Dis. Sci.* **2007**, *52*, 783–788. [CrossRef]
28. Varzaneh, F.N.; Pandey, A.; Ghasabeh, M.A.; Shao, N.; Khoshpouri, P.; Pandey, P.; Zarghampour, M.; Fouladi, D.; Liddell, R.; Anders, R.A.; et al. Prediction of post-TACE necrosis of hepatocellular carcinoma usingvolumetric enhancement on MRI and volumetric oil deposition on CT, with pathological correlation. *Eur. Radiol.* **2018**, *28*, 3032–3040. [CrossRef]
29. Jung, E.S.; Kim, J.H.; Yoon, E.L.; Lee, H.J.; Lee, S.J.; Suh, S.J.; Lee, B.J.; Seo, Y.S.; Yim, H.J.; Seo, T.-S.; et al. Comparison of the methods for tumor response assessment in patients with hepatocellular carcinoma undergoing transarterial chemoembolization. *J. Hepatol.* **2013**, *58*, 1181–1187. [CrossRef]
30. Kudo, M.; Matsui, O.; Izumi, N.; Kadoya, M.; Okusaka, T.; Miyayama, S.; Yamakado, K.; Tsuchiya, K.; Ueshima, K.; Hiraoka, A.; et al. Transarterial chemoembolization failure/refractoriness: JSH-LCSGJ criteria 2014 update. *Oncology* **2014**, *87*, 22–31. [CrossRef]
31. Lee, J.S.; Kim, B.K.; Kim, S.U.; Park, J.Y.; Ahn, S.H.; Seong, J.S.; Han, K.-H.; Kim, D.Y. A survey on transarterial chemoembolization refractoriness and a real-world treatment pattern for hepatocellular carcinoma in Korea. *Clin. Mol. Hepatol.* **2020**, *26*, 24–32. [CrossRef] [PubMed]
32. Zhong, B.-Y.; Wang, W.-S.; Zhang, S.; Zhu, H.-D.; Zhang, L.; Shen, J.; Zhu, X.-L.; Teng, G.-J.; Ni, C.-F. Re-evaluating Transarterial Chemoembolization Failure/Refractoriness: A Survey by Chinese College of Interventionalists. *J. Clin. Transl. Hepatol.* **2021**, *9*, 521–527. [CrossRef] [PubMed]
33. Lu, J.; Zhao, M.; Arai, Y.; Zhong, B.Y.; Zhu, H.D.; Qi, X.L.; de Baere, T.; Pua, U.; Yoon, H.K.; Madoff, D.C.; et al. Clinical practice of transarterial chemoembolization for hepatocellular carcinoma: Consensus statement from an international expert panel of International Society of Multidisciplinary Interventional Oncology (ISMIO). *Hepatobiliary Surg. Nutr.* **2021**, *10*, 661–671. [CrossRef] [PubMed]
34. Ni, J.-Y.; Fang, Z.-T.; Sun, H.-L.; An, C.; Huang, Z.-M.; Zhang, T.-Q.; Jiang, X.-Y.; Chen, Y.-T.; Xu, L.-F.; Huang, J.-H. A nomogram to predict survival of patients with intermediate-stage hepatocellular carcinoma after transarterial chemoembolization combined with microwave ablation. *Eur. Radiol.* **2020**, *30*, 2377–2390. [CrossRef]
35. Ni, J.Y.; Sun, H.L.; Chen, Y.T.; Luo, J.H.; Chen, D.; Jiang, X.Y.; Xu, L.F. Prognostic factors for survival after transarterial chemoembolization combined with microwave ablation for hepatocellular carcinoma. *World J. Gastroenterol.* **2014**, *20*, 17483–17490. [CrossRef]
36. Jaruvongvanich, V.; Sempokuya, T.; Wong, L. Is there an optimal staging system or liver reserve model that can predict outcome in hepatocellular carcinoma? *J. Gastrointest. Oncol.* **2018**, *9*, 750–761. [CrossRef]
37. Chi, C.-T.; Lee, I.-C.; Lee, R.-C.; Hung, Y.-W.; Su, C.-W.; Hou, M.-C.; Chao, Y.; Huang, Y.-H. Effect of Transarterial Chemoembolization on ALBI Grade in Intermediate-Stage Hepatocellular Carcinoma: Criteria for Unsuitable Cases Selection. *Cancers* **2021**, *13*, 4325. [CrossRef]
38. Lin, P.-T.; Teng, W.; Jeng, W.-J.; Chen, W.-T.; Hsieh, Y.-C.; Huang, C.-H.; Lui, K.-W.; Hung, C.-F.; Wang, C.-T.; Chai, P.-M.; et al. Dynamic Change of Albumin-Bilirubin Score Is Good Predictive Parameter for Prognosis in Chronic Hepatitis C-hepatocellular Carcinoma Patients Receiving Transarterial Chemoembolization. *Diagnostics* **2022**, *12*, 665. [CrossRef]
39. Adhoute, X.; Larrey, E.; Anty, R.; Chevallier, P.; Penaranda, G.; Tran, A.; Bronowicki, J.-P.; Raoul, J.-L.; Castellani, P.; Perrier, H.; et al. Expected outcomes and patients' selection before chemoembolization-"Six-and-Twelve or Pre-TACE-Predict" scores may help clinicians: Real-life French cohorts results. *World J. Clin. Cases* **2021**, *9*, 4559–4572. [CrossRef]
40. Wang, Z.-X.; Wang, E.-X.; Bai, W.; Xia, D.-D.; Mu, W.; Li, J.; Yang, Q.-Y.; Huang, M.; Xu, G.-H.; Sun, J.-H.; et al. Validation and evaluation of clinical prediction systems for first and repeated transarterial chemoembolization in unresectable hepatocellular carcinoma: A Chinese multicenter retrospective study. *World J. Gastroenterol.* **2020**, *26*, 657–669. [CrossRef]
41. Reig, M.; Forner, A.; Rimola, J.; Ferrer-Fàbrega, J.; Burrel, M.; Garcia-Criado, Á.; Kelley, R.K.; Galle, P.R.; Mazzaferro, V.; Salem, R.; et al. BCLC strategy for prognosis prediction and treatment recommendation: The 2022 update. *J. Hepatol.* **2022**, *76*, 681–693. [CrossRef] [PubMed]
42. Sieghart, W.; Hucke, F.; Pinter, M.; Graziadei, I.; Vogel, W.; Müller, C.; Heinzl, H.; Trauner, M.; Peck-Radosavljevic, M. The ART of decision making: Retreatment with transarterial chemoembolization in patients with hepatocellular carcinoma. *Hepatology* **2013**, *57*, 2261–2273. [CrossRef] [PubMed]
43. Adhoute, X.; Penaranda, G.; Naude, S.; Raoul, J.L.; Perrier, H.; Bayle, O.; Monnet, O.; Beaurain, P.; Bazin, C.; Pol, B.; et al. Retreatment with TACE: The ABCR SCORE, an aid to the decision-making process. *J. Hepatol.* **2015**, *62*, 855–862. [CrossRef]
44. Iezzi, R.; Casà, C.; Posa, A.; Cornacchione, P.; Carchesio, F.; Boldrini, L.; Tanzilli, A.; Cerrito, L.; Fionda, B.; Longo, V.; et al. Project for interventional Oncology LArge-database in liveR Hepatocellular carcinoma—Preliminary CT-based radiomic analysis (POLAR Liver 1.1). *Eur. Rev. Med. Pharmacol. Sci.* **2022**, *26*, 2891–2899. [CrossRef]

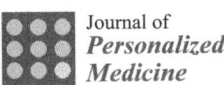

Article

Feasibility of Neovessel Embolization in a Large Animal Model of Tendinopathy: Safety and Efficacy of Various Embolization Agents

Julien Ghelfi [1,2,*], Ian Soulairol [3,4], Olivier Stephanov [5], Marylène Bacle [6], Hélène de Forges [7], Noelia Sanchez-Ballester [3,4], Gilbert Ferretti [1,2], Jean-Paul Beregi [7] and Julien Frandon [7]

1. Faculty of Medicine, University of Grenoble Alpes, 38000 Grenoble, France
2. Department of Radiology, Grenoble-Alpes University Hospital, 38000 Grenoble, France
3. Department of Pharmacy, Nîmes University Hospital, 30900 Nîmes, France
4. ICGM, University of Montpellier, CNRS, ENSCM, 34090 Montpellier, France
5. Anatomopathology Department, Grenoble University Hospital, 38000 Grenoble, France
6. Faculty of Medicine, Montpellier Nîmes University, RAM-PTNIM, 30900 Nîmes, France
7. Department of Medical Imaging, Nîmes University Hospital, Imagine UR UM 103, University of Montpellier, 34090 Montpellier, France
* Correspondence: jghelfi@chu-grenoble.fr

Abstract: Targeting neovessels in chronic tendinopathies has emerged as a new therapeutic approach and several embolization agents have been reported. The aim of this study was to investigate the feasibility of embolization with different agents in a porcine model of patellar tendinopathy and evaluate their safety and efficacy. Eight 3-month-old male piglets underwent percutaneous injection of collagenase type I to induce patellar tendinopathies ($n = 16$ tendons). They were divided into four groups (2 piglets, 4 tendons/group): the control group, 50–100 µm microspheres group, 100–300 µm microspheres group, and the Imipenem/Cilastatin (IMP/CS) group. Angiography and embolization were performed for each patellar tendon on day 7 (D7). The neovessels were evaluated visually with an angiography on day 14. The pathological analysis assessed the efficacy (Bonar score, number of neovessels/mm^2) and safety (off-target persistent cutaneous ischemic modifications and presence of off-target embolization agents). The technical success was 92%, with a failed embolization for one tendon due to an arterial dissection. Neoangiogenesis was significantly less important in the embolized groups compared to the control group angiographies ($p = 0.04$) but not with respect to histology (Bonar score $p = 0.15$, neovessels $p = 0.07$). Off-target cutaneous embolization was more frequently depicted in the histology of the 50–100 µm microspheres group ($p = 0.02$). Embolization of this animal model with induced patellar tendinopathy was technically feasible with different agents and allowed assessing the safety and efficacy of neovessel destruction. Particles smaller than 100 µm seemed to be associated with more complications.

Keywords: tendinopathy; neovessels; embolization; imipenem/cilastatin

1. Introduction

Tendinopathy is a frequent pathology in the general population and especially in athletes. The most significant symptom is pain; analgesic treatments include physical therapy and icing, oral analgesics, peri-tendinous corticosteroid, or intra-tendinous platelet-rich plasma injections [1,2]. They are generally effective, but up to 10% of patients report chronic pain, with an impact on the patient's quality of life and impairment of daily activities. The therapeutic alternative is then surgery, which remains invasive with no guaranteed results.

Chronic tendinopathy is accompanied by neoangiogenesis and neoinnervation [3]. A similar mechanism has been reported in osteoarthritis where it was shown to be a cause of chronic pain resistant to the usual analgesics, as it involves neuropathic signaling pathways [4].

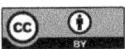

Destruction of these pathological neovessels may help break this neurogenic pain cycle. Ultrasound-controlled injections of sclerosing agents targeting the neovessel area have been reported in patients with patellar tendinopathy, with improvement in some patients [5]. Recently, Okuno et al. [6] have shown that arterial embolization by an endovascular approach in osteoarticular pathologies and tendinopathy, in particular, could be an alternative analgesic therapy by targeting these neovessels [7]. To date, several embolization agents of different sizes have been described [7–9] but no large randomized studies of the embolization technique in osteoarticular pathologies have yet been reported. Among them, an antibiotic that precipitates in the form of crystals, imipenem/cilastatin (IMP/CS), has been reported with very good analgesic efficacy in patients with tendinopathy or knee osteoarthritis [10–14]. Because of its resorbing nature and small size, it allows for the destruction of neovessels without associated complications. Similar studies with definitive microspheres (MS) have shown less conclusive results, with complications including off-target embolization and skin modifications [15].

The identification of the most adequate embolization agents requires the use of animal models that allow arterial catheterization. However, there are only a few large models of tendinopathy allowing angiographic exploration for embolization. A porcine model of patellar tendinopathy with neoangiogenesis was thus developed by our team [16]. A previous study showed the feasibility and reproducibility of induced patellar tendinopathy after collagenase injection. Neovascularization was confirmed by angiographic findings and pathological analyses.

The main objective of the present study was to assess the feasibility of embolization in this model with various embolization agents and to evaluate their safety and efficacy on neovessel destruction via angiography and histology.

2. Materials and Methods

2.1. Patellar Tendinopathy Induction

Eight 3-month-old male piglets underwent percutaneous injection of collagenase type I (Sigma-Aldrich, St. Louis, MO, USA) under ultrasound guidance at a dose of 25 mg, according to the model and protocol previously published [16]. It was performed in accordance with the National Institute of Health guidelines for the use of laboratory animals. Authorization of the local government animal rights protection authorities (Languedoc-Roussillon No 36, ID number Nr 2018011916269335 #13156 v3) was obtained.

2.2. Angiography Explorations

Endovascular explorations were performed 7 days and 14 days after the collagenase injection on a Fluorostar III (GE Healthcare) following the same protocol as previously published [16]. Briefly, a left carotid arterial access was performed under ultrasound guidance using the Seldinger technique. The femoral artery was catheterized with a 4Fr catheter and the genicular arteries with a 2.0 microcatheter. Injections were performed manually with a 5 mL syringe on DSA imaging. Neovascularization was graded as none, mild, or important by two radiologists in consensus, blinded to the treatment group, in a random order, three months after the procedure.

2.3. Embolization Procedure

The piglets were divided into four groups, with four patellar tendons per group (Figure 1):

1. The control group (2 pigs, 4 tendons) underwent diagnostic angiography alone at D7 (no embolization) and D14.
2. Two groups (4 pigs, 8 tendons, 4 tendons in each group) were embolized with calibrated Embosphere® microspheres (Merit Medical, Paris, France) of either 50 to 100 μm (50–100 μm group) or 100 to 300 μm (100–300 μm group) diameter at D7 after collagenase injection. The microspheres were diluted to the 1/20th in NaCl and iodinated contrast was injected 0.1 per 0.1 mL according to the "pruning" technique [17] (Figure 2).

3. The fourth group (2 pigs, 4 tendons) was embolized at D7 using an emulsion of imipenem/cilastatin (IMP/CS group) (500/500 mg) diluted in 10 mL of Visipaque iodinated contrast (GE Healthcare, Marlborough, MA, USA). The mixture was injected 0.1 per 0.1 mL until complete stasis of the feeding artery according to the Martinez et al. technique [18] was achieved (Figure 2).

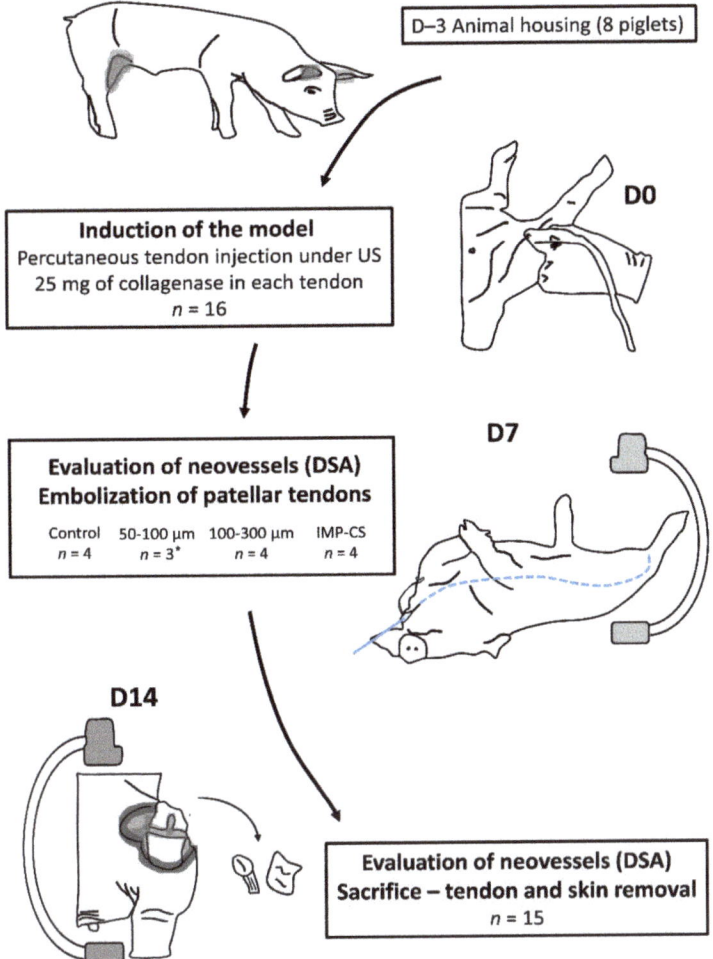

Figure 1. Flowchart of the study. US: ultrasound; D: day; DSA: digital subtraction angiography; *: one tendon was not treated due to femoral artery dissection on D7 angiography.

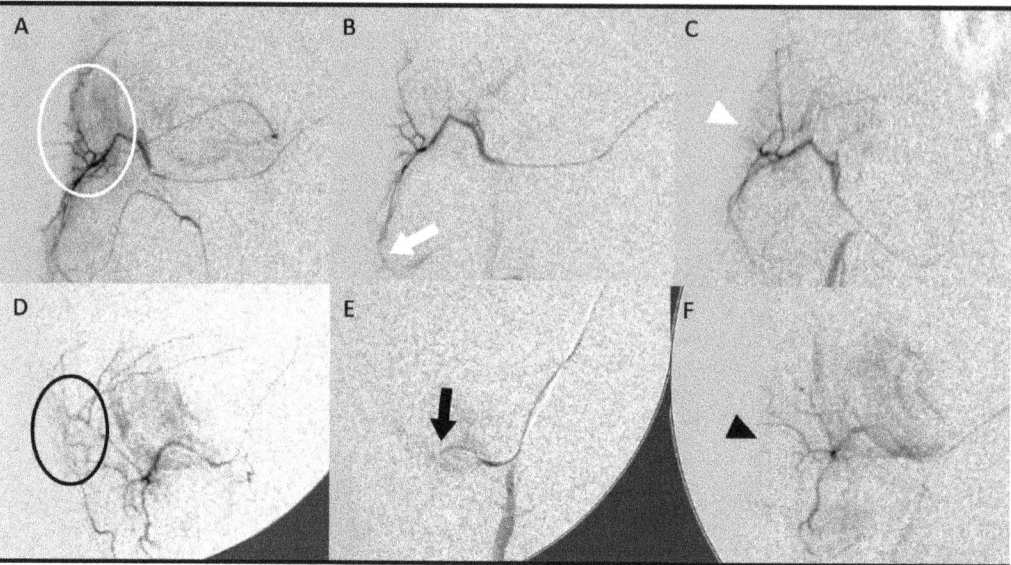

Figure 2. Embolization procedure at D7 using various embolization agents: microspheres (**A–C**) and imipenem/cilastatin (**D–F**). (**A**) Initial digital subtraction angiography (DSA) of a right geniculate artery showing neovascularization-related blush (white circle). (**B**) After embolization using 50–100 µm microspheres according to the "pruning" technique, DSA showed a "dead tree" aspect of the embolized area with a filling area by collaterals (white arrow). (**C**) DSA control at D14 showed no recurrence of neovascularization at the site of tendinopathy (white arrowhead). (**D**) The initial DSA of a right geniculate artery showing a blush related to neovascularization (black circle). (**E**) After embolization with an IMP/CS emulsion in an iodinated contrast medium, opacification revealed a truncated appearance of the geniculate artery (black arrow). (**F**) The DSA control at D14 showed repermeabilization of the native artery with no recurrence of neovessels (black arrowhead).

2.4. Histological Analyses

The analyses were performed following the same protocol as previously published [16]. Briefly, after surgical dissection and sacrifice, tendons and skin samples were taken from the outer side of the thigh, near the tendon, in the area where a livedo was reported in piglets. They were fixed in 4% formaldehyde and embedded in paraffin. A pathologist, blinded to the groups, performed the examination on an Olympus BX51 microscope, with a Bonar score [19–21] characterization focused on the vascularity subclass index. The number of neovessels/mm^2 and the presence of persistent embolization agents in the tendons and the skin were also recorded.

2.5. In Vitro Analysis

A focus on the microscopy study of the crystallization and solubility of IMP/CS was also carried out. Particle size distribution was microscopically evaluated in three samples of 50 mg IMP/CS (Arrow, Lyon, France) suspensions with a mixture of Visipaque iodinated contrast (GE Healthcare, Marlborough, MA, USA) and NaCl using a volume of 1000 µL and a vortex mixing time of 10 s (Scientific Industries SI™ Vortex-Genie™ 2, Fisher Bioblock Scientific).

The longest diameter of the IMP/CS particles was manually measured using a digital microscope (Keyence VHX-700 Digital Microscope) with an image analyzing software (VHX Analyzer; Itasca, IL, USA). The solubility of IMP/CS in formaldehyde was tested with 10 mg of IMP/CS in 10 mL of formaldehyde and stirred for 10 min. The suspension was then filtered through a 0.45 µm syringe filter (Millipore Milliflex®-HV) and UV–Vis spectrophotometrically analyzed in the wavelength range of 200–400 nm using a Specord 200 Plus UV/Vis spectrophotometer (Analytik Jena, Jena, Germany).

2.6. Study Endpoints

The primary endpoint was the technical success of the embolization procedure defined as efficient catheterization and embolization of the patellar artery with no neovessel opacification after embolization, as assessed on angiography imaging just after the procedure and compared to the baseline angiography.

Secondary endpoints were the safety and efficacy of various embolization agents. Efficacy was evaluated on neovessel destruction via angiography and histology on day 14, 7 days after embolization. The angiographic visual evaluation compared neovascularization at day 14 versus controls (none, mild, and severe). In regards to the histology, the evaluation of efficacy compared the number of neovessels/mm^2 and the Bonar score of embolized groups with the control group. Safety was assessed clinically with a behavior scale previously reported [16], weight intake, and screening of off-target embolization using post-embolization immediate clinical cutaneous evaluation (livedo) and delayed histological analysis of the skin around the patellar tendon (inflammatory modifications and persistent embolization agents in the skin). The last objective was to describe the size distribution of the IMP/CS particles as close as possible to the conditions of use as described in the literature in clinical practice [12] (50 mg of IMP/CS and 1 mL of iodinated contrast) as described above.

2.7. Statistical Analyses

Quantitative variables are presented using medians and interquartile ranges (1st–3rd) and qualitative variables with numbers and percentages. Quantitative values were compared using the Kruskal–Wallis test when comparing the four groups and the Mann–Whitney test when comparing two groups. Qualitative values were compared using Pearson's Chi-squared test. Tests were considered significant at the $p < 0.05$ level. Analyses were performed on Excel® (version 16.49) and using Graph Pad Prism version 9.3 (GraphPad Software, San Diego, CA, USA).

3. Results

3.1. Technical Success

Embolization of the neovessels was successfully achieved in 11/12 patellar tendons (92%). One procedure of the 50–100 μm microspheres group failed because of femoral artery dissection without any clinical consequence.

3.2. Safety

No clinical sign of patellar tendinopathy was reported after collagenase injection in all eight piglets. They all reported a walking score of 3/3. No weight loss was reported; the median weight gain between baseline and day 14 was 12% {IQR: 9.3–16}. After embolization, immediate transient livedo was recorded in 7/11 knees (64%), with no difference according to the embolization agent used ($p = 0.76$). On pathological analysis, persistent cutaneous ischemic modifications were more frequently reported in the 50–100 μm microspheres group than in the two other groups ($p = 0.02$) (Table 1). Among the four knees with persistent skin modifications at pathology, persistent embolic agents were depicted in two skin samples (one piglet of the 50–100 μm microspheres group and one piglet of the IMP/CS group) (Figure 3).

Table 1. Safety of various embolization agents.

Groups	Clinical Findings		Pathologic Findings at Day 14			
	Immediate Transient Livedo	p-Value	Persistent Intracutaneous Ischemic Modifications	p-Value	Persistent Intracutaneous Embolization Agent	p-Value
Control (n = 4)	NA		NA		NA	
50–100 (n = 3)	2	0.76	3	0.02	1	0.48
100–300 (n = 4)	3		0		0	
IMP/CS (n = 4)	2		1		1	

IMP/CS: Imipenem/Cilastatin.

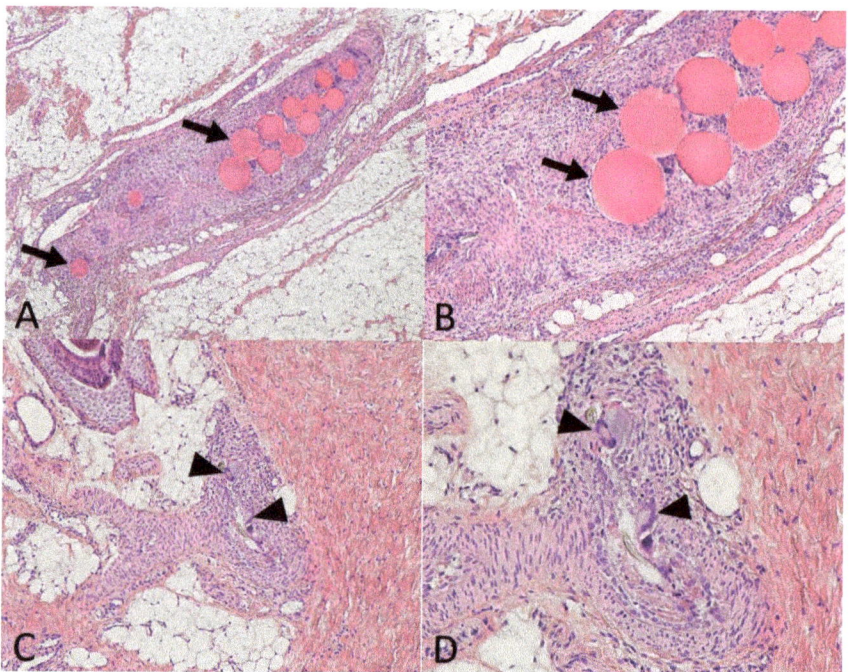

Figure 3. **Histological evaluation of the safety of embolization**. Using a standard stain (Hemathein Eosin Saffron) at ×40 (**A**), ×100 (**B**,**C**), and ×200 (**D**) magnification on tendon and skin samples taken 7 days after embolization. (**A**,**B**) Tendon treated by 50–100 μm microspheres. The peritendinous artery obliterated by the embolization material (arrows) with a granulomatous reaction. (**C**,**D**) Skin samples in the area of a transient livedo episode during embolization with Imipenem/Cilastatin (IMP/CS) emulsion. Dermohypodermal arteriole with granulomatous reaction with giant cells (black arrowheads) resorbing exogenous debris (IMP/CS crystals).

3.3. Efficacy

Neovascularization was similar between the four groups on the baseline angiography (day 7 after collagenase injection, just before embolization) (Table 2). On day 7 after embolization (day 14 after collagenase injection), it was significantly higher in the control group compared to the groups treated with embolization (microspheres groups or IMP/CS group, $p = 0.04$).

Table 2. Efficacy of various embolization agents.

Groups	Angiographic Neovascularization (Visual Evaluation)							
	Day 7				Day 14			
	None	Mild	Severe	p-value	None	Mild	Severe	p-value
Controls (n = 4)	0	1	3		0	1	3	
50–100 (n = 3)	0	1	2	0.87	2	1	0	0.04
100–300 (n = 4)	0	1	3		2	2	0	
IMP/CS (n = 4)	0	2	2		3	1	0	

Groups	Pathologic Findings on Day 14							
	Bonar global score	p-value	Bonar vascularity subclass	p-value	Neovessels/mm^2	p-value	Intratendinous embolization agent	p-value
Controls (n = 4)	12 [10.5–13]		2.5 [1.8–3.0]		33 [29.5–36.8]		NA	
50–100 (n = 3)	6 [6–7.5]	0.15	1 [1.0–1.5]	0.52	17 [16.5–20.5]	0.07	3	0.02
100–300 (n = 4)	9 [6.5–11]		2 [0.8–3.0]		26 [24.8–27.8]		3	
IMP/CS (n = 4)	8.5 [6.8–9.5]		1 [1.0–1.3]		23 [18.3–27.3]		0	

IMP/CS: Imipenem/Cilastatin.

There was no difference in the Bonar score ($p = 0.15$) or the Bonar vascular subclass ($p = 0.52$) between the controls and embolized tendons. The number of neovessels/mm^2 was lower in the embolized groups compared to the control group, although it was not found significant ($p = 0.07$), especially in the 50–100 μm microspheres group (17 neovessels/mm^2 {IQR: 16.5–20.5}) as compared to the control group (33 neovessels/mm^2 {IQR: 29.5–36.8}, $p = 0.06$).

3.4. In Vitro Analysis

Over 1500 particles were measured in each condition of the IMP/CS dilution with contrast. More than 96.8% of IMP/CS particles were <40 μm in all conditions tested (Figure 4). For the solubility of IMP/CS in formaldehyde, no absorption peaks were observed, demonstrating the insoluble character of the IMP/CS at the concentration tested.

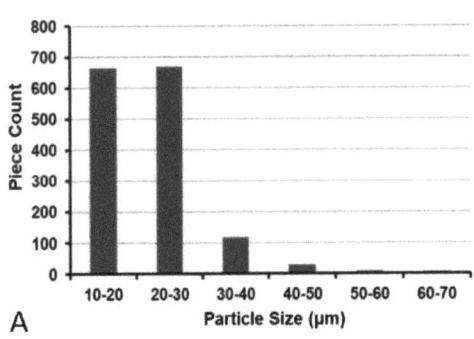
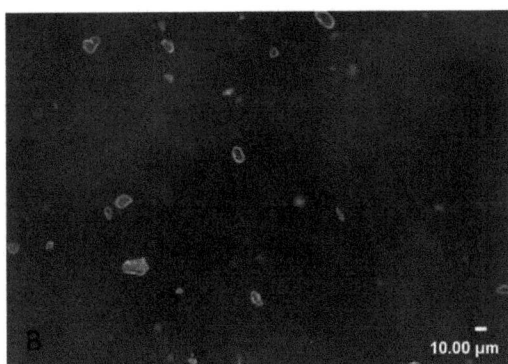

Figure 4. In vitro exploration. (A) Size distribution of 50 mg of imipenem/cilastatin (IMP/CS) particles in 1 mL of iodinated contrast dispersed during 10 s. (B) ×400 magnification of 50 mg/mL IMP/CS in iodinated contrast emulsion.

4. Discussion

Embolization of neovessels in this large animal patellar tendinopathy model was feasible with three different embolization agents. Our results showed the efficacy of the technique in terms of neovessel destruction. Embolization was safer with microspheres larger than 100 µm; with smaller embolization agents, microspheres, or IMP/CS reporting off-target embolization inducing cutaneous ischemia.

4.1. Neoangiogenesis

Our results showed the efficacy of embolization with significant destruction of neovessels in embolized piglets as compared to controls. They are in accordance with a rat model of frozen shoulder treated by embolization with IMP/CS [22]. In their study, a decreased number of mononuclear inflammatory cells was also described, suggesting that transcatheter arterial embolization may also improve the inflammatory reaction in frozen shoulder. Recently, a ram model of knee osteoarthritis was evaluated by intra-arterial injection of mono-iodoacetate. Despite the limited number of treated knees (75 µm calibrated microparticles n = 2 and 250 µm calibrated microparticles n = 2), they showed the slow-down of inflammation progression after embolization on MRI, angiographic, and histologic analyses [23].

The Bonar score, and, in particular, its vascular subclass, has shown discordances and limitations regarding correlation with therapeutic responses [24,25]. Our results add to these limitations, as there was no difference in the vascularity subclass of the Bonar score after embolization, although the number of neovessels was significantly different between controls and embolized piglets. This score does not seem to be optimal in tendinopathy evaluation and another tool to evaluate neoangiogenesis in a more adequate manner, through anatomical imaging (DSA, MRI) or functional imaging (radiotracer), should be considered.

4.2. Safety

Persistent cutaneous ischemia was reported in our study in piglets injected with small microspheres and IMP/CS, but not in those injected with larger microspheres (>100 µm). Although the "pruning" technique was used and emboli were administered slowly and in small amounts at a time, off-target embolization reports suggest that the emboli are passing through the capillary network. The use of skin ice packs near the embolization area has been reported with definitive microspheres to induce the vasoconstriction of collaterals and skin vessels and decrease the risk of off-target embolization [17]. Given the size of the IMP/CS crystals, it is logical that there would be non-target migration but the soluble nature of the crystals makes it transient. Nevertheless, we found residual crystals in a skin territory one week after embolization as reported in a frozen shoulder mouse model [22]. In contrast, a study evaluating rat kidneys 48 h after embolization found no residual crystals in the renal arteries [26]. A Japanese team recently compared IMP/CS embolization (six knees) versus resorbing gel foam (six knees) in a porcine model of knee arthritis. No complication and no off-target embolization agents were found 72 h after the procedure [27].

4.3. In Vitro Analysis

As previously reported [26], almost all IMP/CS particles were found to be smaller than 40 µm. The particle size distribution varied slightly between the emulsion with contrast and NaCl, as it seems to vary with the amount of contrast or with the time after suspension [26]. The transient nature of IMP/CS embolization is related to its solubility, which probably varies with its concentration and flow in the artery. In poorly vascularized terminal territories, or in case of over-embolization (too many injected particles), it is likely that the resorption time would increase. This could expose patients to ischemic complications from definitive microspheres [13]. Furthermore, optimization of the IMP/CS embolization protocol should be performed, such as diluting the IMP/CS in contrast medium as well as the amount and duration of IMP/CS injection, to ensure patient safety and homogenous practices. Indeed, the protocol is likely to be different depending on the embolization indications and the arteries treated, which will have to be clarified for future studies. If the safety of the IMP/CS comes from its transient ischemic character, it is to be noted that in the clinical uses reported, digestive embolization [28] and osteoarticular pathologies [11,12,18], the arterial network is rich in collaterals and the risk of off-target embolization is higher.

On the contrary, although less aggressive than definitive microparticles and despite its transient character, in terminal vascularization, such as the kidney, IMP/CS seems to be responsible for ischemic complications at 48 h [26]. Another hypothesis could be that the endothelium of neovessels may be different from that of normal vessels and are thus more sensitive to even a transient embolic agent and more at risk of thrombosis, whereas healthy vessels would have a greater tendency to recanalization [29].

4.4. Limitations

Our study has some limitations, among which is the small number of piglets. In addition, neovessel evaluation on angiography was performed visually. The use of software to count neovessels induced by collagenase injection and destroyed after embolization may strengthen the results and allow a more objective and reproducible evaluation. Lastly, this piglet model injected with collagenase did not show any clinical signs of tendinopathy [16]. The effect of embolization on pain and the walking score was not assessed. It would be interesting to study the clinical effects of these different embolization agents in other tendinopathy models.

5. Conclusions

Embolization in this porcine model with induced patellar tendinopathy was technically feasible with different embolization agents and allowed for assessing their safety and efficacy on neovessel destruction. The use of particles smaller than 100 μm seems to be associated with more complications than larger particles.

Author Contributions: Conceptualization, J.G., M.B. and J.F.; methodology, J.G. and J.F.; validation, J.F.; formal analysis, J.G.; investigation, J.G., I.S., O.S., M.B., N.S.-B. and J.F.; resources, J.G. and J.F.; data curation, J.G.; writing—original draft preparation, J.G., H.d.F. and J.F.; writing—review and editing, J.G., H.d.F., G.F., J.-P.B. and J.F.; supervision, G.F. and J.-P.B.; project administration, J.F.; funding acquisition, J.G. and J.F. All authors have read and agreed to the published version of the manuscript.

Funding: This research was funded by Merit Medical.

Institutional Review Board Statement: The study was performed with authorization from the local government animal rights protection authorities (Languedoc-Roussillon No 36, ID number Nr 2018011916269335 #13156 v3) in accordance with the National Institute of Health guidelines for the use of laboratory animals.

Informed Consent Statement: Not applicable.

Data Availability Statement: Data will be accessible upon reasonable request to the corresponding author.

Conflicts of Interest: The authors declare no conflict of interest.

References

1. Chen, P.C.; Wu, K.T.; Chou, W.Y.; Huang, Y.C.; Wang, L.Y.; Yang, T.H.; Siu, K.K.; Tu, Y.K. Comparative Effectiveness of Different Nonsurgical Treatments for Patellar Tendinopathy: A Systematic Review and Network Meta-analysis. *Arthroscopy* **2019**, *35*, 3117–3131. [CrossRef] [PubMed]
2. Zayni, R.; Thaunat, M.; Fayard, J.M.; Hager, J.P.; Carrillon, Y.; Clechet, J.; Gadea, F.; Archbold, P.; Sonnery Cottet, B. Platelet-Rich Plasma as a Treatment for Chronic Patellar Tendinopathy: Comparison of a Single versus Two Consecutive Injections. *Muscle Ligaments Tendons J.* **2015**, *5*, 92–98. [CrossRef]
3. Alfredson, H.; Ohberg, L.; Forsgren, S. Is vasculo-neural ingrowth the cause of pain in chronic Achilles tendinosis? An investigation using ultra- sonography and colour Doppler, immunohistochemistry, and diagnostic injections. *Knee Surg. Sports Traumatol. Arthrosc.* **2003**, *11*, 334–338. [CrossRef] [PubMed]
4. Ashraf, S.; Wibberley, H.; Mapp, P.I.; Hill, R.; Wilson, D.; Walsh, D.A. Increased vascular penetration and nerve growth in the meniscus: A potential source of pain in osteoarthritis. *Ann. Rheum. Dis.* **2011**, *70*, 523–529. [CrossRef]
5. Hoksrud, A.S.; Torgalsen, T.; Harstad, H.; Haugen, S.; Andersen, T.; Risberg, M.; Bahr, R. Ultrasound-guided sclerosis of neovessels in patellar tendinopathy: A prospective study of 101 patients. *Am. J. Sports Med.* **2012**, *40*, 542–547. [CrossRef] [PubMed]
6. Okuno, Y.; Matsumura, N.; Oguro, S. Transcatheter arterial embolization using imipenem/cilastatin sodium for tendinopathy and enthesopathy refractory to nonsurgical management. *J. Vasc. Interv. Radiol.* **2013**, *24*, 787–792. [CrossRef] [PubMed]

7. Talaie, R.; Torkian, P.; Clayton, A.; Wallace, S.; Cheung, H.; Chalian, M.; Golzarian, J. Emerging Targets for the Treatment of Osteoarthritis: New Investigational Methods to Identify Neo-Vessels as Possible Targets for Embolization. *Diagnostics* **2022**, *12*, 1403. [CrossRef]
8. Fernández-Martínez, A.M.; Alonso-Burgos, A.; López, R.; Cuesta Marcos, M.T.; Baldi, S. Clinical Outcomes of Transcatheter Arterial Embolization for Secondary Stiff Shoulder. *J. Vasc. Interv. Radiol.* **2021**, *32*, 489–496. [CrossRef]
9. Kim, G.H.; Shin, J.H.; Nam, I.C.; Chu, H.H.; Kim, J.H.; Yoon, H.K. Transcatheter Arterial Embolization for Benign Chronic Inflammatory Joint Pain: A Systematic Review and Meta-Analysis. *J. Vasc. Interv. Radiol.* **2022**, *33*, 538–545. [CrossRef]
10. Okuno, Y.; Korchi, A.M.; Shinjo, T.; Kato, S.; Kaneko, T. Midterm Clinical Outcomes and MR Imaging Changes after Transcatheter Arterial Embolization as a Treatment for Mild to Moderate Radiographic Knee Osteoarthritis Resistant to Conservative Treatment. *J. Vasc. Interv. Radiol.* **2017**, *28*, 995–1002. [CrossRef]
11. Okuno, Y.; Iwamoto, W.; Matsumura, N.; Oguro, S.; Yasumoto, T.; Kaneko, T.; Ikegami, H. Clinical Outcomes of Transcatheter Arterial Embolization for Adhesive Capsulitis Resistant to Conservative Treatment. *J. Vasc. Interv. Radiol.* **2017**, *28*, 161–167. [CrossRef] [PubMed]
12. Iwamoto, W.; Okuno, Y.; Matsumura, N.; Kaneko, T.; Ikegami, H. Transcatheter arterial embolization of abnormal vessels as a treatment for lateral epicondylitis refractory to conservative treatment: A pilot study with a 2-year follow-up. *J. Shoulder Elb. Surg.* **2017**, *26*, 1335–1341. [CrossRef] [PubMed]
13. Inui, S.; Yoshizawa, S.; Shintaku, T.; Kaneko, T.; Ikegami, H.; Okuno, Y. Intra-Arterial Infusion of Imipenem/Cilastatin Sodium through a Needle Inserted into the Radial Artery as a New Treatment for Refractory Trapeziometacarpal Osteoarthritis. *J. Vasc. Interv. Radiol.* **2021**, *32*, 1341–1347. [CrossRef]
14. Hwang, J.H.; Park, S.W.; Kim, K.H.; Lee, S.J.; Oh, K.S.; Chung, S.W.; Moon, S.G. Early Results of Transcatheter Arterial Embolization for Relief of Chronic Shoulder or Elbow Pain Associated with Tendinopathy Refractory to Conservative Treatment. *J. Vasc. Interv. Radiol.* **2018**, *29*, 510–517. [CrossRef] [PubMed]
15. Gremen, E.; Frandon, J.; Lateur, G.; Finas, M.; Rodière, M.; Horteur, C.; Benassayag, M.; Thony, F.; Pailhe, R.; Ghelfi, J. Safety and Efficacy of Embolization with Microspheres in Chronic Refractory Inflammatory Shoulder Pain: A Pilot Monocentric Study on 15 Patients. *Biomedicines* **2022**, *10*, 744. [CrossRef] [PubMed]
16. Ghelfi, J.; Bacle, M.; Stephanov, O.; de Forges, H.; Soulairol, I.; Roger, P.; Ferretti, G.R.; Beregi, J.P.; Frandon, J. Collagenase-Induced Patellar Tendinopathy with Neovascularization: First Results towards a Piglet Model of Musculoskeletal Embolization. *Biomedicines* **2021**, *10*, 2. [CrossRef] [PubMed]
17. Little, M.W.; Gibson, M.; Briggs, J.; Speirs, A.; Yoong, P.; Ariyanayagam, T.; Davies, N.; Tayton, E.; Tavares, S.; MacGill, S.; et al. Genicular artEry embolizatioN in patiEnts with oSteoarthrItiS of the Knee (GENESIS) Using Permanent Microspheres: Interim Analysis. *Cardiovasc. Interv. Radiol.* **2021**, *44*, 931–940. [CrossRef]
18. Fernández Martínez, A.M.; Baldi, S.; Alonso-Burgos, A.; López, R.; Vallejo-Pascual, M.E.; Cuesta Marcos, M.T.; Romero Alonso, D.; Rodríguez Prieto, J.; Mauriz, J.L. Mid-Term Results of Transcatheter Arterial Embolization for Adhesive Capsulitis Resistant to Conservative Treatment. *Cardiovasc. Interv. Radiol.* **2021**, *44*, 443–451. [CrossRef]
19. Fearon, A.; Dahlstrom, J.E.; Twin, J.; Cook, J.; Scott, A. The Bonar Score Revisited: Region of Evaluation Significantly Influences the Standardized Assessment of Tendon Degeneration. *J. Sci. Med. Sport* **2014**, *17*, 346–350. [CrossRef]
20. Khan, K.M.; Cook, J.L.; Bonar, F.; Harcourt, P.; Astrom, M. Histopathology of Common Tendinopathies. Update and Implications for Clinical Management. *Sports Med.* **1999**, *27*, 393–408. [CrossRef]
21. Maffulli, N.; Longo, U.G.; Franceschi, F.; Rabitti, C.; Denaro, V. Movin and Bonar Scores Assess the Same Characteristics of Tendon Histology. *Clin. Orthop. Relat. Res.* **2008**, *466*, 1605–1611. [CrossRef] [PubMed]
22. Taguchi, H.; Tanaka, T.; Nishiofuku, H.; Fukuoka, Y.; Minamiguchi, K.; Taiji, R.; Takayama, K.; Takeda, M.; Hatakeyama, K.; Inoue, T.; et al. A Rat Model of Frozen Shoulder Demonstrating the Effect of Transcatheter Arterial Embolization on Angiography, Histopathology, and Physical Activity. *J. Vasc. Interv. Radiol.* **2021**, *32*, 376–383. [CrossRef] [PubMed]
23. Uflacker, A.B.; Keefe, N.; Bruner, E.T.; Avery, A.; Salzar, R.; Henderson, S.; Spratley, M.; Nacey, N.; Miller, W.; Grewal, S.; et al. Assessing the Effects of Geniculate Artery Embolization in a Nonsurgical Animal Model of Osteoarthritis. *J. Vasc. Interv. Radiol.* **2022**, *33*, 1073–1082. [CrossRef]
24. Zabrzyński, J.; Gagat, M.; Łapaj, Ł.; Paczesny, Ł.; Yataganbaba, A.; Szwedowski., D.; Huri, G. Relationship between long head of the biceps tendon histopathology and long-term functional results in smokers. A time to reevaluate the Bonar score? *Ther. Adv. Chronic Dis.* **2021**, *12*, 2040622321990262. [CrossRef]
25. Szwedowski, D.; Jaworski, Ł.; Szwedowska, W.; Pękala, P.; Gagat, M. Neovascularization in Meniscus and Tendon Pathology as a Potential Mechanism in Regenerative Therapies: Special Reference to Platelet-Rich Plasma Treatment. *Appl. Sci.* **2021**, *11*, 8310. [CrossRef]
26. Yamada, K.; Jahangiri, Y.; Li, J.; Gabr, A.; Anoushiravani, A.; Kumagai, K.; Uchida, B.; Farsad, K.; Horikawa, M. Embolic Characteristics of Imipenem-Cilastatin Particles In Vitro and In Vivo: Implications for Transarterial Embolization in Joint Arthropathies. *J. Vasc. Interv. Radiol.* **2021**, *32*, 1031–1039. [CrossRef] [PubMed]
27. Kamisako, A.; Ikoma, A.; Koike, M.; Makitani, K.; Fukuda, K.; Higashino, N.; Shibuya, M.; Okuno, Y.; Minamiguchi, H.; Sonomura, T. Transcatheter arterial embolization of abnormal neovessels in a swine model of knee arthritis. *Knee* **2022**, *36*, 20–26. [CrossRef] [PubMed]

28. Woodhams, R.; Nishimaki, H.; Ogasawara, G.; Fujii, K.; Yamane, T.; Ishida, K.; Kashimi, F.; Matsunaga, K.; Takigawa, M. Imipenem/cilastatin sodium (IPM/CS) as an embolic agent for transcatheter arterial embolisation: A preliminary clinical study of gastrointestinal bleeding from neoplasms. *Springerplus* **2013**, *26*, 344. [CrossRef]
29. Koucheki, R.; Dowling, K.I.; Patel, N.R.; Matsuura, N.; Mafeld, S. Characteristics of Imipenem/Cilastatin: Considerations for Musculoskeletal Embolotherapy. *J. Vasc. Interv. Radiol.* **2021**, *32*, 1040–1043. [CrossRef]

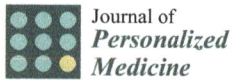

Article

MRI Outcomes Achieved by Simple Flow Blockage Technique in Symptomatic Carotid Artery Stenosis Stenting

Jean-François Hak [1,2,3,*], Caroline Arquizan [4], Federico Cagnazzo [1], Mehdi Mahmoudi [1], Francois-Louis Collemiche [1], Gregory Gascou [1], Pierre-Henry Lefevre [1], Imad Derraz [1], Julien Labreuche [5], Isabelle Mourand [4], Nicolas Gaillard [4], Lucas Corti [4], Mahmoud Charif [4], Vincent Costalat [1] and Cyril Dargazanli [1]

1. Neuroradiology Department, CHRU Gui de Chauliac, Montpellier University Medical Center, 34295 Montpellier, France
2. LIIE, Aix Marseille University, 13005 Marseille, France
3. CERIMED, Aix Marseille University, 13005 Marseille, France
4. Neurology Department, CHRU Gui de Chauliac, Montpellier University Medical Center, 34295 Montpellier, France
5. Biostatistics Department, Centre Hospitalier Universitaire Lille, 59000 Lille, France
* Correspondence: jeanfrancois.hak@gmail.com

Abstract: In this study, we aimed to determine the frequency and clinical impact of new ischemic lesions detected with diffusion-weighted-imaging-MRI (DWI-MRI) as well as the clinical outcomes after carotid artery stenting (CAS) using the simple flow blockage technique (SFB). This is a retrospective study with data extraction from a monocentric prospective clinical registry (from 2017 to 2019) of consecutive patients admitted for symptomatic cervical ICA stenosis or web. Herein, patients benefited from DWI-MRI before and within 48 h of CAS for symptomatic ICA stenosis or web. The primary endpoint was the frequency of new DWI-MRI ischemic lesions and the secondary (composite) endpoint was the rate of mortality, symptomatic stroke or acute coronary syndrome within 30 days of the procedure. All of the 82 CAS procedures were successfully performed. Among the 33 patients (40.2%) with new DWI-MRI ischemic lesions, 30 patients were asymptomatic (90.9%). Irregular carotid plaque surface with ($n = 13$, 44.8%) or without ulceration ($n = 12$, 60.0%) was associated with higher rates of new DWI-MRI lesions by comparison to patients with a regular plaque ($n = 7$, 25%) ($p = 0.048$) using the univariate analysis. Less than half of this CAS cohort using the SFB technique had new ischemic lesions detected with DWI-MRI. Among these patients, more than 90% were asymptomatic. Irregularity of the plaque seems to increase the risk of peri-procedural DWI-MRI lesions.

Keywords: carotid; endovascular; stents; magnetic resonance imaging; diffusion-weighted-imaging

Citation: Hak, J.-F.; Arquizan, C.; Cagnazzo, F.; Mahmoudi, M.; Collemiche, F.-L.; Gascou, G.; Lefevre, P.-H.; Derraz, I.; Labreuche, J.; Mourand, I.; et al. MRI Outcomes Achieved by Simple Flow Blockage Technique in Symptomatic Carotid Artery Stenosis Stenting. J. Pers. Med. 2022, 12, 1564. https://doi.org/10.3390/jpm12101564

Academic Editor: Yoshihiro Noda

Received: 19 July 2022
Accepted: 16 September 2022
Published: 23 September 2022

Publisher's Note: MDPI stays neutral with regard to jurisdictional claims in published maps and institutional affiliations.

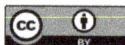

Copyright: © 2022 by the authors. Licensee MDPI, Basel, Switzerland. This article is an open access article distributed under the terms and conditions of the Creative Commons Attribution (CC BY) license (https://creativecommons.org/licenses/by/4.0/).

1. Introduction

Symptomatic carotid stenosis, defined as stenosis of the internal carotid artery (ICA) leading to recent symptoms of amaurosis fugax, transient ischemic attacks or acute ischemic stroke (AIS) ipsilateral to the lesion [1], carries a high risk of early recurrence and stroke and carotid revascularization is recommended [2]. Randomized controlled trials (EVA-3S, SPACE, and ICSS) comparing carotid endarterectomy (CEA) and carotid artery stenting (CAS) have shown a higher periprocedural risk of stroke with CAS than with CEA [3–5]. However, risks of stroke or death in patients younger than 70 years were similar in both treatment groups [6]. Therefore, CAS has been developed during the past two decades to treat symptomatic carotid and is often chosen for anatomic reasons (contralateral occlusion), for patients with high surgical risk (radiation injury, history of prior neck dissection, presence of tracheostomy) or with severe medical comorbidities (high risk for open surgery).

Carotid web (CW) leads to ischemic stroke secondary to blood flow stasis and subsequent embolization. In addition, optimal management strategies for secondary stroke prevention remain unclear. Due to the high stroke recurrence rate in medically managed symptomatic CW patients, carotid revascularization is currently performed, with no periprocedural complications or recurrent strokes in carotid revascularization management with CAS or CEA [7].

Moreover, the recent numerous randomized controlled trials (RCT) established mechanical thrombectomy as the gold standard for the treatment of AIS with large vessel occlusion, with the possibility of emergency carotid stenting in tandem occlusion [8]. This post-thrombectomy era led to an increased number of endovascular treatments of AIS during the past few years. Nevertheless, the current key point is the safety of CAS. During these last years, the technical and medical experience of the operators, as well as new innovative endovascular techniques, devices, and a better management of the antiplatelet therapies could reduce this procedural risk.

Indeed, the embolic protection technique during CAS as proximal balloon occlusion (PBA), and distal filter protection (DFP) can provide similar levels of protection from periprocedural stroke and 30-day mortality [9]. In the dynamic of developing the safest CAS procedure, an innovative approach (simple flow blockage technique [SFB]) was reported as a combination of proximal balloon occlusion and flow blockage, which is inspired from a mechanical thrombectomy technique [10].

Diffusion-weighted-imaging-MRI (DWI-MRI) remains the gold standard to evaluate acute stroke lesions even without any clinical significance. The objective of this study is to report the frequency of new ischemic lesions using DWI-MRI as well as their impact on clinical outcomes after consecutive carotid artery stenting (CAS) is performed with SFB in consecutive patients with AIS (without large vessel occlusion) and symptomatic carotid artery stenosis or carotid web.

2. Materials and Methods

2.1. Study Design

We carried out a retrospective study with data extraction from our prospective clinical registry of consecutive patients admitted for symptomatic ICA atherosclerotic stenosis or carotid web to our Comprehensive Stroke Center (CSC) from January 2017 to September 2019.

This study (reference study RECHMPL 18 0236, No. ID-RCB: 2018-A02651-54) was approved by a local ethics committee (Comité de Protection des Personnes (CPP) SUD-MEDITERRANEE III, UFR MEDECINE 186, chemin du Carreau de Lanes CS 83021 30908 NIMES Cedex 2), and registered on clinicaltrials.gov (NCT04421326).

In the context of carotid stenting using the simple flow blockage technique, we previously reported data from January 2015 to 2018 in 75 patients, focusing on the angiographic pattern [10]. In this previous study, only 40 patients (53.3% of the cohort) benefited from a MRI follow-up [10].

For this current study, focusing on a routine MRI protocol follow-up implemented in our center since January 2017 for CAS, we included 15 patients who were already analyzed in the previous study (from year 2017).

2.2. Inclusion Criteria

Consecutive patients were included if they fulfilled the following criteria: (I) AIS (hemispheric or retinal TIA), cerebral infarct in the anterior circulation without large vessel intracranial occlusion <3 months before admission; (II) pre-procedural (<1 month) brain DWI-MRI (diffusion-weighted-imaging-MRI) showing cytotoxic lesions of AIS and/or perfusion-MRI showing brain hypoperfusion; (III) ipsilateral atheromatous internal carotid artery stenosis >50% or carotid web. The diagnosis of carotid stenosis or web was performed on noninvasive imaging (CT and/or MRI); (IV) CAS for ICA atheromatous stenosis ≤50% was retained in the case of plaque instability as demonstrated by an intraplaque hemorrhage on dedicated black-blood MRI; (V) post-procedural (<48 h) brain DWI-MRI. The decision of endovascular treatment was retained after a multidisciplinary team meeting.

The exclusion criteria were: (1) Patients with intracranial large vessel occlusion; (2) patients with pre-stroke dependency defined as a modified Rankin score > 2; (3) patients with severe or fatal co-morbidities or life expectancy under 6 months; (4) patients treated endovascularly using a DFP device; and (5) patients with carotid artery stenosis at the acute phase of ischemic stroke caused by tandem occlusion.

2.3. Patient Management

2.3.1. Medical Management

All patients were hospitalized in the CSC for maintenance of hemodynamic function (objective of systolic blood pressure > 120 mmHg), and close monitoring of any neurological worsening. Anticoagulants and/or aspirin was left to the discretion of the stroke neurologist.

Clopidogrel (75 mg daily) was given within the days before CAS, with an assessment of platelet inhibition (PRU, Platelet Reactive Units) (VerifyNow, Instrumentation Laboratory, San Diego, CA, USA) before the procedure.

In cases of clopidogrel resistance (230–240 P2Y12 reaction units PRU by the VerifyNow P2Y12 assay or platelet inhibition rate < 20%) [10], prasugrel (20 mg) was given the day before the intervention and platelet inhibition was tested again before the procedure.

All patients had subsequently 3 months of dual antiplatelet medication (aspiring 75 mg), then lifelong aspirin.

In cases of emergency stenting for hemodynamic symptoms or early recurrence, a loading dose of platelet inhibitor (300 mg of clopidogrel or 20 mg of prasugrel) was administered and platelet inhibition was then assessed.

All procedures were performed via a femoral artery approach, and 150 IU/kg heparin was administered intravenously after the placement of the 9-French balloon guiding catheter (Concentric medical, Mountain View, CA, USA) into the targeted common carotid artery. The balloon guiding catheter was prepared according to the instructions provided by the manufacturer, using a combination of contrast agent with saline (50% by volume) to prepare balloon inflation media.

Atropine (0.01–0.02 mg/kg) was administered intravenously at the time of angioplasty, which was performed using a 4.0–7.0 mm balloon (Ultra-soft SV monorail balloon, Boston Scientific, Marlborough, MA, USA).

2.3.2. Simple Flow Blockage (SFB) Technique

All procedures were performed under conscious sedation by experienced interventional neuroradiologists. A baseline angiographic run was performed after the inflation of the balloon guiding catheter in the common carotid artery, and was allowed to determine the different angiographic patterns [10].

In all cases, flushing of the guiding catheter was temporarily interrupted during the critical steps (crossing of culprit lesions, stent deployment, angioplasty) to avoid antegrade embolization.

After a dangerous maneuver (crossing of culprit lesions, stent deployment, angioplasty), two steps were respected: (1) Pump aspiration (Penumbra, Alameda, CA, USA) set on the recommended vacuum pressure of −25.5 inches Hg (−86.4 kPa) via a rotating hemostatic valve (RHV) for approximately 10 s before balloon deflation, to avoid potential embolization from the stagnating column of blood distal to the balloon or from the guiding catheter itself; and (2) after balloon deflation, the RHV is opened for a few seconds and closed progressively during activation of the flushing line, to assure that the RHV is clean (aspiration is performed through it in prevention of the accumulated debris inside the RHV).

A DFP device was not used during any procedures in this study. The type of stent and the use of pre-dilation and post-dilation by balloon angioplasty were performed according to neurointerventionalists' discretion.

Balloon angioplasty was not performed for web cases.

2.3.3. Follow-Up and Outcome

All patients were hospitalized in the CSC for at least 24 h following the intervention, with strict blood pressure monitoring and management (target level of <140/90 mmHg) and close monitoring of any neurological worsening.

Patients with preprocedural severe stenosis (>90%), severe contralateral stenosis or occlusion, or with periprocedural arterial hypertension were considered at high risk of reperfusion syndrome, leading to a stricter blood pressure monitoring and management with a target level of <120/80 mmHg. Patients were treated after the procedure with clopidogrel (75 mg daily) or with prasugrel (10 mg daily) in the case of clopidogrel resistance (in the absence of contraindication). This treatment was delayed by 6 to 24 h for patients treated with intravenous thrombolysis.

A post-procedural (<48 h) follow-up cerebral MRI was systematically performed after stenting.

Patients were discharged 48–72 h post-treatment, after a comprehensive neurological evaluation.

The primary endpoint was the retrospective assessment of new ischemic lesions detected by DWI-MRI by two neurointerventionalists (JFH and CD) blinded to the clinical outcomes and the procedure success (defined as the ability to successfully implant a carotid stent with <30% residual stenosis). The secondary (composite) endpoint was the rate of mortality, symptomatic stroke or acute coronary syndrome within 30 days of the procedure.

The new symptomatic stroke was defined as a neurological deficit, as explained by a new ischemic lesion on DWI.

2.4. MRI Evaluation

MRI scans were performed using a Siemens Avanto 1.5 T.

On the 1.5 T scanner, the sequence parameters were: TR = 24 ms, TE = 6.00 ms, flip angle = 90.3 directions of measurement, 16 cm FOV, 131 × 131 matrix, and 5 mm section thickness. Twelve-channel head coils were used. Foci of diffusion were measured in the longest axial axis. DWI b-value was b = 1000 for all studies. All patients were scanned with the same protocol before CAS and within the 48-h following the CAS procedure.

2.5. Data Collection

Patient's characteristics, imaging data, treatment, and follow-up were prospectively collected at the CSC: (a) Clinical data: Age, gender, medication, and vascular risk factors (hypertension, hypercholesterolemia, diabetes, current smoking); (b) imaging data: Type of initial arterial imaging (MRA, CTA; type of carotid stenosis: Degree of stenosis, web, plaque surface characteristics (ulcerated, irregular)).

Pre- and post-procedural (<48 h) DWI-MRI (diffusion-weighted-MRI) were performed for all patients.

Data supplemental to the main text regarding data collection, patients' management (medical management and SFB technique, follow-up, and outcome) can be found in Appendix A.

2.6. Statistical Analysis

Categorical variables were expressed as frequencies and percentages and continuous as mean (standard deviation) or median (interquartile range, IQR) in the case of non-normal distribution. Normality of distribution was assessed graphically and using the Shapiro-Wilk test. Rates of outcomes were estimated by calculating exact binomial 95% confidence intervals (CIs). Bivariate comparisons in main ICA lesions and treatment characteristics between patients with and without new cerebral lesions at DWI-MRI were conducted using the Chi-Square test (or Fisher's exact test when the expected cell frequency was <5) for categorical variables, and Mann-Whitney U test for continuous variables as appropriate. Statistical testing was conducted at the two-tailed α-level of 0.05. Data were analyzed using the SAS software package, release 9.4 (SAS Institute, Cary, NC, USA).

3. Results

3.1. Patient Characteristics and Angiographic Patterns

From January 2017 to September 2019, 82 patients with symptomatic carotid artery atherosclerotic stenosis ($n = 78$) or symptomatic web ($n = 4$) were treated by CAS using the SFB technique in our CSC and benefited from a DWI-MRI before and within 48 h of the stenting procedure (see flowchart; Figure 1). Patient and treatment characteristics are reported in Table 1. Overall, the median age was 68 years (IQR, 59 to 75), 37 patients (45.1%) were men. Baseline median NIHSS was 5.6 (IQR, 1 to 18). CAS was performed after a median time from symptom of 7 days (IQR, 3 to 30 days). Among the 78 patients with atherosclerotic stenosis (95.1%), the median degree of carotid stenosis was 75% (IQR, 70 to 90), ulcerations were present in 63.7% of cases.

Table 1. Patient and treatment characteristics of the 82 included patients with symptomatic carotid stenosis >50% or symptomatic web treated by CAS using SFB.

Characteristics	n	Values
Demographics		
Age (years), median (IQR)	82	68 (59 to 75)
Men	82	37 (45.1)
Medical history		
Hypertension	82	67 (81.7)
Diabetes mellitus	82	33 (40.2)
Dyslipidemia	82	47 (57.3)
Current smoking	82	45 (54.9)
Long-term antithrombotic use	82	26 (31.7)
Lesion characteristics		
Location of lesion	82	
Right ICA		47 (57.3)
Left ICA		34 (41.5)
Bilateral ICA		1 (1.2)
Degree of carotid stenosis, %, median (IQR)	78	75 (70 to 90)
0 to 49 (including web)		6 (7.7)
50 to 69		13 (16.7)
70 to 99		59 (75.6)
Etiology		
Atherosclerosis	82	78 (95.1)
Web		4 (4.9)
Carotid plaque surface characteristics		
Regular	77	28 (36.4)
Irregular without ulceration		20 (26.0)
Irregular with ulceration		29 (37.7)
Angiographic Pattern		
Pattern 1	82	28 (34.3)
Pattern 2		27 (32.9)
Pattern 3		27 (32.9)
Treatment characteristics		
Onset to endovascular procedure, days, median (IQR)	82	7 (3 to 30)
Duration of endovascular procedure, minutes, median (IQR)	82	35 (25 to 45)
Type of stent [1]		
Casper (Microvention, Aliso Viejo, CA, USA)	95	21 (22.1)
Xact (Abbott Vascular, Santa Clara, CA, USA)		56 (59.6)
Precise (Cordis, Milpitas, CA, USA)		18 (18.9)

[1]: Two patients with three stents (one with three Precise and one with three Xact), and nine patients with two stents (six with Xact and Precise, two with Casper and Xact, and one with Precise). Pattern 1: No anterograde flow; Pattern 2: Wash-out of the internal carotid artery by the external carotid artery; Pattern 3: Retrograde wash-out of the internal carotid artery by the intracranial circulation. Abbreviations: CAS: Carotid artery stenting; ICA: Internal carotid artery; IQR: Interquartile range; SFB: Simple flow blockage.

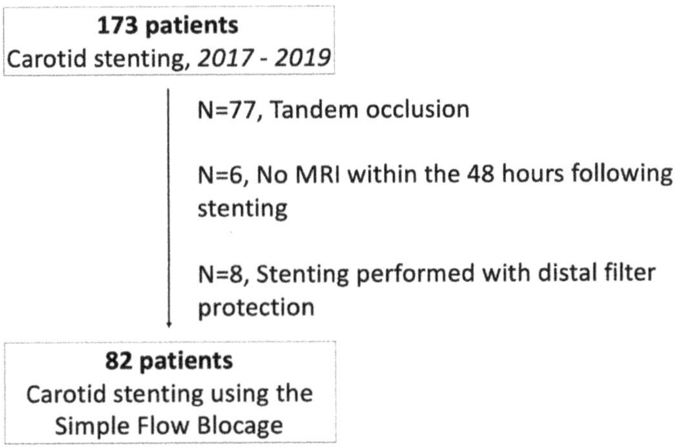

```
173 patients
Carotid stenting, 2017 - 2019
```
　　　　　　　　N=77, Tandem occlusion

　　　　　　　　N=6, No MRI within the 48 hours following stenting

　　　　　　　　N=8, Stenting performed with distal filter protection

```
82 patients
Carotid stenting using the
Simple Flow Blocage
```

Figure 1. Flow-Chart.

No resistance to clopidogrel was observed in this cohort.

Complete stagnation of the contrast column in the ICA (angiographic pattern 1) was observed in 28 patients (34.1%), retrograde wash-out of the internal carotid artery from the intracranial circulation toward the external carotid artery (pattern 2) in 27 patients (32.9%), and antegrade wash-out of contrast toward the intracranial circulation, via the external carotid artery or from the common carotid artery (pattern 3) was observed in the remaining 27 cases (32.9%). CAS was performed using Casper (Carotid Artery Stent designed to Prevent Embolic Release, MicroVention Inc., Tustin, CA, USA) (n = 18), Xact (Abbott Vascular, Abbott Park, IL, USA) (n = 53) or Precise (Cordis, Warren, NJ, USA) (n = 17) stents with a median procedure time of 35 min (IQR, 24 to 45 min). For 11 patients, two or three stents were used (see footnote of Table 1). All the CAS procedures were successfully achieved.

3.2. Clinical and DWI Outcomes

Within the 48 h after CAS, a total of 177 new cerebral lesions (134 punctiform lesions, 32 lesions $\leq$ 10 mm and 11 lesions > 10 mm) were detected by DWI-MRI in 33 patients (40.2%, 95%CI: 29.5 to 51.7%, Table 2). Thirty-one patients (37.8%) had at least one punctiform lesion, thirty-one (37.8%) had at least one ipsilateral lesion, and seven (8.5%) had at least one lesion > 10 mm.

Eight patients (9.8%) had contralateral lesions. Among these 33 patients, the baseline median NIHSS was 7.2 (IQR, 1 to 18). Thirty patients (36.6%) had new ischemic DWI-MRI lesions without new neurological symptoms or modification of the NIHSS during periprocedural follow-up. An example of the new punctiform ischemic DWI-MRI lesions is provided in Appendix B Figure A1.

Three patients had symptomatic ischemic strokes with NIHSS degradation in two patients (respectively from NIHSS 6 and 7 to NIHSS 10 to 9) and death from the reperfusion syndrome in one patient. The latter was known with history of hypertension and hypercholesterolemia, and presented with a symptomatic 75% left ICA stenosis. Baseline NIHSS was 18 and DWI-MRI showed no initial ischemic lesions and no intracranial large vessel occlusion. The CAS procedure was successfully performed 1 day from symptoms onset, but the patient presented pre-procedural hypertension leading to strict blood pressure monitoring after the CAS with a target level of <120/80 mmHg. The DWI-MRI performed 25 h from the CAS revealed symptomatic new cerebral lesions (punctiform and >10 mm) both in the ipsilateral and contralateral side without large intracranial vessel occlusion. Dual antiplatelet medication was continued. A neurologic deterioration occurred, and the 30-h CT revealed an intraparenchymal hemorrhage corresponding to a reperfusion syndrome. The patient died 34 h after the CAS (see Appendix B Figure A2).

Table 2. DWI-MRI new lesions and clinical outcomes in 82 patients with symptomatic carotid stenosis >50% or symptomatic web treated by CAS using SFB.

Outcomes	n (%)	95%CI
DWI-MRI new lesions		
Patients with ≥ 1 lesions	33 (40.2)	29.5 to 51.7
Single	11 (13.4)	
Multiple	22 (26.8)	
Patients with punctiform lesions	31 (37.8)	27.3 to 49.2
Patients with ipsilateral lesions	31 (37.8)	27.3 to 49.2
Patients with contralateral lesions	8 (9.8)	4.3 to 18.3
Patients with lesions > 10 mm	7 (8.5)	3.5 to 16.8
Clinical outcomes		
Composite endpoint at 30 days of intervention	3 (3.7)	1.3 to 12.0
Death	1 (1.2)	
Acute coronary syndrome	0 (0.0)	
Symptomatic ischemic stroke	3 (3.7)	
≥1 Bleeding event	1 (1.2)	
≥1 procedural complications	3 (3.7)	1.3 to 12.0
Cerebral emboli	3 (3.7)	
Groin hematoma	0 (0.0)	
Dissection	0 (0.0)	

No acute coronary syndrome was observed. Overall, the 30-day composite endpoint occurred in three patients (3.7%).

Association of ICA lesion and treatment characteristics with the presence of ≥1 new DWI-MRI lesions are reported in Table 3. Only carotid plaque surface characteristics were significantly associated with the presence of ≥1 new cerebral lesions; patients with irregular plaque with (n = 13, 44.8%) or without ulceration (n = 12, 60.0%) had a higher rate of new cerebral lesions by comparison to patients with regular plaque (n = 7, 25%) (p = 0.048).

Table 3. Comparisons of ICA lesion and treatment characteristics between patients with and without new cerebral lesions detected by DWI-MRI.

	No DWI-MRI Lesions (n = 49)	≥1 DWI-MRI Lesions (n = 33)	p-Value
ICA lesion characteristics			
Stenosis degree, %			
0 to 49	2 (4.4)	4 (12.1)	0.41
50 to 69	7 (15.6)	6 (18.2)	
70 to 99	36 (80.0)	23 (69.7)	
Carotid plaque surface			
Regular	21 (46.7)	7 (21.9)	0.048
Irregular without ulceration	8 (17.8)	12 (37.5)	
Irregular with ulceration	16 (35.6)	13 (40.6)	
Angiographic Pattern			
Pattern 1	18 (40.0)	8 (25.8)	0.30
Pattern 2	15 (33.3)	10 (32.3)	
Pattern 3	12 (26.7)	13 (41.9)	
Treatment characteristics			
Number of stents			
One	43 (87.8)	28 (84.9)	0.75
Two or three	6 (12.2)	5 (15.2)	
Duration of endovascular procedure, minutes, median (IQR)	38 (30 to 45)	29 (24 to 45)	0.17
Delay from symptoms onset to endovascular procedure, days, median (IQR)	11 (3 to 30)	5 (0.8 to 31)	0.17

Values are % (n) unless otherwise as indicated. Abbreviations: DWI-MRI: Diffusion-weighted-imaging-magnetic resonance imaging; ICA: Internal carotid artery; IQR: Interquartile range.

4. Discussion

In this large cohort of 82 consecutive patients with symptomatic severe carotid stenosis or carotid web treated with a standardized procedure of stenting using the SFB technique, less than half of this CAS cohort had new ischemic lesions detected with DWI-MRI (n = 33; 40.2%), asymptomatic in 30 patients (90.9%). Three (3.7%) patients had a newly onset symptomatic ischemic stroke and one (1.2%) had a transient focal neurological deficit. Among the patients with newly onset symptomatic ischemic stroke, one patient (1.2%) experienced reperfusion syndrome.

Both CEA and CAS are known to have increased periprocedural complications in symptomatic patients. However, the risk-benefit balance tilts in favor of treatment, both with CAE [1] and CAS [11].

In a meta-analysis of three RCT (EVA-3S, SPACE, and ICSS), any stroke or death occurred significantly more often in the CAS group compared to the CEA group. Nevertheless, an analysis of individual patient data showed that risk with CAS was twice the risk of CEA in patients greater than age 70 but was the same under 70 [6]. In the same line, the risk for stroke, acute coronary syndrome or death with CAS significantly increased with age according to the CREST investigators [12].

The CREST [13,14] demonstrated equivalent composite outcomes (stroke, myocardial infarction, death) between CEA and CAS. However, the subgroup analysis suggested an increased risk of stroke with CAS. Similarly, a recent meta-analysis (Carotid Artery Stenting Versus Endarterectomy for Stroke Prevention: A Meta-Analysis of Clinical Trials) confirmed these findings [15].

However, over the past two decades, embolic protection devices emerged for CAS and allowed progressive improvements in terms of stroke and mortality rates [16].

More recently, and in contrast to the findings of CREST, Cole et al. suggested that 378,354 patients undergoing CEA had a higher rate of perioperative stroke than 57,273 patients undergoing CAS, primarily among symptomatic patients (8.1% versus 5.6%; odds ratio, 1.47 [CI: 1.29–1.68]; $p < 0.001$) [17].

Current guidelines advise proceeding with CEA for symptomatic carotid only if the surgeon's rate for perioperative stroke or death is <6% [2,18]. In our cohort, perioperative stroke or death occurred for 3.7%, suggesting that progress of CAS, especially using the SFB technique, led to a very attractive approach for symptomatic carotid stenosis.

4.1. DWI Lesions

Clinical series [19] and systematic review [20] showed that patients treated by CAS have about three times more new ischemic lesions on DWI-MRI compared to the CAE group, respectively 37% and 50% in the CAS group, and 10% and 17% in the CAE group ($p < 0.01$).

However, the main weakness of these results is the heterogeneity in the use of the protective device, as well as differences in the used material (balloon, DFP).

Interestingly, in the ICSS-MRI sub-study, Gensicke et al. found that there was no significant difference in total lesion volume per patient between the CAS and CEA groups in the entire study population ($p = 0.18$). Among these patients with silent ischemic DWI-MRI lesions after treatment (CAS, $n = 62$ patients; CEA, $n = 18$), volumes of separate lesions were significantly smaller in the CAS group (median volume, 0.02 mL) than the CEA group (0.08 mL; $p < 0.0001$) [21].

In addition, it is known that a routine diagnostic angiography induces silent ischemic lesions. Bendszus et al. showed that 44% of patients with vasculopathy who benefited from a routine diagnostic angiography had silent embolisms compared to a group without vascular risk factors (13%) [22]. Accordingly, the 40% rate of patients experiencing DWI-MRI lesions after CAS in our cohort is comparable to what was reported in the literature.

4.2. Irregular/Ulcerated Stenosis and Degree of Stenosis

Our study suggests that plaque surface characteristics were significantly associated with the presence of ≥1 new DWI cerebral lesions. Indeed, patients with irregular plaque with ($n = 13$, 44.8%) or without ulceration ($n = 12$, 60.0%) had a higher rate of new cerebral lesions in comparison to patients with regular plaque ($n = 7$, 25%) (Table 3).

This is in accordance with other studies suggesting that the irregular plaque surface was associated with increased incidence of carotid stenting-associated ischemic lesions [23,24].

Exploratory analyses from EVA-3S [3,25], SPACE [26], and ICSS [27] cohorts did not show any significant association between the degree of stenosis and stroke after CAS or CAE with a 70% stenosis [26,27] or a 90% stenosis cut-off [3,25]. Interestingly, the ICSS cohort [27] evaluated fatal or disabling strokes of 3.9% and 6.7% after CAS and 9.6% and 6.2% after CAE, respectively, for an ipsilateral stenosis of 50–69% and 70–99% ($p = 0.155$).

According to our results using SFB and to the literature, the most important point associated with peri-procedural stroke in patients with stenosis > 50% may be the irregularity and not the severity of the stenosis after CAS.

4.3. Timing of Angioplasty

It is interesting to note that the delay from AIS onset and treatment with CAS was not associated with an increased risk of peri-procedural DWI-MRI lesions. Current guidelines are to pursue early revascularization within 14 days of AIS [2]. Due to the increasing risk of recurrence within the first 2 weeks after the first ischemic event of a symptomatic carotid stenosis, Liu et al. showed improved functional outcomes without increasing the rate of new AIS, myocardial infarction or death in the early CAS group (<1 week) compared to the delayed CAS at 1 month [28]. On the contrary, Song et al. evaluated CAS for 206 patients with moderate-to-severe stenosis and found a significantly higher rate of ipsilateral stroke or death (at 30 days) of 12.8% in the early CAS group (within 14 days) compared to only 0.8% in the delayed CAS group (mean timing of CAS was 52.6 ± 36.94 days) [29]. However, this finding did not extend beyond the 30-day follow-up period (31 days to 1 year), wherein there was no significant difference between groups. A post-hoc analysis with the CREST population did not find any relationship between timing and significant adverse events in the 583 patients in the CAS group [30], and this was in agreement to what we found in our study (Table 3).

Transcarotid artery revascularization (TCAR) with flow reversal was developed to mitigate the maneuvers at highest risk for causing stroke during transfemoral CAS.

Comparing TCAR to CEA across different age groups showed no significant differences in outcomes [31,32].

In comparison to transfemoral CAS for patients ≥ 80 years, TCAR was associated with a reduction in stroke risk, reduction in risk of stroke/death, and reduction in the risk of stroke/death/myocardial infarction of respectively 72%, 65%, and 76% [31,32]. However, these results must be set against the advances in the experience of interventional practitioners and their equipment, in particular the famous balloon-guiding-catheters. In addition, aspiration is now possible with mechanical thrombectomy devices and confirms the need to repeat randomized studies.

4.4. Study Limitations

There are several limitations in the current study. The number of patients in our analysis was relatively small and there was no CAE group for comparison.

Moreover, this study only focused on patients who benefited from a DWI-MRI before and within the 48-h following a CAS procedure.

However, this current CAS cohort only included symptomatic patients with symptomatic carotid stenosis or web which carries higher risk than asymptomatic carotid, with a known tendency for more silent ischemic lesions after CAS, suggesting that patients with symptomatic carotid had an increased micro-embolic risk during the CAS procedure [24].

5. Conclusions

In this study, less than half of the CAS cohort using the SFB technique had new ischemic lesions detected with DWI-MRI. Among these patients, more than 90% were asymptomatic. As a result, irregularity of the plaque seems to increase the risk of peri-procedural DWI-MRI lesions.

Author Contributions: Conceptualization, J.-F.H., C.A., F.C. and C.D.; methodology, J.-F.H., V.C. and C.D.; software, J.-F.H. and C.D.; validation, J.-F.H., C.A., V.C. and C.D.; formal analysis, J.-F.H. and C.D.; investigation, J.-F.H., M.M., F.-L.C. and C.D.; resources, V.C.; data curation, J.-F.H., C.A., F.C., M.M., F.-L.C., G.G., P.-H.L., I.D., J.L., I.M., N.G., L.C., M.C., V.C. and C.D.; writing—original draft preparation, J.-F.H., C.A. and C.D.; writing—review and editing, J.-F.H., C.A., F.C., M.M., F.-L.C., G.G., P.-H.L., I.D., J.L., I.M., N.G., L.C., M.C., V.C. and C.D.; visualization, J.-F.H., C.A. and C.D.; supervision, V.C. and C.D.; project administration, V.C. and C.D.; funding acquisition, V.C. All authors have read and agreed to the published version of the manuscript.

Funding: This research received no external funding.

Institutional Review Board Statement: The local ethics committee approved the use of patient data for this retrospective analysis.

Informed Consent Statement: Informed consent was obtained from all subjects involved in the study.

Data Availability Statement: The data presented in this study are available on request from the corresponding author.

Conflicts of Interest: The authors declare no conflict of interest.

Appendix A.

Appendix A.1. Data Collection

On the 1.5 T scanner, the sequence parameters were: TR = 24 ms, TE = 6.00 ms, flip angle = 90.3 directions of measurement, 16 cm FOV, 131 × 131 matrix, and 5 mm section thickness. Twelve-channel head coils were used. Foci of diffusion were measured in the longest axial axis. DWI b-value was b = 1000 for all studies.

Appendix A.2. Patients' Management

Appendix A.2.1. Medical Management and Simple Flow Blockage Technique (SFB)

Clopidogrel (75 mg daily) was given within the days before CAS, with assessment of platelet inhibition (PRU, Platelet Reactive Units) (VerifyNow, Instrumentation Laboratory, San Diego, CA, USA) before the procedure.

In cases of clopidogrel resistance (230–240 P2Y12 reaction units PRU by the VerifyNow P2Y12 assay or platelet inhibition rate <20%), prasugrel (20 mg) was given the day before the intervention and platelet inhibition was tested again before the procedure.

All patients had subsequently 3 months of dual antiplatelet medication (aspiring 75 mg), then lifelong aspirin.

In cases of emergency stenting for hemodynamic symptoms or early recurrence, a loading dose of platelet inhibitor (300 mg of clopidogrel or 20 mg of prasugrel) was administered and platelet inhibition was then assessed.

All procedures were performed via a femoral artery approach, and 150 IU/kg heparin was administered intravenously after the placement of the 9-French balloon guiding catheter (Concentric medical, Mountain View, CA, USA) into the targeted common carotid artery. The balloon guiding catheter was prepared according to the instructions provided by the manufacturer, using a combination of contrast agent with saline (50% by volume) to prepare balloon inflation media.

Atropine (0.01–0.02 mg/kg) was administered intravenously at the time of angioplasty, which was performed using a 4.0–7.0 mm balloon (Ultra-soft SV monorail balloon, Boston Scientific, Marlborough, MA, USA).

All procedures were performed under conscious sedation by experienced interventional neuroradiologists. A baseline angiographic run was performed after the inflation of the balloon guiding catheter in the common carotid artery, and allowed to determine the different angiographic patterns.

In all cases, flushing of the guiding catheter was temporarily interrupted during the critical steps (crossing of culprit lesions, stent deployment, angioplasty) to avoid antegrade embolization.

After a dangerous maneuver (crossing of culprit lesions, stent deployment, angioplasty), two steps were respected: (1) Pump aspiration (Penumbra, Alameda, CA, USA) set on the recommended vacuum pressure of −25.5 inches Hg (−86.4 kPa) via a rotating hemostatic valve (RHV) for approximately 10 s before balloon deflation, to avoid potential embolization from the stagnating column of blood distal to the balloon or from the guiding catheter itself; and (2) after balloon deflation, the RHV is opened for a few seconds and closed progressively during activation of the flushing line, to assure that the RHV is clean (aspiration is performed through it in prevention of accumulated debris inside the RHV).

Appendix A.2.2. Follow-Up and Outcome

Patients with preprocedural severe stenosis (>90%), severe contralateral stenosis or occlusion, or with periprocedural arterial hypertension were considered at high risk of reperfusion syndrome, leading to a stricter blood pressure monitoring and management with a target level of <120/80 mmHg. Patients were treated after the procedure with clopidogrel (75 mg daily) or prasugrel (10 mg daily) in the case of clopidogrel resistance (in the absence of contraindication). This treatment was delayed by 6 to 24 h for patients treated with intravenous thrombolysis.

Appendix B.

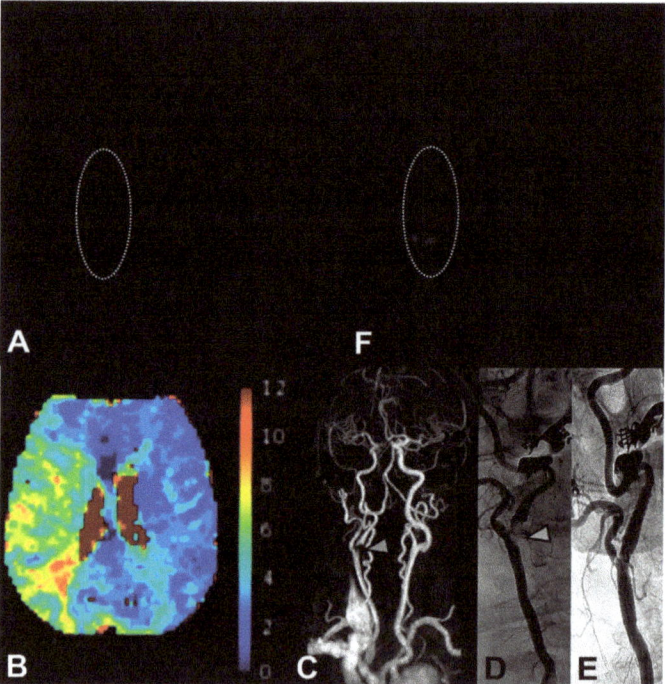

Figure A1. Example of new punctiform ischemic DWI-MRI lesions for a patient with fluctuant left-sided hemiparesis. Initial MRI (5 h from onset) did not find any intracranial large vessel occlusion, but DWI-MRI depicted punctiform ischemic lesions in the right anterior junctional area. (**A**) Perfusion MRI showed a large right sylvian hypoperfusion (TMax > 6 s). (**B**) MR-angiography of supra-aortic arteries objectified a severe proximal ICA stenosis (**C**; white arrow) confirmed by DSA performed (130 h after onset) before (**D**; white arrow) a successful carotid artery stenting (**E**). DWI-MRI performed 24 h after CAS objectified new silent punctiform DWI-MRI lesions in the same right anterior junctional area (**F**).

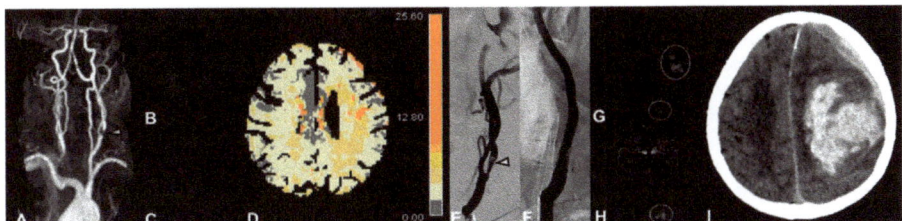

Figure A2. This patient presented right hemiparesis with a symptomatic 75% left ICA stenosis confirmed with angio-MR (**A**) without any ischemic brain lesions on the DWI-MRI performed 8 h from symptom onset (**B,C**), but perfusion MRI showed left sylvian hypoperfusion (TMax > 6 s) (**D**). Carotid artery stenting performed 1 day after symptom onset confirmed the ICA stenosis (**E**) and the stenting was successfully performed (**F**). However, the patient presented pre-procedural hypertension involving strict blood pressure monitoring after the CAS with a target level of <120/80 mmHg. The DWI-MRI performed 25 h from the CAS revealed symptomatic new cerebral lesions (punctiform and >10 mm) in the ipsilateral side (**G,H**) without large intracranial vessel occlusion. Dual antiplatelet medication was continued. However, the 30-h CT performed for a neurologic deterioration revealed an intraparenchymal hemorrhage (**I**) corresponding to a reperfusion syndrome.

References

1. North American Symptomatic Carotid Endarterectomy Trial Collaborators. Beneficial Effect of Carotid Endarterectomy in Symptomatic Patients with High-Grade Carotid Stenosis. *N. Engl. J. Med.* **1991**, *325*, 445–453. [CrossRef] [PubMed]
2. Kernan, W.N.; Ovbiagele, B.; Black, H.R.; Bravata, D.M.; Chimowitz, M.I.; Ezekowitz, M.D.; Fang, M.C.; Fisher, M.; Furie, K.L.; Heck, D.V.; et al. Guidelines for the Prevention of Stroke in Patients With Stroke and Transient Ischemic Attack: A Guideline for Healthcare Professionals From the American Heart Association/American Stroke Association. *Stroke* **2014**, *45*, 2160–2236. [CrossRef]
3. Mas, J.-L.; Chatellier, G.; Beyssen, B.; Branchereau, A.; Moulin, T.; Becquemin, J.-P.; Larrue, V.; Lièvre, M.; Leys, D.; Bonneville, J.-F.; et al. Endarterectomy versus Stenting in Patients with Symptomatic Severe Carotid Stenosis. *N. Engl. J. Med.* **2006**, *355*, 1660–1671. [CrossRef] [PubMed]
4. Ringleb, A.P.; Allenberg, J.R.; Bruckmann, H.; Eckstein, H.H.; Fraedrich, G.; Hartmann, M.; Hennerici, M.G.; Jansen, O.; Klein, E.G.; Kunze, A.; et al. 30 day results from the SPACE trial of stent-protected angioplasty versus carotid endarterectomy in symptomatic patients: A randomised non-inferiority trial. *Lancet* **2006**, *368*, 1239–1247. [CrossRef]
5. International Carotid Stenting Study investigators; Ederle, J.; Dobson, J.; Featherstone, R.L.; Bonati, L.H.; Van Der Worp, H.B.; De Borst, G.J.; Lo, T.H.; Gaines, P.; Dorman, P.J.; et al. Carotid artery stenting compared with endarterectomy in patients with symptomatic carotid stenosis (International Carotid Stenting Study): An interim analysis of a randomised controlled trial. *Lancet* **2010**, *375*, 985–997. [CrossRef] [PubMed]
6. Carotid Stenting Trialists' Collaboration; Bonati, L.H.; Dobson, J.; Algra, A.; Branchereau, A.; Chatellier, G.; Fraedrich, G.; Mali, W.P.; Zeumer, H.; Brown, M.M.; et al. Short-term outcome after stenting versus endarterectomy for symptomatic carotid stenosis: A preplanned meta-analysis of individual patient data. *Lancet* **2010**, *376*, 1062–1073. [CrossRef]
7. Haussen, D.C.; Grossberg, J.A.; Bouslama, M.; Pradilla, G.; Belagaje, S.; Bianchi, N.; Allen, J.W.; Frankel, M.; Nogueira, R.G. Carotid Web (Intimal Fibromuscular Dysplasia) Has High Stroke Recurrence Risk and Is Amenable to Stenting. *Stroke* **2017**, *48*, 3134–3137. [CrossRef]
8. Sivan-Hoffmann, R.; Gory, B.; Armoiry, X.; Goyal, M.; Riva, R.; Lab, C.; Lukaszewicz, A.-C.; Lehot, J.-J.; Derex, L.; Turjman, F. Stent-Retriever Thrombectomy for Acute Anterior Ischemic Stroke with Tandem Occlusion: A Systematic Review and Meta-Analysis. *Eur. Radiol.* **2016**, *27*, 247–254. [CrossRef]
9. Omran, J.; Mahmud, E.; White, C.; Aronow, H.D.; Drachman, D.E.; Gray, W.; Abdullah, O.; Abu-Fadel, M.; Firwana, B.; Mishkel, G.; et al. Proximal balloon occlusion versus distal filter protection in carotid artery stenting: A meta-analysis and review of the literature. *Catheter. Cardiovasc. Interv.* **2016**, *89*, 923–931. [CrossRef]
10. Dargazanli, C.; Mahmoudi, M.; Cappucci, M.; Collemiche, F.-L.; Labreuche, J.; Habza, O.; Gascou, G.; Lefèvre, P.-H.; Eker, O.; Mourand, I.; et al. Angiographic Patterns and Outcomes Achieved by Proximal Balloon Occlusion in Symptomatic Carotid Artery Stenosis Stenting. *Clin. Neuroradiol.* **2019**, *30*, 363–372. [CrossRef]
11. Dietz, A.; Berkefeld, J.; Theron, J.G.; Schmitz-Rixen, T.; Zanella, F.E.; Turowski, B.; Steinmetz, H.; Sitzer, M. Endovascular Treatment of Symptomatic Carotid Stenosis Using Stent Placement. *Stroke* **2001**, *32*, 1855–1859. [CrossRef] [PubMed]
12. Voeks, J.H.; Howard, G.; Roubin, G.S.; Malas, M.B.; Cohen, D.J.; Sternbergh, I.W.C.; Aronow, H.D.; Eskandari, M.K.; Sheffet, A.J.; Lal, B.K.; et al. Age and Outcomes After Carotid Stenting and Endarterectomy. *Stroke* **2011**, *42*, 3484–3490. [CrossRef]

13. Brott, T.G.; Hobson, R.W.; Howard, G.; Roubin, G.S.; Clark, W.M.; Brooks, W.; Mackey, A.; Hill, M.D.; Leimgruber, P.P.; Sheffet, A.J.; et al. Stenting versus Endarterectomy for Treatment of Carotid-Artery Stenosis. *N. Engl. J. Med.* **2010**, *363*, 11–23. [CrossRef]
14. Brott, T.G.; Howard, G.; Roubin, G.S.; Meschia, J.F.; Mackey, A.; Brooks, W.; Moore, W.S.; Hill, M.D.; Mantese, V.A.; Clark, W.M.; et al. Long-Term Results of Stenting versus Endarterectomy for Carotid-Artery Stenosis. *N. Engl. J. Med.* **2016**, *374*, 1021–1031. [CrossRef] [PubMed]
15. Sardar, P.; Chatterjee, S.; Aronow, H.D.; Kundu, A.; Ramchand, P.; Mukherjee, D.; Nairooz, R.; Gray, W.A.; White, C.J.; Jaff, M.R.; et al. Carotid Artery Stenting Versus Endarterectomy for Stroke Prevention. *J. Am. Coll. Cardiol.* **2017**, *69*, 2266–2275. [CrossRef] [PubMed]
16. Knappich, C.; Kuehnl, A.; Tsantilas, P.; Schmid, S.; Breitkreuz, T.; Kallmayer, M.; Zimmermann, A.; Eckstein, H.-H. The Use of Embolic Protection Devices Is Associated With a Lower Stroke and Death Rate After Carotid Stenting. *JACC Cardiovasc. Interv.* **2017**, *10*, 1257–1265. [CrossRef] [PubMed]
17. Cole, T.S.; Mezher, A.W.; Catapano, J.S.; Godzik, J.; Baranoski, J.F.; Nakaji, P.; Albuquerque, F.C.; Lawton, M.T.; Little, A.S.; Ducruet, A.F. Nationwide Trends in Carotid Endarterectomy and Carotid Artery Stenting in the Post-CREST Era. *Stroke* **2020**, *51*, 579–587. [CrossRef]
18. Brott, T.G.; Halperin, J.L.; Abbara, S.; Bacharach, J.M.; Barr, J.D.; Bush, R.L.; Cates, C.U.; Creager, M.A.; Fowler, S.B.; Friday, G.; et al. 2011 ASA/ACCF/AHA/AANN/AANS/ACR/ASNR/CNS/SAIP/SCAI/SIR/SNIS/SVM/SVS Guideline on the Management of Patients With Extracranial Carotid and Vertebral Artery Disease: Executive Summary. *Circulation* **2011**, *124*, 489–532. [CrossRef]
19. Bonati, L.H.; Jongen, L.M.; Haller, S.; Flach, H.Z.; Dobson, J.; Nederkoorn, P.J.; Macdonald, S.; Gaines, A.P.; Waaijer, A.; Stierli, P.; et al. New ischaemic brain lesions on MRI after stenting or endarterectomy for symptomatic carotid stenosis: A substudy of the International Carotid Stenting Study (ICSS). *Lancet Neurol.* **2010**, *9*, 353–362. [CrossRef]
20. Schnaudigel, S.; Gröschel, K.; Pilgram, S.M.; Kastrup, A. New Brain Lesions after Carotid Stenting versus Carotid Endarterectomy. *Stroke* **2008**, *39*, 1911–1919. [CrossRef]
21. Gensicke, H.; Zumbrunn, T.; Jongen, L.M.; Nederkoorn, P.J.; Macdonald, S.; Gaines, P.A.; Lyrer, P.A.; Wetzel, S.G.; van der Lugt, A.; Mali, W.P.T.M.; et al. Characteristics of Ischemic Brain Lesions After Stenting or Endarterectomy for Symptomatic Carotid Artery Stenosis. *Stroke* **2013**, *44*, 80–86. [CrossRef] [PubMed]
22. Bendszus, M.; Koltzenburg, M.; Burger, R.; Warmuth-Metz, M.; Hofmann, E.; Solymosi, L. Silent embolism in diagnostic cerebral angiography and neurointerventional procedures: A prospective study. *Lancet* **1999**, *354*, 1594–1597. [CrossRef]
23. Kastrup, A.; Gröschel, K.; Schnaudigel, S.; Nägele, T.; Schmidt, F.; Ernemann, U. Target lesion ulceration and arch calcification are associated with increased incidence of carotid stenting-associated ischemic lesions in octogenarians. *J. Vasc. Surg.* **2008**, *47*, 88–95. [CrossRef]
24. Spagnoli, L.G.; Mauriello, A.; Sangiorgi, G.; Fratoni, S.; Bonanno, E.; Schwartz, R.S.; Piepgras, D.G.; Pistolese, R.; Ippoliti, A.; Holmes, D.R. Extracranial Thrombotically Active Carotid Plaque as a Risk Factor for Ischemic Stroke. *JAMA* **2004**, *292*, 1845–1852. [CrossRef]
25. Naggara, O.; Touzé, E.; Beyssen, B.; Trinquart, L.; Chatellier, G.; Meder, J.-F.; Mas, J.-L. Anatomical and Technical Factors Associated With Stroke or Death During Carotid Angioplasty and Stenting. *Stroke* **2011**, *42*, 380–388. [CrossRef] [PubMed]
26. Eckstein, H.-H.; Ringleb, P.; Allenberg, J.-R.; Berger, J.; Fraedrich, G.; Hacke, W.; Hennerici, M.; Stingele, R.; Fiehler, J.; Zeumer, H.; et al. Results of the Stent-Protected Angioplasty versus Carotid Endarterectomy (SPACE) study to treat symptomatic stenoses at 2 years: A multinational, prospective, randomised trial. *Lancet Neurol.* **2008**, *7*, 893–902. [CrossRef]
27. Bonati, L.H.; Dobson, J.; Featherstone, R.L.; Ederle, J.; van der Worp, H.B.; de Borst, G.J.; Mali, W.P.T.M.; Beard, J.D.; Cleveland, T.; Engelter, S.T.; et al. Long-term outcomes after stenting versus endarterectomy for treatment of symptomatic carotid stenosis: The International Carotid Stenting Study (ICSS) randomised trial. *Lancet* **2014**, *385*, 529–538. [CrossRef]
28. Liu, H.; Chu, J.; Zhang, L.; Liu, C.; Yan, Z.; Zhou, S. Clinical Comparison of Outcomes of Early versus Delayed Carotid Artery Stenting for Symptomatic Cerebral Watershed Infarction due to Stenosis of the Proximal Internal Carotid Artery. *BioMed Res. Int.* **2016**, *2016*, 6241546. [CrossRef]
29. Song, K.S.; Kwon, O.-K.; Hwang, G.; Bae, H.-J.; Han, M.-K.; Kim, B.J.; Bang, J.S.; Oh, C.W. Early carotid artery stenting for symptomatic carotid artery stenosis. *Acta Neurochir.* **2015**, *157*, 1873–1878. [CrossRef]
30. Meschia, J.F.; Hopkins, L.N.; Altafullah, I.; Wechsler, L.R.; Stotts, G.; Gonzales, N.R.; Voeks, J.H.; Howard, G.; Brott, T.G. Time From Symptoms to Carotid Endarterectomy or Stenting and Perioperative Risk. *Stroke* **2015**, *46*, 3540–3542. [CrossRef]
31. Kwolek, C.J.; Jaff, M.R.; Leal, J.I.; Hopkins, L.N.; Shah, R.M.; Hanover, T.M.; Macdonald, S.; Cambria, R.P.; Flores, A.; Leal, I.; et al. Results of the ROADSTER multicenter trial of transcarotid stenting with dynamic flow reversal. *J. Vasc. Surg.* **2015**, *62*, 1227–1234. [CrossRef] [PubMed]
32. Dakour-Aridi, H.; Kashyap, V.S.; Wang, G.J.; Eldrup-Jorgensen, J.; Schermerhorn, M.L.; Malas, M.B. The impact of age on in-hospital outcomes after transcarotid artery revascularization, transfemoral carotid artery stenting, and carotid endarterectomy. *J. Vasc. Surg.* **2020**, *72*, 931–942. [CrossRef] [PubMed]

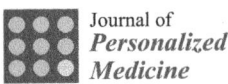

Journal of *Personalized Medicine*

Article

The Safety and Efficacy of Hepatic Transarterial Embolization Using Microspheres and Microcoils in Patients with Symptomatic Polycystic Liver Disease

Alexis Coussy [1], Eva Jambon [1], Yann Le Bras [1], Christian Combe [2], Laurence Chiche [3], Nicolas Grenier [1] and Clément Marcelin [1,*]

[1] Department of Radiology, Pellegrin Hospital, Place Amélie Raba Léon, 33076 Bordeaux, France
[2] Departement of Nephrology, Pellegrin Hospital, Place Amélie Raba Léon, 33076 Bordeaux, France
[3] Department of Digestive surgery, Haut Leveque, 33076 Bordeaux, France
* Correspondence: clement.marcelin@gmail.com; Tel.: +33-556-795-599; Fax: +33-557-821-650

Abstract: Purpose: We investigated the long-term safety and efficacy of hepatic transarterial embolization (TAE) in patients with symptomatic polycystic liver disease (PLD). **Materials and Methods:** A total of 26 patients were included, mean age of 52.3 years (range: 33–78 years), undergoing 32 TAE procedures between January 2012 and December 2019 were included in this retrospective study. Distal embolization of the segmental hepatic artery was performed with 300–500 μm embolic microspheres associated with proximal embolization using microcoils. The primary endpoint was clinical efficacy, defined by an improvement in health-related quality of life using a modified Short Form-36 Health Survey and improvement in symptoms (digestive or respiratory symptoms and chronic abdominal pain), without invasive therapy during the follow-up period. Secondary endpoints were a decrease in total liver volume and treated liver volume and complications. **Results:** Hepatic embolization was performed successfully in 30 of 32 procedures with no major adverse events. Clinical efficacy was 73% (19/26). The mean reduction in hepatic volume was −12.6% at 3 months and −27.8% at the last follow-up 51 ± 15.2 months after TAE (range: 30–81 months; both $ps < 0.01$). The mean visual analog scale pain score was 5.4 ± 2.8 before TAE and decreased to 2.7 ± 1.9 after treatment. Three patients had minor adverse events, and one patient had an adverse event of moderate severity. **Conclusion:** Hepatic embolization using microspheres and microcoils is a safe and effective treatment for PLD that improves symptoms and reduces the volume of hepatic cysts.

Keywords: embolization; polycystic liver disease; safety; efficacy

1. Introduction

Polycystic liver disease (PLD) is a group of genetic disorders that manifest as the progressive development of multiple cysts in the liver parenchyma [1,2]. Autosomal dominant polycystic kidney disease (ADPKD) is the most frequent cause of PLD (80%), liver cysts being the most common extrarenal manifestation [3]. Autosomal dominant polycystic liver disease (ADPLD) is a separate entity with two different mutations, responsible for 20% of PLD, with a cystic disease restricted to the liver [4]. Molecular genetic testing is available to look for mutations in the SEC63, LRP5, PRKCS, GANAB, ALG8, SEC61B PKD1, PKD2, and PKHD1.

Gigot classification is now commonly used to define severity in PLD [5]. Type I is defined by the presence of less than 10 large hepatic cysts measuring more than 10 cm in maximum diameter. Type II is defined by a diffuse involvement of liver parenchyma by multiple cysts with remaining large areas of non-cystic liver parenchyma. Type III is defined by presence of diffuse involvement of liver parenchyma by small- and medium-sized liver cysts with only a few areas of normal liver parenchyma. Cyst puncture, sclerotherapy, or fenestration are used to treat with success for Gigot type I. However, Gigot type II and III are more difficult to treat.

Conversely to ADPLD, ADPKD causes progressive renal dysfunction, whereas liver function remains normal in both diseases. However, up to 20% of patients with PLD may require treatment because the compressive effects of cysts on adjacent structures cause progressive symptoms [6]. Common symptoms include abdominal discomfort, such as early satiety and postprandial fullness, chronic and acute pain, dyspnea, reduced mobility, and fatigue [7]. Severe disease can lead to malnutrition and disability.

Different modalities have been reported for treating PLD, with the objective of reducing the liver volume and relieving symptoms [8]. Treatment with somatostatin analog appears to be insufficient, with a decrease in liver volume of only 1.99% after 2 years [9].

Percutaneous cyst aspiration associated with sclerotherapy and laparoscopic fenestration are indicated in patients with superficial cysts and a limited number of large cysts (Gigot classification type I). These treatments may temporarily relieve symptoms, but there is a high recurrence rate of up to 80% [10].

Hepatic resection has been proposed to treat highly symptomatic patients, with diffuse involvement of the liver parenchyma by multiple cysts and remaining large areas of non-cystic liver parenchyma [8]. However, significant complications can occur, and morbidity and mortality rates associated with this procedure can reach 50% and 3%, respectively [11,12].

Hepatic transplantation has been published in cases of diffuse involvement of the liver parenchyma by small and medium cysts with only a few areas of normal parenchyma with good efficacy but a morbidity rate of 40–50% and a global mortality rate between 8% and 17% at 5 years [12].

Transarterial embolization (TAE) of hepatic arteries in PLD was first described as a promising minimally invasive treatment for patients with abdominal discomfort due to a distended abdomen or gastric compression [13]. Several embolization techniques have been described, including coiling and the use of a mixture of N-butyl cyanoacrylate–iodized oil [14] and polyvinyl alcohol [15], particles tris-acryl gelatin microspheres [16]. The association between distal and proximal embolization was described in renal embolization in cases of ADPKD, with good efficacy [17]. To date no study evaluated quality of life after the TAE.

The present retrospective study was performed to assess the safety and clinical efficacy of TAE using combined embolization with Tris-acryl gelatin microspheres and coils and its long-term impact on reducing liver volume in patients with symptomatic PLD.

2. Patients and Methods

2.1. Patient Population

This retrospective study was approved by the institutional review board, and the requirement for informed consent was waived. A total of 21 patients had PLD and ADPKD (80.7%), whereas 6 had PLD alone. Indication of treatment was based on the following criteria:

Clinically palpable liver hypertrophy responsible for symptomatic mass effects, such as abdominal pain, dyspnea, early satiety, and physical disability

Diffuse disease (Gigot classification type II or III) on imaging precluding surgical resection or percutaneous sclerotherapy

Exclusion criteria included liver cyst infection and the decision of hepatic transplantation taken before TAE.

The decision to perform TAE was made at a multidisciplinary committee based on the patient's degree of clinical discomfort and on liver imaging data on computed tomography (CT).

All patients were followed until June 2020. Quality of life was determined with a modified Short Form-36 Health Survey (SF-36) by mail or e-mail in June 2020 [18,19]. The SF 36 questionnaire is a health survey frequently used on clinical studies to assess health related quality of life. It included 36 questions in 8 domain scores of physical and mental function.

Quality of life and the efficacy of TAE for treating digestive and respiratory symptoms and chronic pain were evaluated retrospectively before and after TAE.

Patients' demographic data, including weight (after dialysis in patients receiving dialysis) and laboratory data were obtained from their electronic medical records. All data were collected before TAE, 3 months after treatment, 2 years, between 2–5 years, and at the last follow-up more than 5 years in June 2020. All medical and surgical treatments undergone by patients before and after TAE were noted.

2.2. Imaging before the Procedure

Pre- and post-TAE total liver volume was calculated on CT with or without contrast injection with validated open source image processing software (Osirix, Pixmeo Sarl, Geneva, Switzerland) [20,21] from the set of contiguous images by the product of liver area, traced manually on each CT with a slice thickness of 5 mm.

2.3. The TAE Procedure

All procedures were performed on two different angiographic units (Allura Xper FD20, Philips, Best, The Netherlands; and Artis Pheno, Siemens Healthcare, Forchheim, Germany) under sedation or general anesthesia. After percutaneous introduction of a 5-Fr sheath (Radifocus Introducer II, Terumo, Tokyo, Japan) into the right or left femoral artery under ultrasound guidance, the celiac trunk and superior mesenteric artery were catheterized with a 4-F artery catheter (SHK 1.0, Cordis, Miami, FL, USA; or Cobra C2 Glidecath, Terumo) and a 0.035" hydrophilic guidewire (Terumo). After contrast injection in each trunk, digital subtraction angiography allowed visualization of the arterial anatomy, and portal hepatography was used to determine the anatomy and permeability of the intra- and extrahepatic portal system (Figure 1). Superselective catheterization of arterial branches vascularizing hepatic segments containing liver cysts was achieved with a 2.7-Fr microcatheter (Progreat, Terumo).

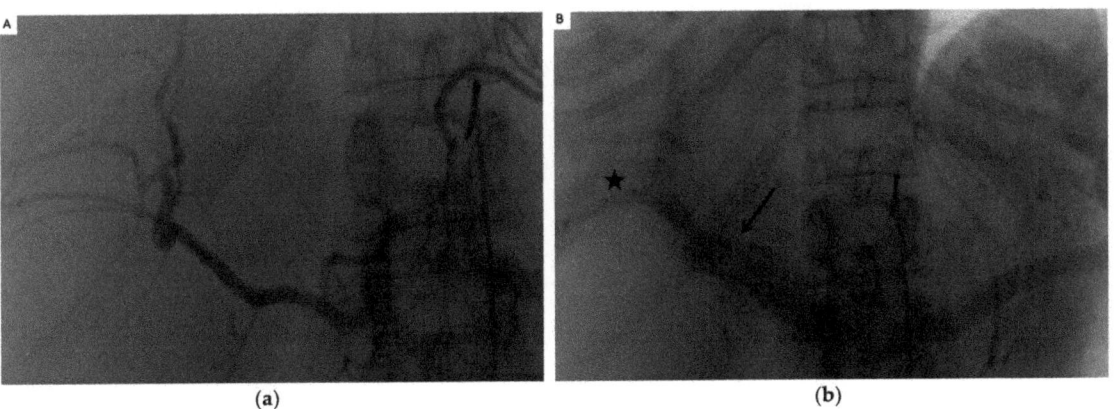

Figure 1. Cont.

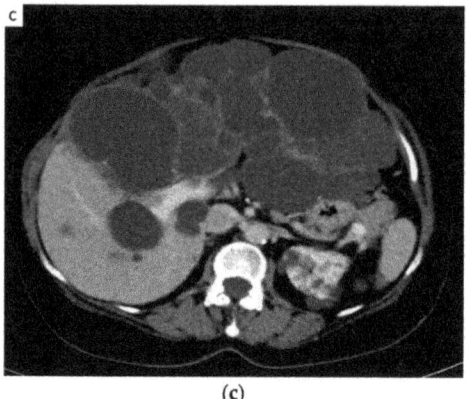 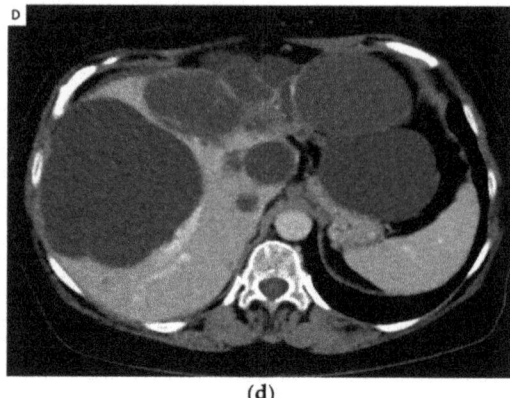

(c) (d)

Figure 1. (a) arteriography of the coeliac artery showing well developed hepatic artery deviated by the cysts without parenchymography of the left liver. (b) Portography showing permeable splenic and portal vein, occlusion of the left portal and right anterior portal vein (arrow), and permeability of the right posterior portal vein (Star). (c,d): CT scan showing good correlation with the arteriography and portography. hepatic parenchyma is completely replaced by cysts in segment II, III and IV.

The hepatic regions for embolization were selected before the TAE procedure based on the distribution of cyst density determined on CT. According to these criteria, total or partial liver embolization was performed. Arterial occlusion of each segmental artery was performed first by distal embolization with 300–500 µm Tris-acryl gelatin microspheres (Embosphere, Merit Medical, South Jordan, UT, USA; or Embogold, Boston Scientific, Natick, MA, USA). Particles were injected through the microcatheter until stasis of feeding arterial flow without reflux. Subsequently, to ensure complete vascular occlusion and prevent revascularization, embolization was completed with one or several microcoils of suitable diameter and length (Tornado or Hilal, Cook Medical, Indiana, IN, USA). Diameter of coils were between 2 and 6 mm. When necessary, extrahepatic collaterals, such as the inferior phrenic or omental arteries, were also embolized.

2.4. Postprocedure Management

To prevent postembolization syndrome (PES), a combination of corticosteroid (methylprednisolone 1 mg/kg) and an analgesic (acetaminophen 1 g) were injected intravenously 2 h before embolization. PES is characterized by moderate to severe epigastric pain, fever, severe nausea, and vomiting that appear early after embolization. Biologically, there is a biological inflammatory syndrome associated with elevated transaminases and bilirubin. All these abnormalities are transient and spontaneously resolved in a few days. During embolization, pain was managed with intravenous nonsteroidal anti-inflammatory drugs and morphinic analgesic titration if necessary. After embolization, patients were admitted to the nephrology department for 2 to 3 days, and analgesic and corticoid treatment was maintained intravenously for at least 24 h. If additional analgesics were needed, morphine was added and administered through a patient-controlled analgesia pump with antiemetic treatment if necessary.

Laboratory data included Creat, Urea, AST, ALT, GGT, Bilirubin, and Alcaline phosphatase were examined on days 1 and 3 after TAE. After discharge, pain was controlled with acetaminophen or tramadol, and prednisolone (20 mg/day) was given for 8 days.

2.5. Endpoints

The primary study endpoint was clinical success, defined as improvement in quality of life (an increase in SF-36 score > 10 points) [22,23] and improvement in abdominal pain, digestive and respiratory symptoms without invasive treatment throughout the follow-up period. The SF-36 was completed in consultation on the follow-up scan was performed. Secondary outcomes were primary technical success, defined by complete occlusion of targeted segmental hepatic arteries; a decrease in liver volume on CT with or without contrast injection and complications according to the guidelines of the Society of Interventional Radiology [24] and Clavien–Dindo [25], including cyst complications, such as hemorrhage or infection during follow-up.

2.6. Statistical Analysis

Data are summarized as proportions and means ± standard deviations as appropriate. Categorical variables were analyzed with the chi-square test, and continuous variables were compared with Student's t test or analysis of variance. In all analyses, $p < 0.05$ was taken to indicate statistical significance. If patients could not visit the hospital at the time of data collection, their data were imputed by linear regression based on the next visit.

3. Results

3.1. Population

From 1 January 2012, to December 2019, a total of 26 consecutive patients (21 women [81%] and 5 men [19%]) with symptomatic PLD underwent a total of 32 TAE procedures at a single institution. Before TAE, 7 patients received treatment with somatostatin for 12–24 months, which was considered ineffective; 11 patients had been treated by cyst puncture and sclerotherapy, but no patients had undergone any previous surgical interventions. Patient characteristics are summarized in Tables 1 and 2. The mean follow-up period was 51 months (range: 6–98 months). In this population, 16 and 10 patients had Gigot liver type II and type III, respectively. Embolization was performed selectively in 23 procedures (72%)—14 in the right liver (44%) and 9 in the left liver (28%)—and was global (right and left) in 9 procedures (28%). The mean number of embolized segments was 4.0 ± 1.7. Extra-hepatic arteries embolized were three left gastric arteries.

Table 1. Patient characteristics.

Patient Characteristics	Mean (Range) or N (%)
Average age in years (range)	52.3 (33–78)
<50 years	10 (39%)
>50 years	16 (61%)
Gender	
-Male	5 (19%)
Weight	86.6 (+/−12.8)
BMI	28.25 (+/−4.1)
-Female	21 (81%)
Weight	63,2 (+/−12.1)
BMI	23.4 (+/−2.4)
Mean time follow-up (months)	51 (6–98)
Type of PLD	
-associated with ADPK	20 (77%)
-PLD isolated	6 (23%)
Laboratory	
Creatinine	117.3 (+/−82)
>60 GFR	10 (38%)
<60 GFR.	13 (50%)
dialysis	3 (11%)
Urea	8.1 (+/−3.6)
AST	39.8 (+/−53)
ALT	33.2 (+/−36.5)
GGT	175.8 (+/−116.8)
Bilirubin	12.3 (+/−9.2)
Alcaline phosphatase	141.6 (+/−106)
TP	92.1 (+/−14)
Hemoglobin	12.7 (+/−1.5)
Platelets	230 (+/−77)

Table 2. Patients characteristics.

Patient Characteristics	Mean (Range) or N (%)
Liver volume	
Total liver volume	6436 cc (2965–13,470)
Right liver	4058 cc (2073–9566)
Left liver	2377 cc (848–5776)
Symptoms	
Abdominal Pain	24 (92%)
Dyspnea	21 (81%)
Dyspepsia	26 (100%)
Previous treatment	
Medical treatment	7 (27%)
Cyst sclerosis	11 (42%)
Fenestration or hepatectomy	0
Anterior complications	13 (50%)
Infection	12 (46%)
Hemorrhage	3 (11%)

3.2. Technical Success

Primary technical success was achieved in 30 of the 32 procedures (93%). TAE was stopped because of difficulty catheterizing segmental branches responsible for a high radiation dose (4 Gy) in one case and dissection of the left liver artery in another case. These two patients underwent a second TAE with effective technical success. Two procedures were necessary in five patients and one patient underwent three procedures because of insufficient reduction in volume. These 6 failures were due to recanalization of hepatic arteries or embolization of insufficient hepatic volume but after the subsequent procedures the secondary technical success rate was 100%.

The mean procedure time was 90.9 ± 28.8 min. The mean quantity of contrast injected during the procedure was 134.5 ± 52 cc, the mean radiation dose area product (DAP) was 1146 ± 935 mGy, and the mean fluoroscopy time was 34.5 ± 14 min.

3.3. Safety

TAE postembolization syndrome occurred after all procedures despite medical preparation, but no patients developed hepatic insufficiency. The mean duration of hospital stay was 4.25 ± 1.9 days (range: 2–10 days). No residual pain was reported after 1 month.

The total complication rate was 12.5%. Three patients presented pain recurrence (grade I) justifying new hospitalization between 1 and 10 days. One patient had a cyst infection (grade III-a) that occurred 20 days after TAE, treated successfully with puncture and intravenous antibiotics over a 5-day hospitalization period.

3.4. Reduction in Hepatic Volume (Figure 2 and Table 3)

The mean decrease in total liver volume at 3 months was -12.6% ($\pm 8.01\%$) compared to the pre-TAE value or a mean loss of -855 cc ($p < 0.01$). CT was performed more than 2 years after TAE in 12 patients, and the mean decrease in total liver volume ratio was -27.8% ($p < 0.01$) (Table 4).

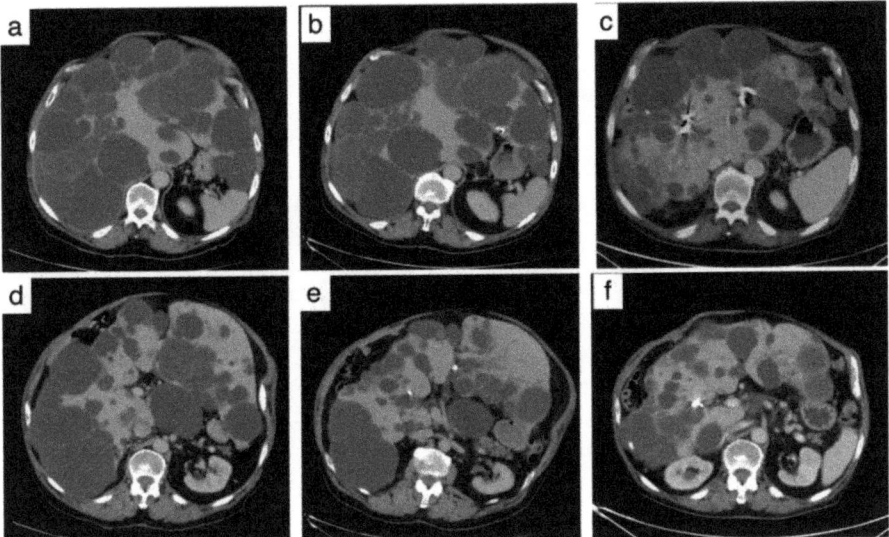

Figure 2. Computed Tomography (CT) from a patient with polycystic liver disease before and after transarterial embolization. (**a**,**b**) Pre-embolization CT showing a voluminous polycystic liver with a compression of the stomach by the cysts. (**c**,**d**) CT at 3 months showing coils and reduction of cysts volume. (**e**,**f**): CT at 4 years showing a significant liver volume reduction of 29% with a decompression of the stomach.

Table 3. Liver volume reduction in sub group analysis.

	Sex	Liver Volume before TAE (mL)	Liver Volume after TAE (mL)	Difference	p
Total liver	men	8808.4	7441.1	−15.2%	$p < 0.01$
	women	5672.4	4932.7	−11.9%	$p < 0.01$
				Qobs = 0.90 IC95% [−4.1169; 10.5965]	$p = 0.37$
Embolized liver	men	5894	4752	−17.8%	$p < 0.01$
	women	3906	3234.7	−24.3%	$p < 0.01$
				Qobs = −1.16 IC95% [−17.4903; 4.7764]	$p = 0.25$
	Disease				
Total liver	ADPLD	8633	7174	−16.8%	$p < 0.01$
	ADPKD	5597	4916	−11.3%	$p < 0.01$
				Qobs = 1.64 IC95 [−1.3294; 12.3023]	$p = 0.11$
Embolized liver	ADPLD	5787	4398	−24%	$p < 0.01$
	ADPKD	3781	3291	−22%	$p < 0.01$
				Qobs = 0.39 IC95 [−8.6315; 12.6986]	$p = 0.69$
	Quality of life				
Total liver	Improved	6313	5322	−15.7%	$p < 0.01$
	Not improved	6420	5878	−8.1%	$p = 0.03$
				Qobs = −2.65 IC95 [−11.7682; −1.5267]	$p < 0.01$
Embolized liver	Improved	4708 cc	3811 cc	−24%	$p < 0.01$
	Not improved	3543 cc	2857 cc	−12%	$p < 0.01$
				Qosb = −3.12 IC95 [−11.7682; −1.5267]	$p < 0.01$

Table 4. Liver volume reduction at 3 months and 2 years after TAE.

	Mean Vol. before TAE (mL)	Mean Vol. after TAE (mL)	Mean Reduction of Volume	p
Scanner 3 months after TAE				
Total liver Volume	6438 (+/−2592)	5567 cc (+/−2122)	−12.6% (+/−8) −855 cc IC95% [570.88; 1140.55]	$p < 0.01$
Liver embolized	4623 (+/−2916)	3692 cc (+/−2460)	−22.7% (+/−12.5) −930 cc IC95% [679.03; 1182.78]	$p < 0.01$
2+ years of follow-up				
Total Liver Volume ($n = 12$ patients)	6275 (+/−2353)	4440 cc (+/−1302)	−27.8% −1863 cc IC95% [757.7333; 2968.4889]	$p < 0.01$
Liver embolized ($n = 12$ patients)	5001(+/−2157)	3546 cc (+/−1769)	−32.5% (+/−17) −1544 cc IC95 [841.9154; 2246.0846]	$p < 0.01$

3.5. Clinical Efficacy

The primary clinical efficacy was 72% (19/26) at the date of evaluation in June 2020, and the average follow-up time was 51 ± 15.2 months (range: 6–98 months). A total of 19 patients (72%) showed a significant improvement in their quality of life with an increase in SF-36 score of >10 points, and 13 (52%) showed an increase of >20 points. No patients reported a worsening of quality of life after embolization. Of the 26 patients, 23 (88%) would recommend TAE for the management of PLD.

Clinical failure occurred in seven patients (27%) who experienced no improvement in quality of life after TAE. Two of these patients (7%) required complementary surgical treatment 7 and 11 months after TAE consisting of a right hepatectomy in one case and a combination of a right hepatectomy and cyst fenestration in the other. Surgery was effective in these two patients. Five patients did not benefit for another treatment. One patient died of metastatic kidney cancer 2 years after treatment unrelated to TAE. The four other patients who did not experience clinical success underwent repeated cyst aspirations or symptomatic treatment and refused a second TAE or surgery.

3.5.1. Chronic Pain

Of the 24 patients (92%) who presented with chronic pain related to liver volume, 20 (83%) noticed an improvement after TAE. Pain evolved from a mean visual analog scale score of 5.4 ± 2.8 before TAE to 2.7 ± 1.9 afterward.

3.5.2. Digestive Symptoms

All patients had digestive symptoms before TAE (moderate in 17 and severe in 9). After TAE, 21/26 patients (81%) showed an improvement in symptoms, including 15 patients (57%) who experienced a complete recovery. Only two patients (11%) had severe persistent digestive symptoms.

3.5.3. Dyspnea

Before TAE, 21 patients (81%) had dyspnea, including 16 with symptoms that caused problems in everyday life. A total of 14 of these patients (66%) reported improvement after TAE.

4. Discussion

TAE using microspheres and coils is a safe and an effective treatment for patients with diffuse and symptomatic PLD. These results confirm the findings of previous studies that used different embolization techniques [14,26–29] (Table 5).

Table 5. Summary of relevant studies on hepatic artery embolization in patients with polycystic liver disease.

Authors	Date	Patient	Embolic Material Used	Reduction in Liver Volume at 6 Months	Reduction in Liver Volume at 1 Year	Reduction in Liver Volume at 2 Years	Mean Liver Volume before Embolization (mL)	Clinical Success
Ubara et al. [13]	2004	1	Coils			−46%	12,364	100%
Takei et al. [27]	2007	30	Coils			−21.2%	7882	80%
Park et al. [15]	2009	3	PVA and Coils		−15%		9490	66%
Wang et al. [14]	2012	21	NBCA and lipiodol	No significative difference	−25.7%		8270	85.3%
Hoshino et al. [26]	2014	221	Coils	−5.3%	−9.2%		7058	-
Yang et al. [29]	2016	18	Coils	−7.6%			7767	31.4%
Zhang et al. [30]	2017	23	NBCA and lipiodol	−16.3%	−29.7%	−29.3%	8070	86%
Sakuhara et al. [16]	2019	5	Tris Acryl Gelatin microsphere	−5.5%	−6.7%		7406	60%

The rate of absence of clinical amelioration and cyst volume reduction was 27% in our cohort compared to 0% reported by Ubara et al. [13], 15% reported by Wang et al. [14], 20% reported by Takei et al. [26], 34% reported by Park et al. [15], 40% reported by Sakuhara et al. [16], and 69.6% reported by Yang et al. [29]. These differences could be due to differences in treatment methodologies, including revascularization of embolized arteries, the development of extrahepatic collaterals stimulated by the cyst and parenchymal ischemia, and the development of intrahepatic collaterals when only one lobe was embolized [16].

These possibilities prompted us to perform a second TAE if the first was ineffective. The second TAE involved meticulously searching for and embolizing extrahepatic collaterals to ensure that there was no residual flow in the embolized artery. Revascularization of the hepatic artery seems to be the principal cause of failure [14,28]. The combination of distal embolization using microspheres and proximal occlusion of the segmental artery using microcoils seems to be very effective for producing irreversible occlusion of the targeted artery.

Selecting the appropriate embolic agent is important. Recanalization is favored by the presence of many intrahepatic collateral vessels (peribiliary vascular plexus) and extrahepatic collateral vessels (omental artery, gastric artery, inferior phrenic artery, etc.) [31].

Different embolic materials have been used in previous studies, with coils being the most common [28]. Liquid adhesives and glue have also been used for distal and proximal embolization with good efficacy [14,30], however, there are risks for polymerization [32] and reflux in non-target areas [14,30], which can cause complications, such as biloma [14]. Calibrated microspheres are more precise and suitable than glue because of their ease of delivery from the inserted microcatheter and the low levels of associated inflammation compared to other liquid embolic agents [33,34].

In this study, the reduction in hepatic volume was −12.6% 3 months after embolization and −27.8% at the last follow-up more than 2 years after TAE are similar to those reported in the literature, that is, −7% to −21% with coils after 1 year [13,26], −25.7% and −29.3% for glue associated with lipiodol [30], and −15% after 1 year for polyvinyl alcohol particles and coils [15].

Neijenhuis et al. [35] showed that symptom reduction is a better outcome parameter than cyst volume reduction for treatment success in patients treated by aspiration sclerotherapy. Indeed, cyst diameter reduction does not reflect treatment success in aspiration sclerotherapy from patients' perspectives, while symptoms measured with the PLD-Q can be used as a reliable outcome measure.

This procedure shows a low rate of complications (12.5%) compared to surgical approaches (50%) [8,36] and good tolerance as soon as postembolization syndrome could be controlled. Cyst infection is a serious but rare complication that occurred in only 4% of our cases and has previously been reported at rates between 0% and 2% [37]. The mean duration of hospitalization for TAE is shorter than that required for hepatic surgery (4.25 days vs. 15 days, respectively) [8,11].

Surgery can be performed after one or two TAE procedures. Indeed, embolization did not complicate surgery, and the reduction in volume permitted better mobilization of the liver and resulted in less risk for arterial bleeding during surgery.

In our study, two patients (7%) underwent partial hepatectomy after TAE because of insufficient clinical results with good efficacy. Partial hepatectomy and cyst fenestration substantially improves symptom burden and quality of life in highly symptomatic polycystic liver disease patients [38] with 11.1% of major complication.

This study is not without limitations. This was a retrospective, single center study with a small population. Additionally, there was an absence of systematic late determination of liver volume, an absence of a surgical control group, and the use of two types of microspheres. Moreover, questionnaire PLD-Q was not used in this study, which was validated by Neijenhuis et al. [39]. Due to the retrospective nature of this investigation, there are missing data.

In conclusion, TAE appears to be a safe and effective noninvasive treatment for patients with symptomatic Gigot 2 and 3 PLD. This study demonstrates a progressive decrease in liver volume with clinical efficacy in 73% of patients after one or two TAE procedures. This approach can improve the standard of care for patients with symptomatic PLD and can be considered before more invasive surgical procedures, even in patients with renal insufficiency.

Author Contributions: Conceptualization, A.C. and C.M.; methodology, A.C., C.M. and N.G.; software, A.C.; validation, Y.L.B., E.J., A.C., C.M. and C.C.; formal analysis, A.C.; investigation, A.C.; data curation, A.C., C.M., L.C. and C.C.; writing—original draft preparation, A.C.; writing—review and editing, A.C. and C.M; visualization, C.M.; supervision, C.M. and N.G.; project administration, C.M. All authors have read and agreed to the published version of the manuscript.

Funding: This research received no external funding.

Institutional Review Board Statement: The study was conducted according to the guidelines of the Declaration of Helsinki, and approved by the Institutional Review Board.

Informed Consent Statement: Informed consent was obtained from all subjects involved in the study.

Data Availability Statement: The data presented in this study are available on request from the corresponding author.

Conflicts of Interest: The authors declare no conflict of interest.

References

1. Cnossen, W.R.; Drenth, J.P.H. Polycystic liver disease: An overview of pathogenesis, clinical manifestations and management. *Orphanet J. Rare Dis.* **2014**, *9*, 69. [CrossRef] [PubMed]
2. Rosenfeld, L.; Bonny, C.; Kallita, M.; Heng, A.E.; Deteix, P.; Bommelaer, G.; Abergel, A. Polycystic liver disease and its main complications. *Gastroenterol. Clin. Biol.* **2002**, *26*, 1097–1106. [PubMed]
3. Wilson, P.D. Polycystic Kidney Disease. *N. Engl. J. Med.* **2004**, *350*, 151–164. [CrossRef] [PubMed]
4. Qian, Q. Isolated Polycystic Liver Disease. *Adv. Chronic Kidney Dis.* **2010**, *17*, 181–189. [CrossRef]
5. Gigot, J.F.; Jadoul, P.; Que, F.; Van Beers, B.E.; Etienne, J.; Horsmans, Y.; Collard, A.; Geubel, A.; Pringot, J.; Kestens, P.J. Adult polycystic liver disease: Is fenestration the most adequate operation for long-term management? *Ann. Surg.* **1997**, *225*, 286–294. [CrossRef]
6. Santos-Laso, A.; Izquierdo-Sánchez, L.; Lee-Law, P.Y.; Perugorria, M.J.; Marzioni, M.; Marin, J.J.G.; Bujanda, L.; Banales, J.M. New Advances in Polycystic Liver Diseases. *Semin. Liver Dis.* **2017**, *37*, 45–55. [CrossRef]

7. Hoevenaren, I.A.; Wester, R.; Schrier, R.W.; McFann, K.; Doctor, R.B.; Drenth, J.P.H.; Everson, G.T. Polycystic liver: Clinical characteristics of patients with isolated polycystic liver disease compared with patients with polycystic liver and autosomal dominant polycystic kidney disease. *Liver Int.* **2008**, *28*, 264–270. [CrossRef]
8. Aussilhou, B.; Dokmak, S.; Dondero, F.; Joly, D.; Durand, F.; Soubrane, O.; Belghiti, J. Treatment of polycystic liver disease. Update on the management. *J. Visc. Surg.* **2018**, *155*, 471–481. [CrossRef]
9. van Aerts, R.M.; Kievit, W.; D'Agnolo, H.M.; Blijdorp, C.J.; Casteleijn, N.F.; Dekker, S.E.; de Fijter, J.W.; van Gastel, M.; Gevers, T.J.; van de Laarschot, L.F.; et al. Lanreotide Reduces Liver Growth in Patients With Autosomal Dominant Polycystic Liver and Kidney Disease. *Gastroenterology* **2019**, *157*, 481–491.e7. [CrossRef]
10. Hahn, S.T.; Han, S.Y.; Yun, E.H.; Park, S.H.; Lee, S.H.; Lee, H.J.; Hahn, H.J.; Hahn, H.M. Recurrence after percutaneous ethanol ablation of simple hepatic, renal, and splenic cysts: Is it true recurrence requiring an additional treatment? *Acta Radiol.* **2008**, *49*, 982–986. [CrossRef]
11. Drenth, J.P.; Chrispijn, M.; Nagorney, D.M.; Kamath, P.S.; Torres, V.E. Medical and surgical treatment options for polycystic liver disease. *Hepatology* **2010**, *52*, 2223–2230. [CrossRef]
12. Abu-Wasel, B.; Walsh, C.; Keough, V.; Molinari, M. Pathophysiology, epidemiology, classification and treatment options for polycystic liver diseases. *World J. Gastroenterol.* **2013**, *19*, 5775–5786. [CrossRef]
13. Ubara, Y.; Takei, R.; Hoshino, J.; Tagami, T.; Sawa, N.; Yokota, M.; Katori, H.; Takemoto, F.; Hara, S.; Takaichi, K. Intravascular embolization therapy in a patient with an enlarged polycystic liver. *Am. J. Kidney Dis.* **2004**, *43*, 733–738. [CrossRef]
14. Wang, M.Q.; Duan, F.; Liu, F.Y.; Wang, Z.J.; Song, P. Treatment of symptomatic polycystic liver disease: Transcatheter superselective hepatic arterial embolization using a mixture of NBCA and iodized oil. *Abdom. Imaging* **2013**, *38*, 465–473. [CrossRef]
15. Park, H.C.; Kim, C.W.; Ro, H.; Moon, J.-Y.; Oh, K.-H.; Kim, Y.; Lee, J.S.; Yin, Y.H.; Jae, H.J.; Chung, J.W.; et al. Transcatheter Arterial Embolization Therapy for a Massive Polycystic Liver in Autosomal Dominant Polycystic Kidney Disease Patients. *J. Korean Med. Sci.* **2009**, *24*, 57–61. [CrossRef]
16. Sakuhara, Y.; Nishio, S.; Hattanda, F.; Soyama, T.; Takahashi, B.; Abo, D.; Mimura, H. Initial experience with the use of tris-acryl gelatin microspheres for transcatheter arterial embolization for enlarged polycystic liver. *Clin. Exp. Nephrol.* **2019**, *23*, 825–833. [CrossRef]
17. Petitpierre, F.; Cornelis, F.; Couzi, L.; Lasserre, A.S.; Tricaud, E.; Le Bras, Y.; Merville, P.; Combe, C.; Ferriere, J.M.; Grenier, N. Embolization of renal arteries before transplantation in patients with polycystic kidney disease: A single institution long-term experience. *Eur. Radiol.* **2015**, *25*, 3263–3271. [CrossRef]
18. McHorney, C.A.; Ware, J.E.; Lu, J.F.; Sherbourne, C.D. The MOS 36-item Short-Form Health Survey (SF-36): III. Tests of data quality, scaling assumptions, and reliability across diverse patient groups. *Med. Care* **1994**, *32*, 40–66. [CrossRef]
19. Ware, J.E., Jr.; Sherbourne, C.D. The MOS 36-item short-form health survey (SF-36). I. Conceptual framework and item selection. *Med. Care* **1992**, *30*, 473–483. [CrossRef]
20. van der Vorst, J.R.; van Dam, R.M.; van Stiphout, R.S.; van den Broek, M.A.; Hollander, I.H.; Kessels, A.G.; Dejong, C.H. Virtual Liver Resection and Volumetric Analysis of the Future Liver Remnant using Open Source Image Processing Software. *World J. Surg.* **2010**, *34*, 2426–2433. [CrossRef]
21. Lodewick, T.M.; Arnoldussen, C.W.; Lahaye, M.J.; van Mierlo, K.M.; Neumann, U.P.; Beets-Tan, R.G.; Dejong, C.H.; van Dam, R.M. Fast and accurate liver volumetry prior to hepatectomy. *HPB* **2016**, *18*, 764–772. [CrossRef]
22. Wyrwich, K.W.; Tierney, W.M.; Babu, A.N.; Kroenke, K.; Wolinsky, F.D. A Comparison of Clinically Important Differences in Health-Related Quality of Life for Patients with Chronic Lung Disease, Asthma, or Heart Disease. *Health Serv. Res.* **2005**, *40*, 577–592. [CrossRef]
23. Brigden, A.; Parslow, R.M.; Gaunt, D.; Collin, S.M.; Jones, A.; Crawley, E. Defining the minimally clinically important difference of the SF-36 physical function subscale for paediatric CFS/ME: Triangulation using three different methods. *Health Qual. Life Outcomes* **2018**, *16*, 202. [CrossRef]
24. Khalilzadeh, O.; Baerlocher, M.O.; Shyn, P.B.; Connolly, B.L.; Devane, A.M.; Morris, C.S.; Cohen, A.M.; Midia, M.; Thornton, R.H.; Gross, K.; et al. Proposal of a New Adverse Event Classification by the Society of Interventional Radiology Standards of Practice Committee. *J. Vasc. Interv. Radiol.* **2017**, *28*, 1432–1437.e3. [CrossRef]
25. Dindo, D.; Demartines, N.; Clavien, P.A. Classification of surgical complications: A new proposal with evaluation in a cohort of 6336 patients and results of a survey. *Ann. Surg.* **2004**, *240*, 205–213. [CrossRef]
26. Takei, R.; Ubara, Y.; Hoshino, J.; Higa, Y.; Suwabe, T.; Sogawa, Y.; Nomura, K.; Nakanishi, S.; Sawa, N.; Katori, H.; et al. Percutaneous Transcatheter Hepatic Artery Embolization for Liver Cysts in Autosomal Dominant Polycystic Kidney Disease. *Am. J. Kidney Dis.* **2007**, *49*, 744–752. [CrossRef]
27. Ubara, Y. New Therapeutic Option for Autosomal Dominant Polycystic Kidney Disease Patients With Enlarged Kidney and Liver. *Ther. Apher. Dial.* **2006**, *10*, 333–341. [CrossRef]
28. Hoshino, J.; Ubara, Y.; Suwabe, T.; Sumida, K.; Hayami, N.; Mise, K.; Hiramatsu, R.; Hasegawa, E.; Yamanouchi, M.; Sawa, N.; et al. Intravascular Embolization Therapy in Patients with Enlarged Polycystic Liver. *Am. J. Kidney Dis.* **2014**, *63*, 937–944. [CrossRef]
29. Yang, J.; Ryu, H.; Han, M.; Kim, H.; Hwang, Y.-H.; Chung, J.W.; Yi, N.-J.; Lee, K.-W.; Suh, K.-S.; Ahn, C. Comparison of volume-reductive therapies for massive polycystic liver disease in autosomal dominant polycystic kidney disease. *Hepatol. Res.* **2016**, *46*, 183–191. [CrossRef]

30. Zhang, J.L.; Yuan, K.; Wang, M.Q.; Yan, J.Y.; Xin, H.N.; Wang, Y.; Liu, F.Y.; Bai, Y.H.; Wang, Z.J.; Duan, F.; et al. Transarterial Embolization for Treatment of Symptomatic Polycystic Liver Disease: More than 2-year Follow-up. *Chin. Med. J.* **2017**, *130*, 1938–1944. [CrossRef]
31. Elsayes, K.M.; Shaaban, A.M.; Rothan, S.M.; Javadi, S.; Madrazo, B.L.; Castillo, R.P.; Casillas, V.J.; Menias, C.O. A Comprehensive Approach to Hepatic Vascular Disease. *RadioGraphics* **2017**, *37*, 813–836. [CrossRef] [PubMed]
32. Pollak, J.S.; White, R.I. The Use of Cyanoacrylate Adhesives in Peripheral Embolization. *J. Vasc. Interv. Radiol.* **2001**, *12*, 907–913. [CrossRef]
33. Spies, J.B.; Cornell, C.; Worthington-Kirsch, R.; Lipman, J.C.; Benenati, J.F. Long-term Outcome from Uterine Fibroid Embolization with Tris-acryl Gelatin Microspheres: Results of a Multicenter Study. *J. Vasc. Interv. Radiol.* **2007**, *18*, 203–207. [CrossRef] [PubMed]
34. Laurent, A.; Beaujeux, R.; Wassef, M.; Rüfenacht, D.; Boschetti, E.; Merland, J.J. Trisacryl gelatin microspheres for therapeutic embolization, I: Development and in vitro evaluation. *AJNR Am. J. Neuroradiol.* **1996**, *17*, 533–540.
35. Neijenhuis, M.K.; Wijnands, T.F.M.; Kievit, W.; Ronot, M.; Gevers, T.J.G.; Drenth, J.P.H. Symptom relief and not cyst reduction determines treatment success in aspiration sclerotherapy of hepatic cysts. *Eur. Radiol.* **2019**, *29*, 3062–3068. [CrossRef]
36. Schnelldorfer, T.; Torres, V.E.; Zakaria, S.; Rosen, C.B.; Nagorney, D.M. Polycystic liver disease: A critical appraisal of hepatic resection, cyst fenestration, and liver transplantation. *Ann. Surg.* **2009**, *250*, 112–118. [CrossRef]
37. Suwabe, T.; Ubara, Y.; Hayami, N.; Yamanouchi, M.; Hiramatsu, R.; Sumida, K.; Sawa, N.; Sekine, A.; Kawada, M.; Hasegawa, E.; et al. Factors Influencing Cyst Infection in Autosomal Dominant Polycystic Kidney Disease. *Nephron Exp. Nephrol.* **2019**, *141*, 75–86. [CrossRef]
38. Bernts, L.H.; Neijenhuis, M.K.; Edwards, M.E.; Sloan, J.A.; Fischer, J.; Smoot, R.L.; Nagorney, D.M.; Drenth, J.P.; Hogan, M.C. Symptom relief and quality of life after combined partial hepatectomy and cyst fenestration in highly symptomatic polycystic liver disease. *Surgery* **2020**, *168*, 25–32. [CrossRef]
39. Neijenhuis, M.K.; Gevers, T.J.; Hogan, M.C.; Kamath, P.S.; Wijnands, T.F.; Ouweland, R.C.V.D.; Edwards, M.E.; Sloan, J.A.; Kievit, W.; Drenth, J.P. Development and Validation of a Disease-Specific Questionnaire to Assess Patient-Reported Symptoms in Polycystic Liver Disease. *Hepatology* **2016**, *64*, 151–160. [CrossRef]

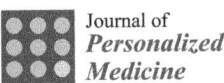

Journal of Personalized Medicine

Article

Retrospective Analysis of Doses Delivered during Embolization Procedures over the Last 10 Years

Joël Greffier [1,2,*], Djamel Dabli [1,2], Tarek Kammoun [1], Jean Goupil [1], Laure Berny [1], Ghizlane Touimi Benjelloun [1], Jean-Paul Beregi [1] and Julien Frandon [1]

1. IMAGINE UR UM 103, Department of Medical Imaging, Montpellier University, Nîmes University Hospital, 30029 Nîmes, France
2. Department of Medical Physics, Nîmes University Hospital, 30029 Nîmes, France
* Correspondence: joel.greffier@chu-nimes.fr; Tel.: +33-466-683-309

Abstract: Background: This study aimed to retrospectively analyze dosimetric indicators recorded since 2012 for thoracic, abdominal or pelvic embolizations to evaluate the contribution of new tools and technologies in dose reduction. Methods: Dosimetric indicators (dose area product (DAP) and air kerma (AK)) from 1449 embolizations were retrospectively reviewed from August 2012 to March 2022. A total of 1089 embolizations were performed in an older fixed C-Arm system (A1), 222 in a newer fixed C-Arm system (A2) and 138 in a 4DCT system (A3). The embolization procedures were gathered to compare A1, A2 and A3. Results: DAP were significantly lower with A2 compared to A1 for all procedures (median $-50\% \pm 5\%$, $p < 0.05$), except for uterine elective embolizations and gonadal vein embolization. The DAP values were significantly lower with A3 than with A1 ($p < 0.001$). CT scan was used for guidance in 90% of embolization procedures. Conclusions: The last C-Arm technology allowed a median reduction of 50% of the X-ray dose. The implementation of a CT scan inside the IR room allowed for more precise 3D-guidance with no increase of the dose delivered.

Keywords: embolization; dose optimization; interventional radiology; CT scan

1. Introduction

Thoracic, abdominal or pelvic embolizations represent an important proportion of all procedures performed in interventional radiology (IR), with many indications [1–4]. Embolizations may be long and complex procedures, with high radiation doses delivered to the patients, and it is possible that the patient skin dose may exceed the threshold of deterministic effects (2 to 3 Gy), leading to radiodermatitis or alopecia [5–8]. Another issue, even when relatively low doses are delivered in IR, is the risk of long-term stochastic effects, including induced cancer [9,10]. Optimization of IR practices is thus needed to reduce these risks [11].

The International Commission on Radiological Protection (ICRP) has recommended the collection and monitoring of dose indicators for each patient exposed to ionizing radiation [11]. In IR, this collection allows for improved detection and follow-up of patients at risk of a deterministic effect to improve their therapeutic management. In addition, an evaluation of the skin dose can be performed when the air kerma at the interventional reference point (AK) or the dose area product (DAP) are high [12,13].

To reduce the doses delivered during interventional procedures, the optimization principle must be applied with great rigor. Dose optimization consists in reducing radiation doses as low as reasonably achievable while maintaining sufficient image quality. For this purpose, the protocols are often optimized by the medical physicists and the resulting image quality for each protocol is validated by the interventional radiologists [14]. Medical physicists may also train radiologists on good patient radiation protection practices. Finally, manufacturers develop new equipment to reduce the dose delivered to the patients, with a sufficient image quality, using new tools or new modalities to facilitate guidance and improve patient management [15–21].

In our institution, dosimetric indicators have been collected daily by medical physicists for all IR procedures since 2012 and methods to calculate or measure the skin dose have been implemented since 2013 [22,23]. Between 2012 and 2020, all embolizations were performed in a single vascular room equipped with a fixed C-arm. In 2020, this room was replaced by two new IR rooms: a room with a fixed C-arm and equipped with the ClarityIQ technology, which allows reducing the dose while maintaining an equivalent image quality, and a second room with a fixed C-arm coupled with a CT-scan. The use of the CT-scan in this new room allows improving percutaneous and vascular guidance, controlling the environment of the treated area and performing a control at the end of the procedure. For these two new equipped rooms, the protocols and practices have also been optimized. We therefore assumed that the new features introduced in these two rooms may modify the doses delivered and the management of the patients.

The purpose of our study was to retrospectively analyze the dosimetric indicators recorded since 2012 and evaluate the contribution of the new tools and new rooms in dose reduction and patient management.

2. Materials and Methods

2.1. Patient Study

The present retrospective study was approved by the local institutional review board (Interface Recherche Bioethique Institutional Review Board, number 22.04.03) and patient approval was waived due to the study retrospective character. The study was carried out in accordance with current guidelines and regulations. Patients (or their legal guardians) were systematically informed that their data were collected in an anonymous manner for a retrospective study and that they could refuse at any time to participate in the study (non-opposition statement).

Data were acquired consecutively for all adult participants undergoing thoracic or abdomen-pelvic embolization from August 2012 to March 2022 in our institute. Ten embolization procedures were studied (Table 1):

- Bronchial artery embolizations (BE);
- Abdominal elective embolizations for scheduled treatment and visceral aneurysm (except for renal artery) treatments (AEE);
- Abdominal urgent embolizations for active bleedings or vascular injuries of digestive arteries (AUE);
- Hepatic chemoembolizations (HCE);
- Radioembolization for primary and metastatic liver cancers (RaE);
- Renal artery embolizations (RE);
- Pelvic embolizations for planned prostatic embolizations (PE);
- Uterine elective embolizations for leiomyomas or vascular malformations (UEE);
- Uterine urgent embolizations for postpartum hemorrhages (UUE);
- Gonadal vein embolizations (GVE).

Patients were not included in the study if they were under 18 years old or if they refused to participate in the study (opposition statement).

For all patients, the age, total dose area product (DAP), air kerma (AK), total fluoroscopy time (FT) and number of fluorography images were collected. The total dose length product (DLP) was collected only for patients who had undergone a CT scan during the procedure. For all procedures, the dosimetric indicators were collected daily from the dose reports available in the Picture Archiving and Communication System (PACS) or in the Dose Archiving and Communication System (DACS) by the medical physicists and were archived in a database.

Table 1. Patients' characteristics.

Procedures	Allura FD 20 (A1)			Azurion 7 M20 (A2)			Alphenix 4DCT (A3)		
	Number of Patients	Sex (F/M)	Age (Years)	Number of Patients	Sex (F/M)	Age (Years)	Number of Patients	Sex (F/M)	Age (Years)
AEE	203	58/145	60.4 ± 18.9	58	19/39	64.5 ± 17.7	-	-	-
AUE	123	38/85	66.5 ± 16.4	38	16/22	64.5 ± 17.3	-	-	-
GVE	156	32/124	36.4 ± 13.3	30	13/17	40.7 ± 13.1	-	-	-
RE	99	50/49	63.4 ± 18.0	25	6/19	67.7 ± 15.8	-	-	-
UEE	81	81/0	41.2 ± 12.4	18	18/0	46.9 ± 16.5	-	-	-
BE	44	9/35	61.9 ± 16.2	36	10/26	64.2 ± 15.9	-	-	-
UUE	60	60/0	31.8 ± 6.2	17	17/0	31.4 ± 7.8	-	-	-
HCE	158	22/136	70.3 ± 9.8	-	-	-	67	12/55	72.2 ± 9.6
PE	142	0/142	76.5 ± 10.1	-	-	-	47	0/47	76.5 ± 12.1
RaE	23	1/22	70.6 ± 6.8	-	-	-	24	10/14	66.8 ± 10.9
Total	1089	351/738	58.7 ± 20.2	222	99/123	57.6 ± 19.7	138	22/116	72.7 ± 11.2

Age values are expressed as means ± standard deviations. AEE: abdominal elective embolizations for tumors and visceral aneurysms; AUE: abdominal urgent embolizations for active bleeding or vascular injuries of digestive arteries; BE: bronchial artery embolizations; HCE: hepatic chemoembolizatiosn; PE: pelvic embolizations for planned prostatic embolizations; RaE: radioembolisations; RE: renal artery embolizations; UEE: uterine elective embolizations for leiomyomas or vascular malformations; UUE: uterine urgent embolizations for postpartum hemorrhages; GVE: gonadal vein embolizations.

2.2. X-ray Sources

From August 2012 to September 2020, all embolization procedures were performed on the fixed C arm Allura® Xper FD 20 (Philips Healthcare Systems, Best, The Netherlands) system (A1). Since September 2020, the embolization procedures were performed on the fixed C-arm Azurion 7 M20 (Philips Healthcare Systems, Best, The Netherlands) system (A2) or on the Alphenix 4DCT (Canon Medical Systems, Otawara, Japan) system (A3), which combines a flat-panel Angio C-arm (Alphenix) and a CT unit (Aquilion One Genesis). Seven embolization procedures studied were preferentially performed using the A2 system (BE, AEE, AUE, RE, UEE, UUE and GVE) and the three others preferentially using the A3 system (HCE, PE and RaE).

For the two Philips systems, the pulsed fluoroscopy mode (7.5 pulses) with an additional filtration of 0.9 mm Cu and 0.1 mm for the Al system were used. Digital subtraction angiography images were used for all embolization procedures with a frame rate of 2 or 3 frames according to the procedure performed and an additional filtration of 0.1 mm Cu and 0.1 mm for the Al system. Cone-beam CT acquisition was used for all PEs but not for the other procedures.

For the C-arm of the 4DCT, the low-pulsed fluoroscopy mode (5 or 7.5 pulses) and the additional filtration were used (from 0.2 to 0.5 mm Cu) depending on the procedure type, the difficulties encountered and the operator. For all embolization procedures, digital subtraction angiography images were used at a 3-frames rate and an additional 0.2 mm-Cu filtration. CT acquisitions were usually performed during the procedure to assess the proper vascular targeting of the embolization. CT acquisitions were initially performed for planning, guidance or post-embolization control [15,22].

For the A1 and A2 systems, the detector was rectangular with a diagonal length of 48 cm while in A3, the diagonal length was 40 cm. Eight electronic zooms were available in A1 and A2 (diagonals of 48/42/37/31/27/22/19/15 cm) and six in A3 (diagonals of 40/30/20/15/11/8 cm).

For the A1 and A2 systems, the AK was measured in air at a distance of 66 cm from the X-ray tube. For A3, the AK was measured in air at 55 cm from the X-ray tube but took into account the table and mattress attenuation. To compare the AK of the different systems, for A3, AK was corrected to be obtained at a 66-cm distance from the X-ray tube (correction factor of 0.694) and its measurement was performed in the air without taking into account the table and mattress attenuation (correction factor of 1.225).

The average field size during each procedure was calculated as the ratio of the total DAP to the total AK (in air at 66 cm from the X-ray tube). The proportion of fluoroscopy in the total dose was also calculated as the ratio of fluoroscopy DAP to total DAP.

2.3. Statistical Analysis

Statistical analyses were performed using the 3.5.1 version of R (R Core Team (2017); R: A language and environment for statistical computing; R Foundation for Statistical Computing, Vienna, Austria). For all quantitative data, normality was tested using the Shapiro–Wilk test. Data are presented as means and standard deviations or medians and 1st and 3rd quartiles, according to the variable statistical distribution.

The comparison of dosimetric indicators between the A1 and A2 systems was performed for the following embolization procedures: BE, AEE, AUE, RE, UEE, UUE and GVE, and for HCE, PE and RaE for the comparison between the A1 and A3 systems. The comparison between all dosimetric indicators was performed using the paired Mann–Whitney–Wilcoxon test. A p-value less than 0.05 was considered significant.

3. Results

3.1. Patients

During the study period, 1449 procedures were performed. There were 472 women and 977 men, of mean age 59.9 ± 19.9 (SD) (range: 18.0–99.8) years old (Table 1). A total of 1089 embolization procedures of all 10 procedure types were performed with the A1 system, 222 embolization procedures were performed with the A2 system, including 7 types of procedures (BE, AEE, AUE, RE, UEE, UUE and GVE), and 138 procedures of 3 different types (HCE, PE, and RaE) were performed with the A3 system. No adult patients objected to their participation in the study but 26 pediatric patients were excluded.

3.2. Comparison of the Dosimetric Indicators between the Allura FD 20 (A1) and the Azurion 7 M20 (A2) Systems

The dosimetric indicator values obtained with the A1 and A2 systems for the 7 embolization procedures performed with A2 are depicted in Table 2. The DAP values were significantly lower with A2 compared to A1 for all procedures ($p < 0.05$), except for GVE and UEE. For these two procedures, the differences between the medians were −32% for GVE ($p = 0.09$) and −26% for UEE ($p = 0.481$) while they were on average of −50% ± 5% for the 5 other procedures. AK values were lower with A2 compared to A1 for all procedures ($p < 0.05$), except for UUE ($p = 0.224$). The average difference between the medians for the 6 procedures were −56% ± 8% but −23% for UEE. The average field size was higher with A2 than with A1 (Figure 1A).

Table 2. Comparison of the dosimetric indicators between the Allura FD20 (A1) and Azurion 7 M20 (A2) C-arms systems for 7 embolization procedures.

Procedures	Dosimetric Indicators	Allura FD20 (A1)	Azurion 7 M20 (A2)	p-Values
AEE	Dose Area Product (Gy.cm^2)	110.9 (54.6; 186.4)	48 (29.3; 85.9)	***p < 0.001***
	Air Kerma (mGy)	510 (264; 959)	207 (130; 337)	***p < 0.001***
	Fluoroscopy Time (min)	17 (11; 28)	17 (11; 23)	0.676
	Number of graphy images	133 (84; 246)	109 (70; 190)	0.063
AUE	Dose Area Product (Gy.cm^2)	126.0 (65.2; 238.9)	61.3 (36.5; 103.4)	***p < 0.001***
	Air Kerma (mGy)	566 (278; 1097)	216 (132; 375)	***p < 0.001***
	Fluoroscopy Time (min)	19 (9; 29)	17 (12; 27)	0.550
	Number of graphy images	157 (93; 330)	148 (88; 216)	0.316

Table 2. Cont.

Procedures	Dosimetric Indicators	Allura FD20 (A1)	Azurion 7 M20 (A2)	p-Values
GVE	Dose Area Product (Gy.cm^2)	31.4 (20.1; 63.2)	21.5 (14.3; 52.5)	0.09
	Air Kerma (mGy)	141 (87; 258)	66 (36; 105)	***p < 0.001***
	Fluoroscopy Time (min)	16 (11; 24)	29 (20; 38)	***p < 0.001***
	Number of graphy images	41 (22; 77)	66 (35; 107)	0.153
RE	Dose Area Product (Gy.cm^2)	83.8 (41.7; 125.2)	42.8 (35.5; 98.3)	***0.019***
	Air Kerma (mGy)	461 (273; 808)	207 (148; 381)	***0.001***
	Fluoroscopy Time (min)	17 (11; 25)	16 (8; 22)	0.542
	Number of graphy images	151 (91; 223)	105 (73; 182)	0.166
UEE	Dose Area Product (Gy.cm^2)	92.1 (49; 161.9)	68.1 (35.5; 158.6)	0.481
	Air Kerma (mGy)	417 (239; 862)	319 (189; 661)	0.224
	Fluoroscopy Time (min)	17 (11; 27)	30 (20; 43)	***0.001***
	Number of graphy images	112 (79; 208)	186 (133; 313)	***0.022***
BE	Dose Area Product (Gy.cm^2)	49.4 (29.9; 79.6)	29.7 (20.5; 47.3)	***0.010***
	Air Kerma (mGy)	288 (148; 478)	166 (114; 235)	***0.012***
	Fluoroscopy Time (min)	24 (17; 40)	31 (21; 43)	0.319
	Number of graphy images	131 (93; 196)	128 (101; 252)	0.315
UUE	Dose Area Product (Gy.cm^2)	166.9 (86.3; 273.4)	80.3 (51.8; 130.4)	***0.009***
	Air Kerma (mGy)	710 (423; 1092)	249 (161; 497)	***0.002***
	Fluoroscopy Time (min)	14 (9; 22)	18 (9; 24)	0.815
	Number of graphy images	108 (59; 182)	175 (121; 260)	***0.032***

p-values in bold italics are significant p-values (<0.05). AEE: abdominal elective embolizations for tumors and visceral aneurysms; AUE: abdominal urgent embolizations for active bleedings or vascular injuries of digestive arteries; BE: bronchial artery embolizations; RE: renal artery embolizations; UEE: uterine elective embolizations for leiomyomas or vascular malformations; UUE: uterine urgent embolizations for postpartum hemorrhages; GVE: gonadal vein embolization.

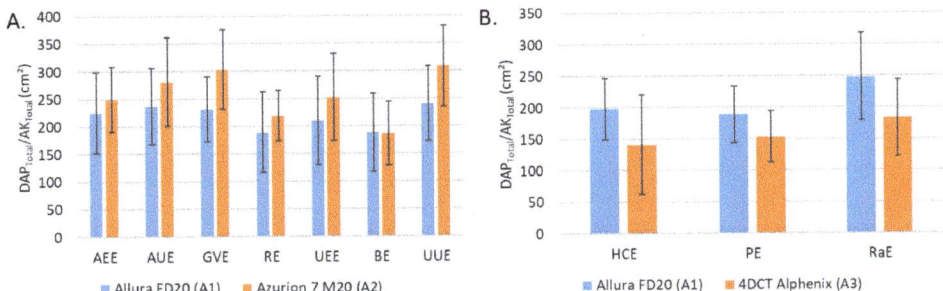

Figure 1. Average field size corresponding to the total dose area product (DAP) on total air kerma at 66 cm ratio (**A**) between Allura FD20 (A1) and Azurion 7 M20 (A2) for 7 embolization procedures and (**B**) between Allura FD20 (A1) and 4DCT Alphenix (A3) for 3 embolization procedures (**B**). Values are expressed as means ± standard deviations (error bars). DAP: dose area product; AK: air kerma; AEE: abdominal elective embolizations for tumors and visceral aneurysms; AUE: abdominal urgent embolizations for active bleedings or vascular injuries of digestive arteries; BE: bronchial artery embolizations; HCE: hepatic chemoembolizations; PE: pelvic embolizations for planned prostatic embolizations; RaE: radioembolisations; RE: renal artery embolizations; UEE: uterine elective embolizations for leiomyomas or vascular malformations; UUE: uterine urgent embolizations for postpartum hemorrhages; GVE: gonadal vein embolization.

For the fluoroscopy time, similar values were found between the A1 and A2 systems for AEE, AUE and RE. FT were higher with A2 compared to A1 for the other 4 procedures with significant differences for GVE ($p < 0.001$) and UEE ($p = 0.001$).

The number of fluorographies was significantly lower with A2 compared to A1 for AEE, AUE and RE but the opposite for the other embolization procedures (GVE, UEE, BE and UUE). The differences were significant for UEE ($p = 0.022$) and UUE ($p = 0.032$). The proportion scopy DAP in the total DAP was greater with A2 than with A1 (Figure 2A).

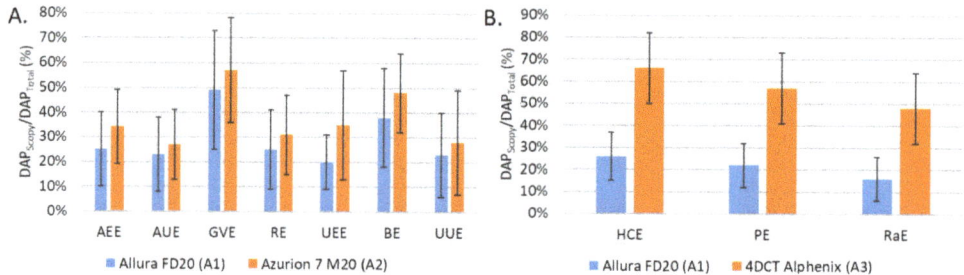

Figure 2. Comparison of the fluoroscopy dose area product (DAP) to total DAP ratio (**A**) between the Allura FD20 (A1) and Azurion 7 M20 (A2) systems for 7 embolization procedures and (**B**) between the Allura FD20 (A2) and 4DCT Alphenix (A3) systems for 3 embolization procedures. Values are expressed as means ± standard deviations (error bars). DAP: dose area product; AEE: abdominal elective embolizations for tumors and visceral aneurysms; AUE: abdominal urgent embolizations for active bleedings or vascular injuries of digestive arteries; BE: bronchial artery embolizations; HCE: hepatic chemoembolizations; PE: pelvic embolizations for planned prostatic embolizations; RaE: radioembolisations; RE: renal artery embolizations; UEE: uterine elective embolizations for leiomyomas or vascular malformations; UUE: uterine urgent embolizations for postpartum hemorrhages; GVE: gonadal vein embolization.

3.3. Comparison of the Dosimetric Indicators between the Allura FD20 (A1) and the 4DCT Alphenix (A3) Systems

The dosimetric indicator values obtained with the A1 and A3 systems for HCE, PE and RaE procedures are depicted in Table 3. The DAP values were significantly lower with A3 than with A1 ($p < 0.001$). The corrected AK with the A3 system were significantly lower than with A1 for PE and RaE ($p < 0.001$) but the opposite for HCE ($p = 0.827$). The average field size was lower with A3 compared with A1, 120 ± 67 cm^2 vs. 198 ± 49 cm^2 for HCE, 130 ± 35 cm^2 vs. 189 ± 45 cm^2 for PE, 156 ± 52 cm^2 vs. 248 ± 69 cm^2 for RaE (Figure 1B).

Table 3. Comparison of the dosimetric indicators between the Allura FD20 (A1) and 4DCT Alphenix (A3) C-arms systems for 3 embolization procedures.

Procedures	Dosimetric Indicators	Allura FD20 (A1)	Alphenix 4DCT (A3)	*p*-Values
HCE	Dose Area Product (Gy.cm^2)	126.9 (72.7; 188.6)	91.4 (44; 127.5)	*p < 0.001*
	Air Kerma (mGy)	672 (365; 1074)	**699 (391; 1005)**	0.827
	Fluoroscopy Time (min)	24 (16; 34)	37 (26; 48)	*p < 0.001*
	Number of graphy images	403 (144; 760)	80 (58; 139)	*p < 0.001*
	Dose Length Product (mGy.cm) ($n = 61$)	-	267 (185; 629)	-
PE	Dose Area Product (Gy.cm^2)	239.1 (135.1; 322.7)	134.1 (96.2; 161.7)	*p < 0.001*
	Air Kerma (mGy)	1314 (735; 1849)	**874 (629; 1306)**	0.012
	Fluoroscopy Time (min)	43 (30; 54)	50 (40; 60)	0.024
	Number of graphy images	1018 (638; 1345)	191 (155; 280)	*p < 0.001*
	Dose Length Product (mGy.cm) ($n = 43$)	-	228 (139; 392)	-
RaE	Dose Area Product (Gy.cm^2)	103.4 (78; 156.4)	36.6 (19.1; 56.1)	*p < 0.001*
	Air Kerma (mGy)	498 (305; 657)	**258 (130; 319)**	0.001
	Fluoroscopy Time (min)	11 (8; 20)	20 (12; 25)	0.140
	Number of graphy images	783 (662; 1067)	83 (48; 114)	*p < 0.001*
	Dose Length Product (mGy.cm) ($n = 21$)	-	282 (189; 530)	-

HCE: Hepatic chemoembolizations; PE: Pelvic embolizations for planned prostatic embolizations; RaE: Radioembolisations.

The fluoroscopy time was higher with A3 than with A1 for the 3 procedures and the differences were significant for HCE ($p < 0.001$) and PE ($p = 0.024$). The number of graphy images was significantly lower with A3 than with A1 for all procedures. The proportion was higher for A2 than for A1 (Figure 1B).

With the A3 system, the CT-scan was used for 91% of HCE and PE procedures and 88% for RaE (Table 4). The median DLP were 267 (185; 629) mGy.cm for HCE, 228 (139; 392) mGy.cm for PE and 282 (189; 530) mGy.cm for RaE. The median number of CT acquisitions were 3 (2; 4) for HCE, 3 (2; 3) for PE and 2 (2; 4) for RaE.

Table 4. Dose length product and number of CT acquisitions.

Dosimetric Indicators	HCE	PE	RaE
Number of embolizations	67	47	24
Number of procedures	61	43	21
Dose Length Product (mGy.cm)	267 (185; 629)	228 (139; 392)	282 (189; 530)
Number of CT acquisitions	3 (2; 4)	3 (2; 3)	2 (2; 4)

HCE: hepatic chemoembolizations; PE: pelvic embolizations for planned prostatic embolizations; RaE: radioembolisations.

The proportion of CT acquisition types for the three embolization procedures studied are depicted in Figure 3. Volumic CT acquisitions represented 65% of the total CT acquisitions for HCE, 44% for PE and 52% for RaE. Perfusion CT acquisitions were used for HCE (1%) and PE (9%).

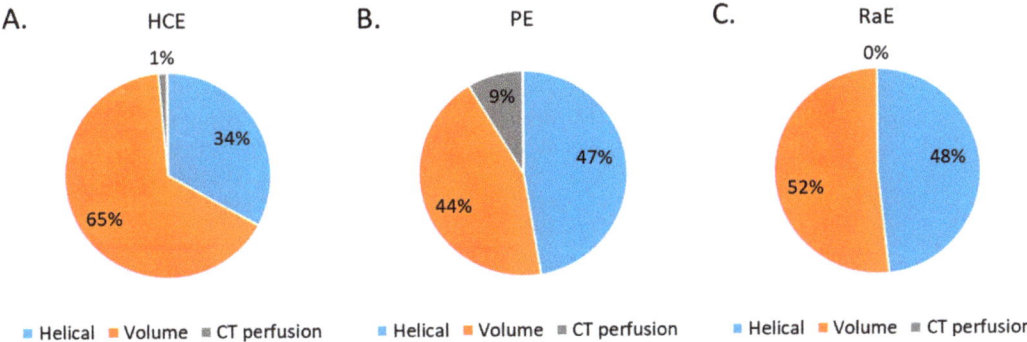

Figure 3. Percentage of CT acquisition types for all 3 embolization procedures. (**A**) HCE: hepatic chemoembolizations; (**B**) PE: pelvic embolizations for planned prostatic embolizations; (**C**) RaE: radioembolisations.

3.4. Comparison of the Dosimetric Indicators with the Litterature

The dosimetric indicator values for the 5 embolization procedures studied (BE, UEE, UUE, RE, HCE) were lower than the proposed DRL, except for the fluoroscopic time of BE with A2 and that of HCE with A3, and for the number of graph images of HCE with A3 (Table 5).

Table 5. Comparison of dosimetric indicators with the reference levels proposed by Etard et al. [10].

Dosimetric Indicators	Systems	BE	UEE	UUE	RE	HCE
Dose Area Product (Gy.cm^2)	Allura FD 20 (A1)	49	92	167	84	127
	Azurion 7 M20 (A2)	30	68	80	43	-
	4DCT Alphenix (A3)	-	-	-	-	91
	DRL	135	175	255	325	250
Air Kerma (mGy)	Allura FD 20 (A1)	288	417	710	461	672
	Azurion 7 M20 (A2)	166	319	249	207	-
	4DCT Alphenix (A3)	-	-	-	-	699
	DRL	830	800	930	1700	990

Table 5. *Cont.*

Dosimetric Indicators	Systems	BE	UEE	UUE	RE	HCE
Fluoroscopy time (min)	Allura FD 20 (A1)	24	17	14	17	24
	Azurion 7 M20 (A2)	31	30	18	16	-
	4DCT Alphenix (A3)	-	-	-	-	37
	DRL	38	29	25	22	28
Number of graphy images	Allura FD 20 (A1)	131	112	108	151	403
	Azurion 7 M20 (A2)	128	186	175	105	-
	4DCT Alphenix (A3)	-	-	-	-	80
	DRL	240	160	260	210	200

BE: bronchial artery embolizations; RE: renal artery embolizations; UEE: uterine embolizations for leiomyomas or vascular malformations; UUE: uterine urgent embolizations for postpartum hemorrhages; HCE: hepatic chemoembolizations. DRL: dose reference levels proposed by Etard et al. corresponding to the third quartile rounded to the nearest integer [10].

4. Discussion

A retrospective analysis of the doses delivered during 1449 thoracic, abdominal and/or pelvic embolization procedures was performed over a 10-year period during which three IR systems were used. The doses delivered in an older and a newer version of the IR system were compared. The contribution of CT in a multimodal room equipped with a scanner and a fixed C-arm was also compared to the older IR system.

The results of this study showed that the dosimetric indicator values collected for 7 embolization procedures were lower with the Azurion 7 M20 system (newer version) than with the Allura FD20 system (older version). AK values measured at the same interventional reference point were lower for the 7 embolization procedures studied. These differences were not related to differences in additional filtration or cadence for scopy (pulses/s) and graphy (images/s) as the same values were used with the two IR systems. They were directly related to the use of the ClarityIQ technology available in the new IR system. This technology was shown to reduce the image noise that improves image quality, and therefore reduces the dose while keeping the same image quality [16–20]. In this study, we found that the ClarityIQ technology reduced the AK by an average of 52% (24–65%), and the DAP to a lesser extent. Similar outcomes were found for AK reductions in different studies on uterine fibroid embolizations [16,18,19], bronchial artery embolization [20] and transarterial chemoembolization [17]. However, the reductions in DAP were smaller than those found in these studies [16–20]. This can be explained by the fact that the DAP variation was related to the increase in mean field size values, which may be related to the new service organization replacing a single room by two newly equipped rooms. Indeed, the room with the C-arm alone, which was mainly dedicated to the emergency embolizations and short-term endovascular procedures, was mostly used by junior radiologists (fellows and trainees). The complex and time-consuming procedures were usually performed in the 4DCT room by the senior radiologists. In the older IR room, the procedures were performed by both junior and senior radiologists. Junior radiologists often tend to use larger fields of exposure and increase the number of X-ray control, which resulted in an increased number of graphy images and a longer fluoroscopy time. This was reported for BE, UEE, UUE and GVE procedures while the other studies found similar or decreased fluoroscopy times using a C-arm system equipped with the ClarityIQ technology [16–18]. Training junior radiologists to good patient radiation protection practices is therefore essential to harmonize and improve practices, and thus reduce the doses delivered to the patients. Furthermore, the DAP and AK values obtained in this study for these two IR systems were lower than the national DRL values [10], which shows that the practices in our institution were already optimized [14] and were even more so with the arrival of this new IR system. Last, the median DAP values of UEE and BE for both C-arm systems used in our study were lower than the DAP values found in the literature [16,18–20]. For these procedures, our fluoroscopy times were within the range of those found in these studies [16,18,20].

The variations in dosimetric indicators obtained between the older IR system and the 4DCT room depended on the procedure performed. The AK values were lower with the 4DCT than with the older IR system for PE and RaE procedures but for HCE AK values were slightly higher with the 4DCT. These results are directly related to the use of CT acquisitions during the procedure, which changes patient management. For PE and RaE procedures, the helical and volume angiographic CT acquisitions were performed at the beginning, during and at the end of the procedure. These images provide a more accurate anatomy and a 3D artery volume, which could be merged with the IR images to improve treatment planning and simplify the procedure. Conversely, for HCE procedures, the use of CT angiography allows the treatment of several targets that could not be treated with standard IR systems and CBCT acquisitions. An ancillary study could be carried out to correlate the AK values with the number of targets treated. Additionally, the use of CT during the procedure changed the operators' practices. Compared to the older IR system, the fluoroscopy times were increased but the number of graphy images were significantly reduced. The radiologists do their planning under CT and their follow-up with fluoroscopy with a sufficient and adapted image quality. This reduces the radiologist's need for digital subtraction angiography acquisitions, which significantly reduces the number of graphy images. It should also be noted that the average field size was reduced using the Alphenix C-arm. In contrast to Azurion 7 M20, the most complex procedures were performed in the 4DCT system with the help of CT and were performed by senior radiologists who were more aware of the good practices. The AK and DAP values obtained for HCE were lower than the national DRL values [10]. However, the DAP, AK and fluoroscopy time values were higher in our study than those found by Piron et al. [15] for HCE. Although this result may be explained by the differences in the complexity of the procedures and the number of targets treated (not evaluated in this study), optimization of the procedure is required to be implemented in our 4DCT system to reduce the dose delivered to patients. Additionally, the dose reduction tools proposed by Canon "Live Zoom" and "Spot fluoro" were rarely used in the 4DCT room whereas they were used for all HCE procedures in the Piron et al. study [15]. Awareness of the use of these tools in the 4DCT room should be performed by the interventional radiologists. On the other hand, the DLP values found in our study were lower than those found by Piron et al. [15]. This result may be linked to the use of a deep-learning image reconstruction algorithm (AiCE) in our CT system compared to the iterative reconstruction algorithm (AIDR 3D) used in their study [24]. Indeed, this new algorithm was shown to improve the image quality and have a high potential for dose reduction compared to the iterative reconstruction algorithm.

This study has some limitations. It reflects the practices of a single center, with a 10-year experience of thorough optimization processes and the presence of two medical physicists. As the two new IR systems were installed in September 2020, the patient samples may be different from the older IR system. However, the number of patients was sufficient to perform a statistical analysis. In addition, this study only focused on the dosimetric indicators; clinical factors were not taken into account. Another limitation is that the experience of the operators was only indirectly taken into account in the study of the new organization with two new rooms dedicated to the junior and senior radiologists, unlike the older room. The 4DCT, with its much higher anatomical precision, allows carrying out more complex procedures which should impact the dose received by the patients [25]. Furthermore, we did not evaluate the differences in image quality between the different rooms for the different procedures studied. Also, the acquisition protocols were defined by the medical physicist and the application engineer and the resulting image quality was validated by the interventional radiologists in each room. However, for some patients and some complex procedures, the image quality proposed may not have been sufficient and adapted, especially in scopy, which may explain the higher scopy time in the 4DCT room. Further targeted studies will be carried out to validate the image quality. Last, ancillary studies may now be performed to correlate the dose indicators with the number of targets or with the type of arteries/veins or organs treated.

5. Conclusions

This monocentric retrospective analysis of the doses delivered during thoracic, abdominal and pelvic embolization procedures over a 10-year period showed the contribution of the new IR tools in dose reduction and patient management. The last C-arm technology reduced the image noise and improved image quality, allowing a 50% reduction of the air kerma and showing a significant dose reduction. The implementation of a CT scan inside the IR room allowed a more precise 3D guidance without increasing the dose delivered to the patients.

Author Contributions: Conceptualization, J.G. (Joël Greffier) and J.F.; methodology, J.G. (Joël Greffier), D.D. and J.F.; validation, J.G. (Joël Greffier) and J.F.; formal analysis, J.G. (Joël Greffier) and J.F.; investigation, J.G. (Joël Greffier) and J.F.; resources, J.-P.B. and J.F.; data curation, J.G. (Joël Greffier), D.D. and J.F.; writing—original draft preparation, J.G. (Joël Greffier) and J.F.; writing—review and editing, all authors; visualization, J.G. (Jean Goupil), T.K., G.T.B., L.B., J.F. and J.-P.B.; supervision, J.F. and J.-P.B.; project administration, J.-P.B. and J.F.; funding acquisition, no funding. All authors have read and agreed to the published version of the manuscript.

Funding: This research received no external funding.

Institutional Review Board Statement: The study was conducted in accordance with the Declaration of Helsinki, and approved by the Institutional Review Board of the Nîmes University Hospital (number 22.04.03, approved on 22 April 2022).

Informed Consent Statement: Patient consent was waived due to the retrospective character of the study. According to the current national regulation, patients (or their legal guardian when necessary) were systematically informed that their data were collected for an anonymous retrospective study and could refuse at any time to participate in the study (non-opposition statement).

Data Availability Statement: The data presented in this study are available on request from the corresponding author.

Acknowledgments: The authors would like to thank Hélène de Forges for her help in writing and editing the manuscript.

Conflicts of Interest: The authors declare no conflict of interest.

References

1. Szemitko, M.; Golubinska-Szemitko, E.; Warakomski, M.; Falkowski, A. Evaluation of CRC-Metastatic Hepatic Lesion Chemoembolization with Irinotecan-Loaded Microspheres, According to the Site of Embolization. *J. Pers. Med.* **2022**, *12*, 414. [CrossRef] [PubMed]
2. Talaie, R.; Torkian, P.; Moghadam, A.D.; Tradi, F.; Vidal, V.; Sapoval, M.; Golzarian, J. Hemorrhoid embolization: A review of current evidences. *Diagn. Interv. Imaging* **2022**, *103*, 3–11. [CrossRef] [PubMed]
3. Chevallier, O.; Comby, P.O.; Guillen, K.; Pellegrinelli, J.; Mouillot, T.; Falvo, N.; Bardou, M.; Midulla, M.; Aho-Glele, S.; Loffroy, R. Efficacy, safety and outcomes of transcatheter arterial embolization with N-butyl cyanoacrylate glue for non-variceal gastrointestinal bleeding: A systematic review and meta-analysis. *Diagn. Interv. Imaging* **2021**, *102*, 479–487. [CrossRef]
4. Young, S. Prostate artery embolization for benign prostatic hyperplasia: The hunt for the ideal patient population. *Diagn. Interv. Imaging* **2021**, *102*, 119–120. [CrossRef]
5. Balter, S.; Hopewell, J.W.; Miller, D.L.; Wagner, L.K.; Zelefsky, M.J. Fluoroscopically guided interventional procedures: A review of radiation effects on patients' skin and hair. *Radiology* **2010**, *254*, 326–341. [CrossRef] [PubMed]
6. Koenig, T.R.; Wolff, D.; Mettler, F.A.; Wagner, L.K. Skin injuries from fluoroscopically guided procedures: Part 1, characteristics of radiation injury. *AJR Am. J. Roentgenol.* **2001**, *177*, 3–11. [CrossRef] [PubMed]
7. Miller, D.L.; Balter, S.; Cole, P.E.; Lu, H.T.; Berenstein, A.; Albert, R.; Schueler, B.A.; Georgia, J.D.; Noonan, P.T.; Russell, E.J.; et al. Radiation doses in interventional radiology procedures: The RAD-IR study: Part II: Skin dose. *J. Vasc. Interv. Radiol.* **2003**, *14*, 977–990. [CrossRef] [PubMed]
8. Valentin, J. Avoidance of radiation injuries from medical interventional procedures. *Ann. ICRP* **2000**, *30*, 7–67. [CrossRef]
9. Pearce, M.S.; Salotti, J.A.; Little, M.P.; McHugh, K.; Lee, C.; Kim, K.P.; Howe, N.L.; Ronckers, C.M.; Rajaraman, P.; Sir Craft, A.W.; et al. Radiation exposure from CT scans in childhood and subsequent risk of leukaemia and brain tumours: A retrospective cohort study. *Lancet* **2012**, *380*, 499–505. [CrossRef]
10. Etard, C.; Bigand, E.; Salvat, C.; Vidal, V.; Beregi, J.P.; Hornbeck, A.; Greffier, J. Patient dose in interventional radiology: A multicentre study of the most frequent procedures in France. *Eur. Radiol.* **2017**, *27*, 4281–4290. [CrossRef] [PubMed]

11. ICRP Publication 103: The 2007 Recommendations of the International Commission on Radiological Protection. *Ann. ICRP* **2007**, *37*, 1–332.
12. Stecker, M.S.; Balter, S.; Towbin, R.B.; Miller, D.L.; Vano, E.; Bartal, G.; Angle, J.F.; Chao, C.P.; Cohen, A.M.; Dixon, R.G.; et al. Guidelines for patient radiation dose management. *J. Vasc. Interv. Radiol.* **2009**, *20*, S263–S273. [CrossRef] [PubMed]
13. Miller, D.L.; Balter, S.; Schueler, B.A.; Wagner, L.K.; Strauss, K.J.; Vano, E. Clinical radiation management for fluoroscopically guided interventional procedures. *Radiology* **2010**, *257*, 321–332. [CrossRef] [PubMed]
14. Greffier, J.; Goupil, J.; Larbi, A.; Stefanovic, X.; Pereira, F.; Moliner, G.; Ovtchinnikoff, S.; Beregi, J.P.; Frandon, J. Assessment of patient's peak skin dose during abdominopelvic embolization using radiochromic (Gafchromic) films. *Diagn. Interv. Imaging* **2018**, *99*, 321–329. [CrossRef]
15. Piron, L.; Le Roy, J.; Cassinotto, C.; Delicque, J.; Belgour, A.; Allimant, C.; Beregi, J.P.; Greffier, J.; Molinari, N.; Guiu, B. Radiation Exposure During Transarterial Chemoembolization: Angio-CT Versus Cone-Beam CT. *Cardiovasc. Interv. Radiol.* **2019**, *42*, 1609–1618. [CrossRef] [PubMed]
16. Schernthaner, R.E.; Haroun, R.R.; Nguyen, S.; Duran, R.; Sohn, J.H.; Sahu, S.; Chapiro, J.; Zhao, Y.; Radaelli, A.; van der Bom, I.M.; et al. Characteristics of a New X-ray Imaging System for Interventional Procedures: Improved Image Quality and Reduced Radiation Dose. *Cardiovasc. Interv. Radiol.* **2018**, *41*, 502–508. [CrossRef]
17. Schernthaner, R.E.; Duran, R.; Chapiro, J.; Wang, Z.; Geschwind, J.F.; Lin, M. A new angiographic imaging platform reduces radiation exposure for patients with liver cancer treated with transarterial chemoembolization. *Eur. Radiol.* **2015**, *25*, 3255–3262. [CrossRef]
18. Kohlbrenner, R.; Kolli, K.P.; Taylor, A.G.; Kohi, M.P.; Lehrman, E.D.; Fidelman, N.; Conrad, M.; LaBerge, J.M.; Kerlan, R.K.; Gould, R. Radiation Dose Reduction during Uterine Fibroid Embolization Using an Optimized Imaging Platform. *J. Vasc. Interv. Radiol.* **2017**, *28*, 1129–1135 e1121. [CrossRef]
19. Thomaere, E.; Dehairs, M.; Laenen, A.; Mehrsima, A.; Timmerman, D.; Cornelissen, S.; Op de Beeck, K.; Bosmans, H.; Maleux, G. A new imaging technology to reduce the radiation dose during uterine fibroid embolization. *Acta Radiol.* **2018**, *59*, 1446–1450. [CrossRef]
20. Spink, C.; Avanesov, M.; Schmidt, T.; Grass, M.; Schoen, G.; Adam, G.; Koops, A.; Ittrich, H.; Bannas, P. Noise reduction angiographic imaging technology reduces radiation dose during bronchial artery embolization. *Eur. J. Radiol.* **2017**, *97*, 115–118. [CrossRef]
21. Spink, C.; Avanesov, M.; Schmidt, T.; Grass, M.; Schoen, G.; Adam, G.; Bannas, P.; Koops, A. Radiation dose reduction during transjugular intrahepatic portosystemic shunt implantation using a new imaging technology. *Eur. J. Radiol.* **2017**, *86*, 284–288. [CrossRef]
22. Greffier, J.; Belaouni, A.; Dabli, D.; Goupil, J.; Perolat, R.; Akessoul, P.; Kammoun, T.; Hoballah, A.; Beregi, J.P.; Frandon, J. Comparison of peak skin dose and dose map obtained with real-time software and radiochromic films in patients undergoing abdominopelvic embolization. *Diagn. Interv. Imaging* **2022**, *103*, 338–344. [CrossRef]
23. Greffier, J.; Grussenmeyer-Mary, N.; Hamard, A.; Goupil, J.; Miller, D.E.; Cayla, G.; Ledermann, B.; Demattei, C.; Beregi, J.P.; Frandon, J. Clinical evaluation of a dose management system-integrated 3D skin dose map by comparison with radiochromic films. *Eur. Radiol.* **2020**, *30*, 5071–5081. [CrossRef]
24. Greffier, J.; Dabli, D.; Frandon, J.; Hamard, A.; Belaouni, A.; Akessoul, P.; Fuamba, Y.; Le Roy, J.; Guiu, B.; Beregi, J.P. Comparison of two versions of a deep learning image reconstruction algorithm on CT image quality and dose reduction: A phantom study. *Med. Phys.* **2021**, *48*, 5743–5755. [CrossRef]
25. Schembri, V.; Piron, L.; Le Roy, J.; Hermida, M.; Lonjon, J.; Escal, L.; Pierredon, M.A.; Belgour, A.; Cassinotto, C.; Guiu, B. Percutaneous ablation of obscure hypovascular liver tumours in challenging locations using arterial CT-portography guidance. *Diagn. Interv. Imaging* **2020**, *101*, 707–713. [CrossRef]

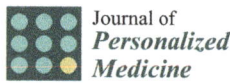

Article

Transarterial Embolization for Active Gastrointestinal Bleeding: Predictors of Early Mortality and Early Rebleeding

Chloé Extrat [1], Sylvain Grange [1], Alexandre Mayaud [1], Loïc Villeneuve [1], Clément Chevalier [1], Nicolas Williet [2], Bertrand Le Roy [3], Claire Boutet [1] and Rémi Grange [1,*]

[1] Department of Radiology, University Hospital of Saint-Etienne, 42270 Saint-Priest-en-Jarez, France
[2] Department of Gastro-Enterology, University Hospital of Saint-Etienne, 42270 Saint-Priest-en-Jarez, France
[3] Department of Oncologic and Digestive Surgery, University Hospital of Saint-Etienne, 42270 Saint-Priest-en-Jarez, France
* Correspondence: remgrange1@gmail.com

Abstract: Background: The aim of this study was to determine predictive factors of early mortality and early rebleeding (≤30 days) following transarterial embolization (TAE) for treatment of acute gastrointestinal bleeding. Methods: All consecutive patients admitted for acute gastrointestinal bleeding to the interventional radiology department in a tertiary center between January 2012 and January 2022 were included. Exclusion criteria were patients: (1) aged < 18-year-old, (2) referred to the operation room without TAE, (3) treated for hemobilia, (4) with mesenteric hematoma, (5) lost to follow-up within 30 days after the procedure. We evaluated pre and per-procedure clinical data, biological data, outcomes, and complications. Results: Sixty-eight patients were included: 55 (80.9%) experienced upper gastrointestinal bleeding and 13 (19.1%) lower gastrointestinal bleeding. Median age was 69 (61–74) years. There were 49 (72%) males. Median hemoglobin was 7.25 (6.1–8.3) g/dL. There were 30 (50%) ulcers. Coils were used in 46 (67.6%) procedures. Early mortality was 15 (22.1%) and early rebleeding was 17 (25%). In multivariate analysis, hyperlactatemia (≥2 mmol/L) were predictive of early mortality (≤30 days). A high number of red blood cells units was associated with early rebleeding. Conclusion: This study identified some predictive factors of 30-day mortality and early rebleeding following TAE. This will assist in patient selection and may help improve the management of gastrointestinal bleeding.

Keywords: gastrointestinal bleeding; embolization; rebleeding; mortality; lactate

Citation: Extrat, C.; Grange, S.; Mayaud, A.; Villeneuve, L.; Chevalier, C.; Williet, N.; Le Roy, B.; Boutet, C.; Grange, R. Transarterial Embolization for Active Gastrointestinal Bleeding: Predictors of Early Mortality and Early Rebleeding. J. Pers. Med. 2022, 12, 1856. https://doi.org/10.3390/jpm12111856

Academic Editors: Julien Frandon and Emilio González-Jiménez

Received: 10 August 2022
Accepted: 4 November 2022
Published: 7 November 2022

Publisher's Note: MDPI stays neutral with regard to jurisdictional claims in published maps and institutional affiliations.

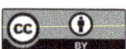

Copyright: © 2022 by the authors. Licensee MDPI, Basel, Switzerland. This article is an open access article distributed under the terms and conditions of the Creative Commons Attribution (CC BY) license (https://creativecommons.org/licenses/by/4.0/).

1. Introduction

Acute gastrointestinal bleeding (GIB) is a clinical situation that can lead to significant mortality and morbidity without urgent care. Lower Gastrointestinal Bleeding (LGIB) originates downstream of the Treitz ligament, while Upper Gastrointestinal Bleeding (UGIB) originates upstream of the Treitz ligament. Despite advances in endoscopic hemostasis and adjuvant pharmacologic treatment, the hospital mortality rate from UGIB remains 10% and has not significantly improved over the past 50 years [1]. Although surgery is the historical treatment for GIB, it is associated with a high risk of complications and an estimated mortality of 10–30% [2]. Immediate endoscopy is the examination of choice for the diagnosis and treatment of gastrointestinal bleeding and should not be delayed for more than 24 h following admission [3]. Rebleeding in UGIB occurs in 7–16% of cases despite endoscopic therapy [4].

In patients with clinical evidence of rebleeding following successful initial endoscopic hemostasis, the European Society of Gastroenterology recommends repeat upper endoscopy with hemostasis if indicated. In the case of failure of this second attempt at hemostasis, transarterial embolization (TAE) or surgery should be considered (strong recommendation, high-quality evidence) [5,6]. For LGIB, TAE should be reserved for the treatment of acute potentially life-threatening GIB in hemodynamically unstable patients or in patients not amenably treated by endoscopic interventions [5].

Studies on the efficacy of endovascular treatments have mainly focused on one location [7] or on a type of embolic agent [8,9] by assessing clinical success. Evaluation of prognostic factors is lacking. Additionally, few published series have analyzed factors predicting early death after TAE. In addition, studies on predictive factors of early rebleeding show contradictory results. Loffroy et al. reported that the use of coils in patients with coagulation disorders is associated with rebleeding [10]. Mohan et al. reported that patients with a history of malignancy were more likely to rebleed within 30 days and that younger patients (<60 years) were significantly less likely to experience rebleeding within 30 days [11]. Finally, the rate of rebleeding varies between the studies, from 13% [12] to 46.8% [11].

The aim of this monocentric retrospective study was to determine predictive factors of early mortality ($\leq$30 days) and early rebleeding ($\leq$30 days) following TAE in the treatment of acute GIB during a 10-year period.

2. Materials and Methods

2.1. Study Population

All of the patients referred to our hospital for GIB who were treated by TAE based on clinical decisions in emergency and CT scan between January 2012 and January 2022 were retrospectively reviewed. GIB was defined as intra luminal hemorrhage of the gastrointestinal tractus diagnosed by endoscopy and/or CT scan. Inclusion criteria were all patients with GIB who were treated by emergency TAE. Exclusion criteria were patients (1) aged < 18 years old, (2) referred to the operating room and who did not have TAE, (3) treated for hemobilia without associated GI lumen bleeding, (4) with isolated mesenteric hematoma, and (5) lost to follow-up within 30 days of the procedure.

2.2. Clinical Data

The following data were collected from electronic medical records. The patient demographics included age, gender, and comorbid conditions prior to TAE. Comorbid conditions included diabetes, coronaropathy, high blood pressure (HBP), chronic renal failure (CRF), active cancer, cancer in remission, and anticoagulation or antiplatelet treatments. Biological data included prior coagulopathy, lactate rate, transfusion requirements, and number of RBC units transfused. Imaging data included endoscopic or angiographic findings, causes of GIB, and CT findings (active bleeding, pseudoaneurysm, and location of bleeding).

Procedure data included angiographic findings, embolization material, vessel embolized, and duration of procedure. The post-procedure data included the occurrence of minor and major complications, rebleeding, type of management for rebleeding, length of hospitalization, hospital admission, length of hospitalization in an intensive care unit, and mortality.

2.3. Pre-Procedure

Pre-angiographic investigations sometimes involved an endoscopy performed at the onset of acute gastrointestinal bleeding. We therefore recorded the number of gastroscopies and colonoscopies performed before embolization. The endoscopy was considered positive if acute bleeding was observed. Endoscopic treatment was considered as a failure if active bleeding was not stopped.

Patients underwent an abdominal CT scan (SOMATOM DEFINITION AS 64, Siemens AG, Medical Solution, Erlangen, Germany). Patients received $\geq$90 mL contrast medium (Xenetix 350, Guerbet, Villepinte, France) with a flow rate $\geq$3 mL/s. Unenhanced and contrast-enhanced liver CT at the arterial and portal phases were performed according to the standard-of-care protocol of our hospital. A bleed was considered active when iodine contrast was present at the arterial phase and increased at the portal phase. Pseudoaneurysm was considered as a rupture of arterial caliber without an increase in the portal phase.

2.4. Transarterial Embolization Methods and Techniques

TAE procedures were performed by 1 of the 10 interventional radiologists whose experience ranged from 2 to 30 years after multidisciplinary consultation (surgeon, clinician, and radiologist). After local anesthesia with lidocaine, the right common femoral artery was accessed routinely. Celiac, superior mesenteric, and/or inferior mesenteric angiograms were performed to determine the focus of mesenteric injury using a 4F catheter and a hydrophilic guidewire (Terumo®, Tokyo, Japan). Supraselective catheterization was systematically performed using a 2.7F microcatheter (Progreat®, Terumo, Tokyo, Japan). TAE was performed under fluoroscopic monitoring using fibered microcoils (Interlock®, Boston Scientific, Marlborough, MA, USA), N-butyl-2-cyanoacrylate-NBCA (Glubran2®, GEM, Viareggio, Italy), gelatine sponge (Gelitaspon®, Gelita Medical, Amsterdam, Holland), or microparticles (Embosphere® Microspheres, BioSphere Medical, Rockland) depending on the vascular wound and at the discretion of the radiologist. After the procedure, complete angiograms were performed to confirm that bleeding had been successfully controlled.

When angiography remained negative despite active bleeding in CT scans or endoscopy, "empiric" TAE of the suspected bleeding artery was performed at the discretion of the interventional radiologist. No spasmolytic agents to reduce bowel peristaltic were administered, and no provocation test was conducted.

2.5. Patient Follow Up

After TAE, all the patients were closely monitored for clinical signs and symptoms suggestive of ischemic complications or recurrent bleeding until discharge or death. These clinical findings were supplemented by laboratory studies.

Patients' long-term outcomes, specifically incidence of rebleeding, mortality, and procedure-related complications, were collected from patient charts. CT follow-up and endoscopic examination were not routine practices performed following TAE in our unit.

2.6. Definitions

Technical success was defined as the cessation of angiographic extravasation immediately after TAE based on angiographic findings. Clinical success was defined as resolution of signs and symptoms of bleeding during the 30-day follow-up after TAE and without required endoscopic treatment, surgery, or repeat TAE or death related to massive blood loss during this period of time. Prior coagulopathy was defined as INR > 1.5, PT < 50%, or PC < 150 G/L. Acute renal failure was defined as a rapid and reversible decline in the glomerular filtration rate. Endoscopic treatment failure was defined as failure to stop bleeding or early recurrence within 48 h of endoscopy. The number of RBDs transfused was calculated from the day of embolization to 48 h after embolization.

Rebleeding events were classified as early events if they occurred ≤30 days following TAE and as late events if they occurred >30 days following TAE. Complications were defined as per operative complications if they occurred during TAE and as post-operative complications if they occurred during follow-up. Minor and major complications were separated using the CIRSE classification [13]. Grades I and II were considered minor complications, and grades III, IV, and V were considered major complications.

2.7. Outcomes

The primary endpoint of our study was to identify any predictors of early death (≤30 days) after TAE.

Secondary endpoints were to identify predictive factors of early rebleeding (≤30 days) and clinical failure after TAE.

2.8. Statistical Analysis

Results are presented as median and inter-quartile for continuous variables and as number and frequency for categorical variables. Categorical variables were compared with the Chi-squared test, and continuous variables were compared with Student's t-test. A univariate analysis was performed to assess the association between early mortality and predictive factors. A multivariate regression analysis was performed using the backward stepwise selection model. Variables with a p value < 0.1 in the univariate analysis were entered into the multivariate analysis. The odds ratio (OR) and 95% confidence intervals were reported. A statistically significant difference was considered for $p < 0.05$. Statistical analyses were performed using the R software.

2.9. Ethical Considerations

This study was approved by the ethics committee of our institute (CHU de Saint-Etienne "Terre d'Ethique", IRBN112021).

3. Results

Between January 2012 and January 2022, 789 patients were referred for TAE in our institute. A flowchart of the patient sample population is presented in Figure 1.

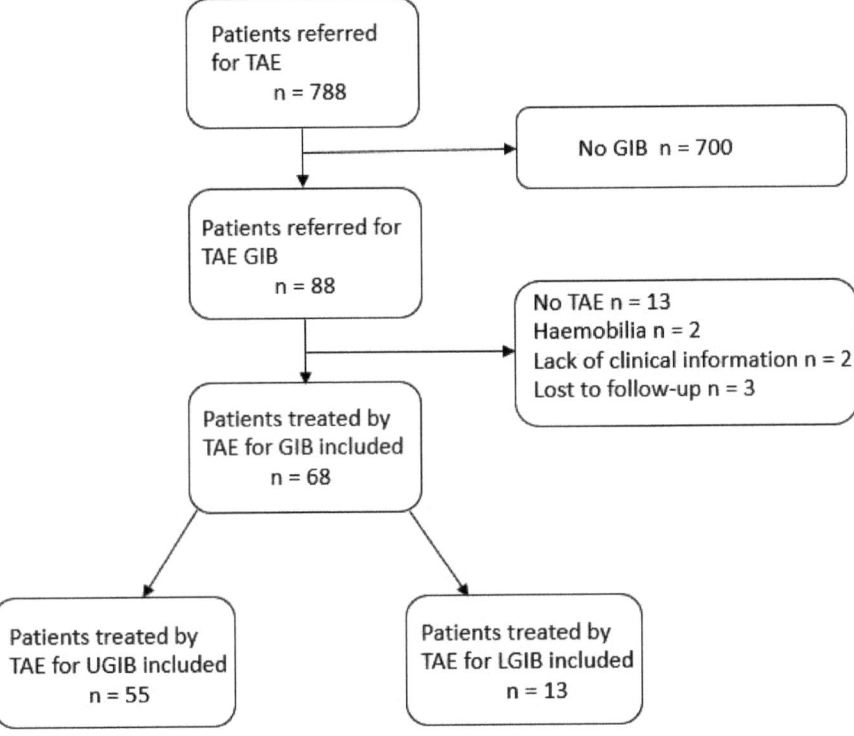

Figure 1. Flow chart of the study population.

3.1. Patient Characteristics

Sixty-eight patients admitted to our interventional department for GIB requiring TAE were included. The detailed patient characteristics are presented in Table 1. The median age was 69 (61–74) years, including 49/68 (72%) males. Regarding previous treatments, 14/68 (20.6%) patients had received antiplatelet therapy, and 19/68 (27.9%) had received anticoagulation therapy. There were 7/68 (10.3%) patients with a history of cancer, and 25/68 (36.8%) patients had an active cancer. There were 55/68 (80.9%) patients with UGIB (Figure 2), including 45 with duodenal and 10 with gastric bleeding, and 13/68 (19.1%) patients with LGIB, including six with colonic bleeding, four with jejunal bleeding, and three with rectal bleeding (Figure 3).

The clinical presentation of the patients was hematemesis in 22/68 (32.4%) patients, melena in 31/68 (45.6%) patients, and rectorragia in 27/68 (39.7%) patients. The main causes of bleeding were ulcer (50%) and post-operative (20.6%). The causes of bleeding are detailed in Table 2.

Table 1. Characteristics of the 68 patients included in the study.

Variable		n = 68
	Age, years	69 (61–74)
Male n (%)		49 (72)
Comorbidities n (%)		
	Diabetes	12 (17.6)
	Coronaropathy	13 (19.1)
	HBP	39 (57.3)
	CRF	7 (10.3)
	Cancer in remission	7 (10.3)
	Active cancer	25 (36.8)
	Anticoagulation therapy	19 (27.9)
	Antiplatelet therapy	14 (20.6)
Clinical presentation n (%)		
	Melena	31 (45.6)
	Rectorragia	27 (39.7)
	Hematemesis	22 (32.4)
Biology n (%)		
	Lactate $\geq$ 2 mmol/L	25 (36.8)
	Prior coagulopathy	24 (35.3)
	Hb nadir	7.25 (6.1–8.3)
	Acute renal failure	14 (20.5)
Pre-operative CT n (%)		62 (91.1)
	Active bleeding	41 (60.3)
	Pseudoaneurysm	9 (13.2)
Localization of bleeding n (%)		
UGIB		55 (80.9)
	Duodenal	45 (66.2)
	Gastric	10 (14.7)
LGIB		13 (19.1)
	Colon	6 (8.8)
	Jejunum	4 (5.9)
	Rectum	3 (4.4)
	Ileum	0
Pre-operative gastroscopy n (%)		40 (58.8)
	Active bleeding	38 (55.8)
	Failure of endoscopic treatment	35 (51.4)
Pre-operative coloscopy		8 (11.8)
	Positive coloscopy	4 (5.9)
	Failure of endoscopic treatment	4 (5.9)
Transfusion n (%)		62 (91.2)
	RBC units	5 (3–8)

Quantitative parameters are presented as median and interquartile range (IQR, 25th–75th percentile). RBC: Red blood cell, CRF: Chronic renal failure, Hb: Hemoglobin.

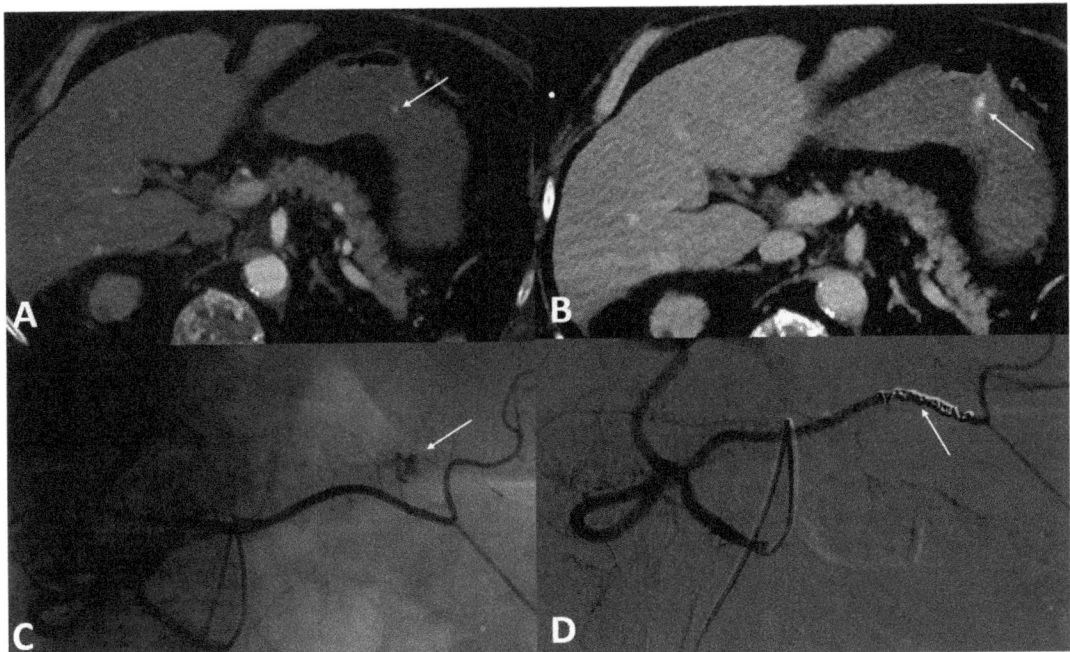

Figure 2. A 56-year-old male was referred to the emergency room for profuse hematemesis. Gastroscopy confirmed the presence of antral bleeding, with no possibility of stopping the bleeding. (**A**) Axial section CT scan injected at the arterial phase, confirming the active contrast extravasation. (**B**) Axial section abdominal CT scan injected at portal phase showing an increase of the leak of iodine contrast. (**C**) Angiography performed within the superior mesenteric artery using a Cobra probe showed an active contrast leak from a branch of the right gastroepiploic artery. (**D**) After embolization with three coils, the angiographic control showed a clear stop of the bleeding.

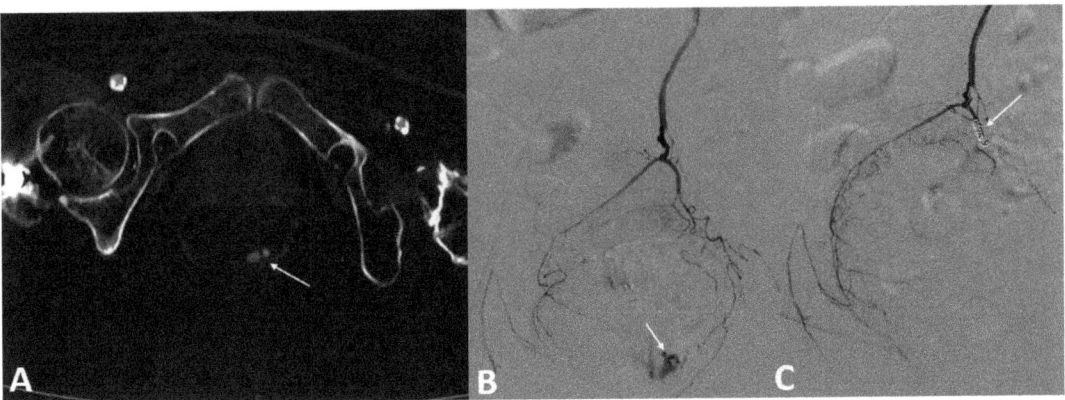

Figure 3. A 73-year-old patient on anticoagulation was referred for profuse rectal bleeding. Colonoscopy failed to stop the bleeding. (**A**) Axial section CT scan injected at arterial time confirming the active contrast extravasation in the rectal lumen. (**B**) Arteriography of the inferior mesenteric artery confirmed the presence of active bleeding from the left superior rectal artery. (**C**) Embolization with three fibered coils allowed a complete stop of the bleeding.

Table 2. Causes of bleeding in the study population.

Variable		n = 68
Ulcer		**34 (50)**
Post operative		**14 (20.6)**
	Duodeno pancreatectomy	7 (10.3)
	Sphincterotomy	5 (7.4)
	Gastrectomy	2 (2.9)
Cancer		**13 (19.1)**
	Gastric cancer	8 (11.8)
	Pancreatic cancer	4 (5.9)
	Rectal Cancer	1 (1.5)
Pancreatitis		**2 (2.9)**
Idiopathic		**2 (2.9)**
Diverticulosis		**2 (2.9)**
Angiodysplasia		**1 (1.5)**

3.2. Pre-Procedure

Regarding pre-procedure investigations of the patients, 62/68 (91.1%) patients had a pre-operative angiographic CT: active bleeding was detected in 41/68 (60.3%) patients, and pseudoaneurysm was detected in 9/68 (13.2%) patients. In total, 40/68 (58.8%) patients had a gastroscopy, of which 38 showed active bleeding; 35 experienced failure of endoscopic treatment. On the three patients treated for rectal bleeding, two experienced failure of endoscopy. The third patient had abundant active bleeding, which pushed us to perform treatment by TAE directly. The embolized vessels were in the superior rectal artery in all three cases.

3.3. Procedure Data

The details of the per-procedure data are presented in Table 3. Out of the patients, 12/68 (17.6%) had no abnormalities on fluoroscopic angiogram and were treated by empiric embolization. Among the 12 patients treated by empiric TAE, seven patients had active bleeding on CT, and three patients had active bleeding on endoscopy. These elements made it possible to orientate TAE. Two patients had neither active bleeding on endoscopy nor on CT but did have a duodenal ulcer: an occlusion of the gastroduodenal artery using coils was performed.

TAE was performed using coils in 46/68 (67.6%) patients, NCBA in 8/68 (11.8%) patients, a combination of coils and resorbable gelatine in 5/68 (7.4%) patients, gelatine sponge in 3/68 (4.4%) patients, microparticles in 4/68 (5.9%) patients, and a combination of microparticles and gelatine sponge in 2/68 (2.9%) patients.

The main artery embolized was the gastroduodenal artery, which was embolized in 43/68 (63.2%) patients. The median time for the procedure was 60 (40–87) min.

3.4. Post-Angiography Course

Detailed clinical outcomes after TAE are presented in Table 4. Technical success was achieved in 68/68 patients. There were 7/68 (10.3%) complications per procedure, including 3/68 (4.4%) non-target embolizations, 1 (1.5%) coil migration, and 3 (4.4%) hematomas at the puncture site. There were 13/68 (19.1%) post-operative complications. The most common post-operative complication was acute renal failure in 9/68 (13.2%) patients, which did not require dialysis.

Table 3. Per procedure characteristics of the 68 patients.

Variable	n = 68
Angiographic data. (%)	
Pseudoaneurysm	11 (16.2)
Empirical Embolization	12 (17.6)
Arteries Embolized n. (%)	
Gastroduodenal	43 (63.2)
Upper Mesenteric	8 (11.8)
Inferior mesenteric	5 (7.4)
Left colic	2 (2.9)
Superior rectal	3 (4.4)
Left Gastric	4 (5.9)
Splenic	2 (2.9)
Gastroepiploic	2 (2.9)
Pancreaticoduodenal	1 (1.5)
Left Hepatic	1 (1.5)
Right Gastric	1 (1.5)
Right Hepatic	1 (1.5)
Embolic Agents n. (%)	
Coils	46 (67.6)
NCBA	8 (11.8)
Coils + Gelatine Sponge	5 (7.4)
Microparticles	4 (5.9)
Gelatine Sponge	3 (4.4)
Microparticles + gelatine sponge	2 (2.9)
Duration of procedure (min)	60 (40–87)

Quantitative parameters are presented as median and interquartile range (IQR, 25th–75th percentile). NBCA: N-butyl Cyanoacrylate.

Table 4. Outcome of the 68 patients included in the study.

Variable	n = 68
Technical Success n (%)	**68 (100)**
Clinical Success n (%)	**50 (73)**
Mortality during follow-up n (%)	**32 (47)**
Day-30 mortality n (%)	**15 (22.1)**
Per-operative Complications n (%)	**7 (10.3)**
Non-target embolization	3 (4.4)
Coil Migration	1 (1.5)
Hematoma at puncture site	3 (4.4)
Post-Operative Complications n (%)	**13 (19.1)**
Acute renal failure without dialysis	9 (13.2)
Bowel Ischemia	2 (2.9)
Splenic Ischemia	2 (2.9)
Recurrence of Bleeding n (%)	**19 (27.9)**
Early ≤ 30 days	17 (25)
Delayed > 30 days	2 (2.9)
Management of Early Rebleeding n (%)	**17 (25)**
Surgery	3 (4.4)
Repeat TAE	2 (2.9)
Endoscopy followed by Surgery	4 (5.9)
Endoscopy	3 (4.4)
TAE followed by endoscopy followed by surgery	2 (2.9)
Conservative treatment	3 (4.4)
Length of hospital stay (days)	**12 (6–24)**
Length of stay in intensive units (days)	**3 (1–6)**
Duration of follow-up (months)	**5 (1–11)**

Quantitative parameters are presented as median and interquartile range (IQR, 25th–75th percentile).

The median length of stay in intensive care units was 3 (1–6) days. The median length of hospital stay was 12 (6–24) days. The median follow-up time was 5 (1–11) months. During the follow-up period, 32/68 (47.0%) patients died, including 15/68 (22.1%) patients who died during the 30 days following the procedure. The clinical success rate was 50/68 (73%) patients, and 17/68 (25%) patients experienced early rebleeding. Among these 17 patients, 3 were treated by surgery, 3 were treated by endoscopy, 2 were treated by repeat TAE, 4 were treated by endoscopy followed by surgery, 2 were treated by repeat TAE followed by endoscopy followed by surgery, and 3 were treated by conservative treatment; 9/17 (53%) died within 30 days.

3.5. Predictors of Early Mortality

In the univariate analysis (Table 5), acute renal failure (OR = 3.75 CI = 1.02–13.7 $p < 0.05$), lactate $\geq$ 2 mmol/L (OR = 6.8 CI = 1.37–33.2 $p < 0.01$), and ulcers (OR = 3.59 CI = 1.01–12.73 $p < 0.05$) were statistically associated with early mortality. Early mortality was not predicted by age, sex, coagulopathy disorders, symptoms, location of bleeding, or any type of embolic agent.

Table 5. Univariate and multivariate regression analysis for early death and early rebleeding.

	Early Death $\leq$ 30 Days				Early Rebleeding $\leq$ 30 Days			
	Univariate Analysis		Multivariate Analysis		Univariate Analysis		Multivariate Analysis	
Characteristics	OR	p Value	OR	p Value	OR	p Value	OR	p Value
Demographics data								
Age $\geq$ 70	0.99 (0.94–1.03)	0.64	–	–	0.71 (0.23–2.25)	0.57	–	–
Male	0.72 (0.21–2.47)	0.6	–	–	0.62 (0.19–2.04)	0.43	–	–
HBP	1.15 (0.36–3.69)	0.81	–	–	1.5 (0.48–4.69)	0.48	–	–
Diabetes	0.66 (0.13–3.41)	0.62	–	–	1 (0.24–4.22)	1	–	–
Chronic renal failure	1.48 (0.26–8.50)	0.66	–	–	1.23 (0.21–6.99)	0.82	–	–
Active cancer	0.55 (0.16–1.97)	0.36	–	–	0.28 (0.07–1.1)	0.07	–	–
Coagulation disorder								
Prior coagulopathy	0.38 (0.12–1.22)	0.1			0.51 (0.17–1.68)	0.25		
Curative Anticoagulation	0.31 (0.06–1.52)	0.15	–	–	0.70 (0.19–2.49)	0.58	–	–
Antiplatelet	0.20 (0.02–1.70)	0.14	–	–	1.16 (0.31–4.37)	0.81	–	–
Lactates $\geq$ 2mmol/L	6.3 (1.7–23.2)	**0.006**	6.10 (1.54–24.2)	**0.01**	2.76 (0.87–9.71)	0.08	–	–
Clinical Presentation								
Duodenal Bleeding	1.54 (0.43–5.50)	0.51	–	–	1.92 (0.55–6.78)	0.31	–	–
Hematemesis	1.41 (0.43–4.66)	0.57	–	–	0.86 (0.26–2.87)	0.8	–	–
Active infection	3.35 (0.77–14.56)	0.11	–	–	2.7 (0.63–11.58)	0.18	–	–
Acute renal failure	3.75 (1.02–13.7)	**0.043**	–	–	1.94 (0.55–6.91)	0.3	–	–
Pre-operative data								
Active bleeding on CT	2.11 (0.59–7.48)	0.25	–	–	0.92 (0.30–2.81)	0.89	–	–
Failed pre-operative gastroscopy	1.56 (0.49–5.00)	0.46	–	–	1.08 (0.36–3.25)	0.89	–	–
Hb and transfusion requirement								
Hb < 8	2.9 (0.89–9.48)	0.07	–	–	2.86 (0.93–8.83)	0.07	–	
Number of RBC	1.07 (0.94–1.2)	0.31	–	–	1.19 (1.04–1.38)	**0.011**	1.17 (1.01–1.35)	**0.037**
Causes and arteries embolized								
Ulcer	3.59 (1.01–12.73)	**0.048**	–	–	3.16 (0.97–10.3)	0.056	–	–
Gastroduodenal Artery	0.35 (0.09–1.40)	0.14	–	–	2.74 (0.75–5.48)	0.91	–	–
Procedure								
Empiric Embolization	0.66 (0.13–3.41)	0.62	–	–	1 (0.23–4.2)	1	–	–
Embolization with Coils only	0.29 (0.06–1.48)	0.138	–	–	0.42 (0.11–1.68)	0.22	–	–

HBP: High Blood Pressure Hb: Hemoglobin.

In multivariate analysis, lactate $\geq$ 2 mmol/L (OR = 6.10 CI = 1.54–24.2 $p = 0.03$) was associated with early mortality.

3.6. Predictors of Early Rebleeding

In univariate analysis (OR = 1.19 CI = 1.04–1.38, $p = 0.011$) and multivariate analysis (OR = 1.92 CI = 1.01–1.35, $p = 0.037$), higher red blood cell (RBC) units administered in a transfusion was associated with early rebleeding. Early rebleeding was not predicted by age, sex, comorbidities, symptoms, hemostasis anomalies, source of bleeding, embolized artery, or embolic agent.

4. Discussion

Several authors have studied the prognosis of patients treated with TAE for gastrointestinal bleeding. However, most of these studies have focused on LGIB or UGIB [14], on a particular embolizing agent [8], or a particular clinical situation [15] or have had limited pre- or per-procedural clinical information [11,16]. Some studies include patients with arterial splanchnic bleeding without intraluminal bleeding [9]. There is a lack of a uniform reporting system because of the variety of definitions for clinical success. For example, the Society of Interventional Radiology defined clinical success as resolution of symptoms within 30 days after TAE, whereas other authors use 7 days after TAE as their time cut-off [17–19]. Furthermore, studies do not systematically report the number of patients lost to follow-up [20], nor do they report if these patients are excluded from the study or included in the final statistical analysis. We believe that the study of rebleeding and early mortality are the most appropriate to evaluate the effectiveness of TAE for GIB.

Causes of early death following TAE are multifactorial and include acute renal failure, infection, multiorgan failure, and bleeding. The early mortality rate (21.1%) is comparable to other previous studies [10,16]. Lactate level is known to be a useful and rapid tool for assessing severity of disease in critically ill patients [21]. It is also known as a predictor of post-operative infection, cardiopulmonary dysfunction, renal impairment, and increased mortality after elective cardiac surgery [22]; aortic dissection [23]; and liver transplantation [24]. Cellular stress, tissue hypoxemia, infection, and various critical illnesses are triggers for the accumulation of serum lactate [25]. In the critically ill patient, normal blood lactate is less than 2 mmol/L. Lactate $\geq$ 2 mmol/L was the only predictor of early mortality $\leq$30 days in the present study. To our knowledge, these biological data have never been investigated in prognostic studies of TAE for GIB. To our knowledge, no previous study has shown that hyperlactatemia is a predictor of early mortality after TAE. The advantage of these data is that they are easy to use, are quickly accessible, and represent an objective measure in patient assessment. They would allow clinicians to closely monitor patients with GIB treated by TAE with hyperlactatemia $\geq$ 2 mmol/L.

In the present study, the early rebleeding rate (25%) was comparable to previous studies and was approximately 33% (range 9–66%) for UGIB [26]. This is in line with other studies, such as the study of Loffroy et al. in 2009 [10], in which among the 16 patients who presented with early rebleeding, 3 (18.8%) were treated by repeat TAE, with a secondary clinical success of 77.2%. The influence of rebleeding on patient outcomes is contradictory. Mohan et al. [11] showed that rebleeding within 30 days was associated with increased odds of 30-day mortality that were more than 45 times higher than normal. On the other hand, Loffroy et al. [10] reported 28.1% (16/57 patients) mortality within 30 days of TAE, with only three deaths caused by early rebleeding.

Regarding early rebleeding, a greater amount of RBC transfusion has been found as a predictive factor. However, we did not find that the presence of coagulopathy was associated with early rebleeding, contrary to previous studies in the literature [20]. Lee et al. [27] showed that coagulopathy is associated with rebleeding. In a retrospective study of 114 patients, Mohan et al. [11] identified two predictive factors of rebleeding: age > 60 years and patients with known malignancy. A longer time to angiography, a greater number of RBCs, the use of coils as the only embolic agent, and previous surgery have also been found [28–30] to be predictive factors for early rebleeding in some studies.

We have shown that TAE can be performed successfully, even when angiography fails to visualize active bleeding. Indeed, among the 12 empiric TAE, only 1/12 (8.3%) patients died early from bleeding, with no statistical differences between empiric and targeted TAE in terms of early rebleeding and mortality. This result is consistent with the meta-analysis by Yu et al. [31], which found a clinical success rate of 74.7% for empiric TAE and no statistically difference between empiric and targeted TAE in terms of rebleeding. However, this result can also be explained by the potential spontaneous drying up of the bleeding, explaining the absence of active bleeding.

In our study, embolic agents were not predictive of early rebleeding or early mortality. Coils were the most common embolic agents used in this study. Several studies have demonstrated a statistically significant association between the use of coils and higher rebleeding rates [10,28,32]. In contrast, Kim et al. [33] showed a clinical success rate of 82% for UGIB TAE using NCBA. Despite this, NBCA was used less frequently than coils because NBCA can be challenging to use, especially in high-flow arteries such as the gastroduodenal artery, and it requires extensive experience to be used successfully. The results of our study temper the results of these previous studies, highlighting the influence of an embolic agent on the risk of recurrent bleeding. This study shows that no single embolic agent should be preferred in principle. However, the technical skill of all embolic agents, including NBCA, allows the operator to adapt to all clinical situations and to avoid complications such as non-target embolization or coil migration. Only two transient bowel ischemia occurred in this study sample among patients with LGIB. Neither case required surgical resection. This is in line with the systematic review of Beggs et al. [2], who did not report any ischemic complications for UGIB, which can be explained by the rich collateral blood supply of the gastro duodenal artery. In contrast, studies on LGIB showed higher rates of ischemic complications in relation to a less developed anastomotic network. For instance, Bua-Ngam et al. [34] showed an ischemic complication rate of 13%. Recently, interventional teams have even used pre-operative splanchnic or inferior mesenteric artery TAE before surgery for rectal cancer [35] or esophagus cancer [36] as pre-ischemic conditioning to prevent post-operative anastomosis leakage. In addition, our study confirms the safety profile of TAE for GIB, and no major complications were noted. The main complications were acute renal failure, the causes of which were multifactorial and related to the contrast injection and volume depletion.

This study has several limitations. First, this study was retrospective. Second, our investigation represents the experience of a single institution. Third, because the patients in this study were reviewed over a 10-year period, very minor technical differences in TAE among the primary interventional operators as well as differences in medical care during the study period could have contributed to disparities in clinical outcomes over time. Additionally, there was no systematic scanning or endoscopic follow-up after the operation to assess ischemic complications. Finally, the number of events, such as early death and early rebleeding, are relatively small to ensure the robustness of our multivariate analyses.

In conclusion, this retrospective study suggests hyperlactatemia as a potential and previously undocumented predictor for early mortality after TAE for GIB. As the blood lactate level is easily evaluated in clinical practice, these findings have practical implications for clinicians' early assessments of GIB so that they can adjust patient management accordingly. Further prospective and larger multicenter studies are needed to support these data. In addition, large-scale studies comparing risk factors for early mortality of TAE with endoscopic and surgical treatment for GIB seem necessary.

Author Contributions: Conceptualization, R.G.; Methology, C.E., R.G.; Software, C.E., R.G.; Validation, S.G., B.L.R., N.W.; Formal analysis, C.E., R.G.; Investigation, C.E., R.G.; Resources and data curation, C.E., S.G., A.M., L.V., C.C., N.W., B.L.R., C.B., R.G.; Writing-Original draft preparation, C.E., R.G.; Writing-review and editing, R.G., S.G., B.L.R., N.W., C.B.; Supervision, S.G., C.B., N.W., B.L.R. All authors have read and agreed to the published version of the manuscript.

Funding: This study was not supported by any funding.

Institutional Review Board Statement: This study was conducted in accordance with the Declaration of Helsinki and approved by the Institutional Review Board of the University Hospital of Saint-Etienne.

Informed Consent Statement: This study has obtained IRB approval form the University of Saint-Etienne, and informed consent have been obtained.

Data Availability Statement: The data presented in this study are available on request from the corresponding author.

Acknowledgments: The authors thank Michael J.Deml, for proofreading the manuscript.

Conflicts of Interest: The authors declare that they have no conflict of interest.

Abbreviations

CT	Computed Tomography
GIB	Gastrointestinal bleeding
INR	International Normalized Ratio
ICU	Intensive Care Unit
LGIB	Lower Gastrointestinal Bleeding
NBCA	N-butyl-2-cyanoacrylate
PC	Platelet count
PT	Prothrombin Time
TAE	Transarterial Embolization
UGIB	Upper Gastrointestinal Bleeding

References

1. Oakland, K.; Guy, R.; Uberoi, R.; Hogg, R.; Mortensen, N.; Murphy, M.F.; Jairath, V.; UK Lower GI Bleeding Collaborative. Acute lower GI bleeding in the UK: Patient characteristics, interventions and outcomes in the first nationwide audit. *Gut* 2018, *67*, 654–662. [CrossRef] [PubMed]
2. Beggs, A.; Dilworth, M.; Powell, S.; Atherton, H.; Griffiths, E. A systematic review of transarterial embolization versus emergency surgery in treatment of major nonvariceal upper gastrointestinal bleeding. *Clin. Exp. Gastroenterol.* 2014, *7*, 93–104. [CrossRef] [PubMed]
3. Bardou, M.; Benhaberou-Brun, D.; Le Ray, I.; Barkun, A.N. Diagnosis and management of nonvariceal upper gastrointestinal bleeding. *Nat. Rev. Gastroenterol. Hepatol.* 2012, *9*, 97–104. [CrossRef]
4. van Leerdam, M.E. Epidemiology of acute upper gastrointestinal bleeding. *Best Pract. Res. Clin. Gastroenterol.* 2008, *22*, 209–224. [CrossRef] [PubMed]
5. Gralnek, I.; Dumonceau, J.-M.; Kuipers, E.; Lanas, A.; Sanders, D.; Kurien, M.; Rotondano, G.; Hucl, T.; Dinis-Ribeiro, M.; Marmo, R.; et al. Diagnosis and management of nonvariceal upper gastrointestinal hemorrhage: European Society of Gastrointestinal Endoscopy (ESGE) Guideline. *Endoscopy* 2015, *47*, a1–a46. [CrossRef]
6. Greenspoon, J.; Barkun, A. A summary of recent recommendations on the management of patients with nonvariceal upper gastrointestinal bleeding. *Pol. Arch. Intern. Med.* 2010, *120*, 341–346. [CrossRef]
7. Huang, C.-C.; Lee, C.-W.; Hsiao, J.-K.; Leung, P.-C.; Liu, K.-L.; Tsang, Y.-M.; Liu, H.-M. N-butyl Cyanoacrylate Embolization as the Primary Treatment of Acute Hemodynamically Unstable Lower Gastrointestinal Hemorrhage. *J. Vasc. Interv. Radiol.* 2011, *22*, 1594–1599. [CrossRef]
8. Huang, Y.-S.; Chang, C.-C.; Liou, J.-M.; Jaw, F.-S.; Liu, K.-L. Transcatheter arterial embolization with N-butyl cyanoacrylate for nonvariceal upper gastrointestinal bleeding in hemodynamically unstable patients: Results and predictors of clinical outcomes. *J. Vasc. Interv. Radiol.* 2014, *25*, 1850–1857. [CrossRef]
9. Mensel, B.; Kühn, J.-P.; Kraft, M.; Rosenberg, C.; Ivo Partecke, L.; Hosten, N.; Puls, R. Selective microcoil embolization of arterial gastrointestinal bleeding in the acute situation: Outcome, complications, and factors affecting treatment success. *Eur. J. Gastroenterol. Hepatol.* 2012, *24*, 155–163. [CrossRef]
10. Loffroy, R.; Guiu, B.; D'Athis, P.; Mezzetta, L.; Gagnaire, A.; Jouve, J.; Ortega–Deballon, P.; Cheynel, N.; Cercueil, J.-P.; Krausé, D. Arterial Embolotherapy for Endoscopically Unmanageable Acute Gastroduodenal Hemorrhage: Predictors of Early Rebleeding. *Clin. Gastroenterol. Hepatol.* 2009, *7*, 515–523. [CrossRef]
11. Mohan, P.; Manov, J.; Diaz-Bode, A.; Venkat, S.; Langston, M.; Naidu, A.; Howse, R.; Narayanan, G. Clinical Predictors of Arterial Extravasation, Rebleedingand Mortality Following Angiographic Interventions in Gastrointestinal Bleeding. *J. Gastrointest. Liver Dis.* 2018, *27*, 221–226. [CrossRef] [PubMed]
12. Lai, H.-Y.; Wu, K.-T.; Liu, Y.; Zeng, Z.-F.; Zhang, B. Angiography and transcatheter arterial embolization for non-variceal gastrointestinal bleeding. *Scand. J. Gastroenterol.* 2020, *55*, 931–940. [CrossRef]

13. AssesSurgery GmbH. The Clavien-Dindo Classification [Internet]. Available online: https://www.assessurgery.com/claviendindo-classification/ (accessed on 3 February 2021).
14. Kwon, J.H.; Kim, M.-D.; Han, K.; Choi, W.; Kim, Y.S.; Lee, J.; Kim, G.M.; Won, J.Y.; Lee, D.Y. Transcatheter arterial embolisation for acute lower gastrointestinal haemorrhage: A single-centre study. *Eur. Radiol.* **2019**, *29*, 57–67. [CrossRef] [PubMed]
15. Lee, S.M.; Jeong, S.Y.; Shin, J.H.; Choi, H.C.; Na, J.B.; Won, J.H.; Park, S.E.; Chen, C.S. Transcatheter arterial embolization for gastrointestinal bleeding related to pancreatic adenocarcinoma: Clinical efficacy and predictors of clinical outcome. *Eur. J. Radiol.* **2020**, *123*, 108787. [CrossRef] [PubMed]
16. Fontana, F.; Piacentino, F.; Ossola, C.; Coppola, A.; Curti, M.; Macchi, E.; De Marchi, G.; Floridi, C.; Ierardi, A.M.; Carrafiello, G.; et al. Transcatheter Arterial Embolization in Acute Non-Variceal Gastrointestinal Bleedings: A Ten-Year Single-Center Experience in 91 Patients and Review of the Literature. *J. Clin. Med.* **2021**, *10*, 4979. [CrossRef] [PubMed]
17. Angle, J.F.; Siddiqi, N.H.; Wallace, M.J.; Kundu, S.; Stokes, L.; Wojak, J.C.; Cardella, J.F. Quality Improvement Guidelines for Percutaneous Transcatheter Embolization. *J. Vasc. Interv. Radiol.* **2010**, *21*, 1479–1486. [CrossRef] [PubMed]
18. Defreyne, L.; De Schrijver, I.; Decruyenaere, J.; Van Maele, G.; Ceelen, W.; De Looze, D.; Vanlangenhove, P. Therapeutic Decision-Making in Endoscopically Unmanageable Nonvariceal Upper Gastrointestinal Hemorrhage. *Cardiovasc. Interv. Radiol.* **2008**, *31*, 897–905. [CrossRef]
19. Ang, D.; Teo, E.K.; Tan, A.; Ibrahim, S.; Tan, P.S.; Ang, T.L.; Fock, K.M. A comparison of surgery versus transcatheter angiographic embolization in the treatment of nonvariceal upper gastrointestinal bleeding uncontrolled by endoscopy. *Eur. J. Gastroenterol. Hepatol.* **2012**, *24*, 929–938. [CrossRef]
20. Yap, F.Y.; Omene, B.O.; Patel, M.N.; Yohannan, T.; Minocha, J.; Knuttinen, M.G.; Owens, C.A.; Bui, J.T.; Gaba, R.C. Transcatheter Embolotherapy for Gastrointestinal Bleeding: A Single Center Review of Safety, Efficacy, and Clinical Outcomes. *Dig. Dis. Sci.* **2013**, *58*, 1976–1984. [CrossRef]
21. Drolz, A.; Horvatits, T.; Rutter, K.; Landahl, F.; Roedl, K.; Meersseman, P.; Wilmer, A.; Kluwe, J.; Lohse, A.W.; Kluge, S.; et al. Lactate Improves Prediction of Short-Term Mortality in Critically Ill Patients With Cirrhosis: A Multinational Study: Liver Failure, Cirrhosis, and Portal Hypertension. *Hepatology* **2019**, *69*, 258–269. [CrossRef]
22. Minton, J.; Sidebotham, D.A. Hyperlactatemia and Cardiac Surgery. *J. Extra-Corpor. Technol.* **2017**, *49*, 7–15. [PubMed]
23. Zindovic, I.; Luts, C.; Bjursten, H.; Herou, E.; Larsson, M.; Sjögren, J.; Nozohoor, S. Perioperative Hyperlactemia Is a Poor Predictor of Outcome in Patients Undergoing Surgery for Acute Type-A Aortic Dissection. *J. Cardiothorac. Vasc. Anesth.* **2018**, *32*, 2479–2484. [CrossRef] [PubMed]
24. Cheong, Y.; Lee, S.; Lee, D.-K.; Kim, K.-S.; Sang, B.-H.; Hwang, G.-S. Preoperative hyperlactatemia and early mortality after liver transplantation: Selection of important variables using random forest survival analysis. *Anesth. Pain Med.* **2021**, *16*, 353–359. [CrossRef] [PubMed]
25. Levy, B. Lactate and shock state: The metabolic view. *Curr. Opin. Crit. Care* **2006**, *12*, 315–321. [CrossRef]
26. Loffroy, R.; Rao, P.; Ota, S.; De Lin, M.; Kwak, B.-K.; Geschwind, J.-F. Embolization of Acute Nonvariceal Upper Gastrointestinal Hemorrhage Resistant to Endoscopic Treatment: Results and Predictors of Recurrent Bleeding. *Cardiovasc. Interv. Radiol.* **2010**, *33*, 1088–1100. [CrossRef]
27. Lee, H.H.; Park, J.M.; Chun, H.J.; Oh, J.S.; Ahn, H.J.; Choi, M.-G. Transcatheter arterial embolization for endoscopically unmanageable non-variceal upper gastrointestinal bleeding. *Scand. J. Gastroenterol.* **2015**, *50*, 809–815. [CrossRef]
28. Aina, R.; Oliva, V.L.; Therasse, É.; Perreault, P.; Bui, B.T.; Dufresne, M.-P.; Soulez, G. Arterial Embolotherapy for Upper Gastrointestinal Hemorrhage: Outcome Assessment. *J. Vasc. Interv. Radiol.* **2001**, *12*, 195–200. [CrossRef]
29. Poultsides, G.A.; Kim, C.J.; Orlando, R.; Peros, G.; Hallisey, M.J.; Vignati, P.V. Angiographic Embolization for Gastroduodenal Hemorrhage: Safety, Efficacy, and Predictors of Outcome. *Arch. Surg.* **2008**, *143*, 457. [CrossRef]
30. Walsh, R.M.; Anain, P.; Geisinger, M.; Vogt, D.; Mayes, J.; Grundfest-Broniatowski, S.; Henderson, J.M. Role of angiography and embolization for massive gastroduodenal hemorrhage. *J. Gastrointest. Surg.* **1999**, *3*, 61–66. [CrossRef]
31. Yu, Q.; Funaki, B.; Navuluri, R.; Zangan, S.; Zhang, A.; Cao, D.; Leef, J.; Ahmed, O. Empiric Transcatheter Embolization for Acute Arterial Upper Gastrointestinal Bleeding: A Meta-Analysis. *Am. J. Roentgenol.* **2021**, *216*, 880–893. [CrossRef]
32. Loffroy, R.; Guiu, B. Role of transcatheter arterial embolization for massivebleeding from gastroduodenal ulcers. *World J. Gastroenterol.* **2009**, *15*, 5889–5897. [CrossRef] [PubMed]
33. Kim, P.H.; Tsauo, J.; Shin, J.H.; Yun, S.-C. Transcatheter Arterial Embolization of Gastrointestinal Bleeding with N-Butyl Cyanoacrylate: A Systematic Review and Meta-Analysis of Safety and Efficacy. *J. Vasc. Interv. Radiol.* **2017**, *28*, 522–531.e5. [CrossRef] [PubMed]
34. Bua-ngam, C.; Norasetsingh, J.; Treesit, T.; Wedsart, B.; Chansanti, O.; Tapaneeyakorn, J.; Panpikoon, T.; Vallibhakara, S.-O. Efficacy of emergency transarterial embolization in acute lower gastrointestinal bleeding: A single-center experience. *Diagn. Interv. Imaging* **2017**, *98*, 499–505. [CrossRef]
35. Frandon, J.; Berny, L.; Prudhomme, M.; de Forges, H.; Serrand, C.; de Oliveira, F.; Beregi, J.-P.; Bertrand, M.M. Inferior mesenteric artery embolization ahead of rectal cancer surgery: AMIREMBOL pilot study. *Br. J. Surg.* **2022**, *109*, 650–652. [CrossRef] [PubMed]
36. Ghelfi, J.; Brichon, P.-Y.; Frandon, J.; Boussat, B.; Bricault, I.; Ferretti, G.; Guigard, S.; Sengel, C. Ischemic Gastric Conditioning by Preoperative Arterial Embolization Before Oncologic Esophagectomy: A Single-Center Experience. *Cardiovasc. Interv. Radiol.* **2017**, *40*, 712–720. [CrossRef] [PubMed]

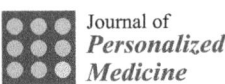

Article

Angio Cone-Beam CT (Angio-CBCT) and 3D Road-Mapping for the Detection of Spinal Cord Vascularization in Patients Requiring Treatment for a Thoracic Aortic Lesion: A Feasibility Study

Pierre-Antoine Barral [1], Mariangela De Masi [2,3], Axel Bartoli [1,4,*], Paul Beunon [1], Arnaud Gallon [5], Farouk Tradi [1], Jean-François Hak [6], Marine Gaudry [2,3] and Alexis Jacquier [1,4]

1. Department of Radiology, CHU Timone, AP-HM, 264, Rue Saint-Pierre, 13005 Marseille, France
2. Department of Vascular Surgery, CHU Timone, AP-HM, 264, Rue Saint-Pierre, 13005 Marseille, France
3. Aortic Center, CHU Timone, AP-HM, 264, Rue Saint-Pierre, 13005 Marseille, France
4. CRMBM-UMR CNRS 7339, Aix-Marseille University, 27, Boulevard Jean Moulin, CEDEX 05, 13385 Marseille, France
5. Department of Visceral and Vascular Radiology, Centre Hospitalier Universitaire de Clermont-Ferrand, Clermont-Ferrand, France Aortic Center, CHU Timone, AP-HM, 264, Rue Saint-Pierre, CEDEX 1, 13005 Marseille, France
6. Department of Neuroradiology, CHU Timone, AP-HM, 264, Rue Saint-Pierre, 13005 Marseille, France
* Correspondence: axel.bartoli@ap-hm.fr; Tel.: +33-6-64-53-16-82

Abstract: Background: Spinal cord ischemia is a major complication of treatment for descending thoracic aorta (DTA) disease. Our objectives were (1) to describe the value of angiographic cone-beam CT (angio-CBCT) and 3D road-mapping to visualize the Adamkiewicz artery (AA) and its feeding artery and (2) to evaluate the impact of AA localization on the patient surgical strategy. Methods: Between 2018 and 2020, all patients referred to our institution for a surgical DTA disorder underwent a dedicated AA evaluation by angio-CBCT. If the AA feeding artery was not depicted on angio-CBCT, selective artery catheterization was performed, guided by 3D road-mapping. Intervention modifications, based on AA location and one month of neurologic follow-up after surgery, were recorded. Results: Twenty-one patients were enrolled. AA was assessable in 100% of patients and in 15 (71%) with angio-CBCT alone. Among them, 10 patients needed 3D road-mapping-guided DSA angiography to visualize the AA feeding artery. The amount of contrast media, irradiation dose, and intervention length were not significantly different whether the AA was assessable or not by angio-CBCT. AA feeding artery localization led to surgical sketch modification for 11 patients. Conclusions: Angio-CBCT is an efficient method for AA localization in the surgical planning of DTA disorders.

Keywords: interventional radiology; preconditioning; endovascular

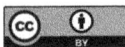

1. Introduction

Neurological complications, such as spinal cord injury, remain a major concern in the treatment of descending thoracic aortic (DTA) disease. Spinal cord ischemia arises in between 1% and 8% of patients after treatment with DTA [1–3]. Several methods to decrease the spinal cord injury rate have been described, including cerebrospinal fluid (CSF) drainage, motor somatosensory-evoked potential, or surgical reimplantation of the feeding artery of the Adamkiewicz artery (AA) [4,5].

The need for assessing the anatomical location of the feeding artery of the AA before DTA treatment is debated in the literature for several reasons. The variability of its anatomical origin is high, most commonly found between T8 and L1, and originates from the left intercostal or lumbar artery in 70% to 85% of cases [6,7]. Additionally, the feeding artery of the AA is a small artery, and its anatomical location might be hidden with the deformation of the aneurysmal aorta and aortic thrombus. However, a lower rate of postoperative neurologic complications is observed in patients with DTA surgical repair if they benefit from previous AA detection and preservation [8]. If the AA feeding artery is covered in TEVAR, CSF drainage is associated with a lower incidence of symptomatic spinal cord ischemia [9]. There is no consensus regarding spinal cord ischemia prevention before surgical treatment of the descending thoracic aorta. The anatomical location of the AA might help in decision-making before treatment. Selective DSA of each patent intercostal artery could be very challenging in the case of large aortic aneurysms. New angiographic techniques such as angio-CBCT might help in detecting small arteries such as the AA in large aneurismal vessels.

Several invasive and noninvasive techniques to assess the AA location have been described [10–14]. Noninvasive assessment methods involving the use of magnetic resonance (MR) angiography and multidetector row CT angiography have recently been employed [15–17]. However, their wide adoption can be limited because of patient morphology. On the other hand, digital subtraction angiography (DSA) is challenging to perform, as it is difficult to catheterize the intercostal artery ostium in an aneurysmal sac.

The periprocedural use of cone beam CT (CBCT) has been described in many interventional radiology procedures [18]. The arm of the angio-suite can perform localized CT acquisition by rotating around the patient in a cone-shaped beam. The acquisition, coupled with vessel angiography, is called angio-CBCT. It allows small vessel detection with a higher spatial resolution than CT–angiography and MRI acquisition. Additionally, angio-CBCT acquisition can be used as a 3D road-mapping mask for the rest of the procedure. It was found to be efficient in the detection of injured vessels for emergency embolization, transarterial chemoembolization guidance, or the evaluation of spinal arteriovenous fistulas [19–21]. However, there is no evaluation of this technique in the preprocedural visualization of the AA feeding arteries before DTA disease treatment. Therefore, our goals were to (1) describe the value of contrast angio-CBCT and 3D road-mapping in locating the feeding artery of the AA in patients with DTA disease requiring surgical treatment; (2) quantify the total amount of contrast media, irradiation dose and intervention length required to locate the feeding artery of the AA; (3) assess the impact of the preprocedural location of the feeding artery of the AA on the treatment strategy; and (4) report the rate of one month postprocedural neurologic complications.

2. Materials and Methods

2.1. Study Design

This single-center nonrandomized retrospective study included all patients being followed in our center for DTA disorders with planned thoracic or thoracoabdominal aortic repair with a risk of spinal cord infarction from February 2018 to April 2020 in the Centre Aorte Timone. The exclusion criteria were patients referred for emergency and contraindications for iodine injection. All patients included during this period underwent angiography with angio-CBCT acquisition after iodine injection and, if needed, selective opacification of selected patent intercostal artery-guided 3D road-mapping to detect AA and AA feeding arteries. In the second phase, we evaluated our attitude toward surgical treatment modification after AA detection. Ethical review and approval were not applicable for this retrospective study.

2.2. Diagnostic Angiography Procedure

All angiographic procedures were performed in an angiography room (Discovery IGS 730, General Electric, Buc, France) under local anesthesia. The first phase of the intervention was always angio-CBCT aortic acquisition. We performed a femoral approach with the Seldinger technique (5F introducer sheath, Terumo Cardiovascular Systems Corporation, MI, USA). A multipurpose 5F pig tail catheter was placed at the level of T9. Angio-CBCT acquisition was then performed during a breath hold at a rotation speed of $40°/s$ and during contrast media injection. A diluted bolus was used with 50% saline and 50% iodixanol 320 (Visipaque, Gerbet, Aulnay-sous-Bois, France). Seventy cc of this mixture was injected with the following parameters: injection speed = 10 cc/s, delay between injection and angio-CBCT acquisition: between 3 to 4 s, according to the volume of the aneurysm and left to the judgment of the radiologist (Figure 1). In the case of a lack of opacification of the feeding artery of the AA, a second angio-CBCT was performed at a different level of the aorta depending on the aortic lesion anatomy (mostly involving a thoracic or abdominal disorder). Following the acquisition, images were processed on a dedicated work station AW Volume Share 4.6 (GE Healthcare, Chicago, IL, USA) to detect the feeding artery of the AA using a double oblique view within MPR reconstruction and Volume Rendering (Figure 1).

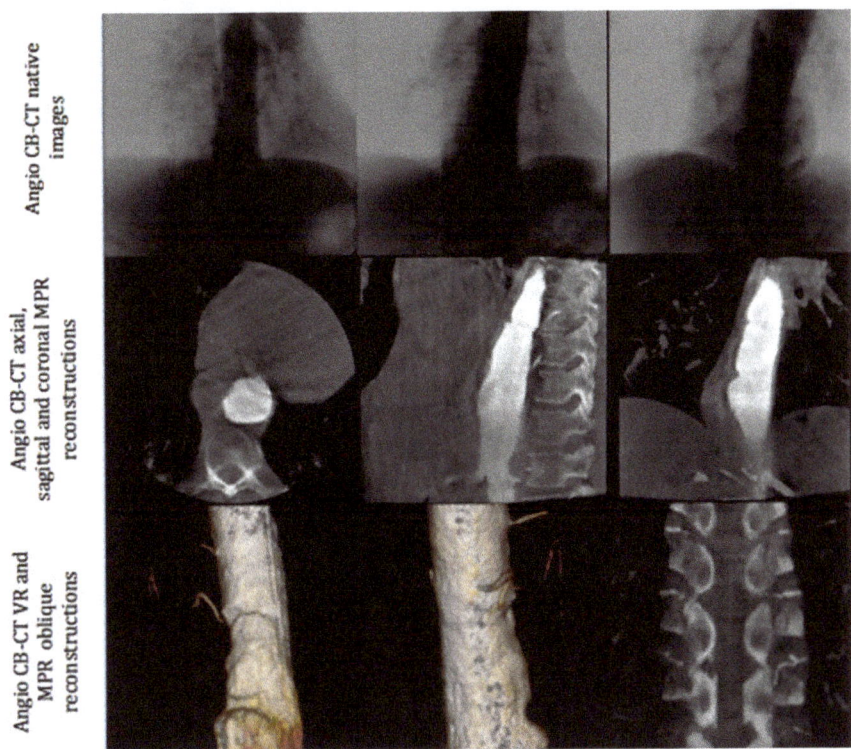

Figure 1. Different phases of angio-CBCT image acquisition: native images (upper section), MPR reconstructions (middle section), and volume rendering and oblique reconstructions (lower section).

The AA was considered assessable on angio-CBCT and angio-CBCT positive if we visualized an AA artery defined as "a collateral artery of the radiculomedullary artery running obliquely along the anterior surface of the spinal cord with a classic hairpin turn connection to the anterior spinal artery" (Figure 2).

If the feeding artery of the AA was clearly defined, exploration was considered complete.

The definition of the feeding artery of the AA was a continuous vascular route for the anterior spinal artery, the AA, the radiculomedullary artery, the posterior branch of the intercostal (or lumbar) artery, the intercostal (or lumbar) artery and the aorta.

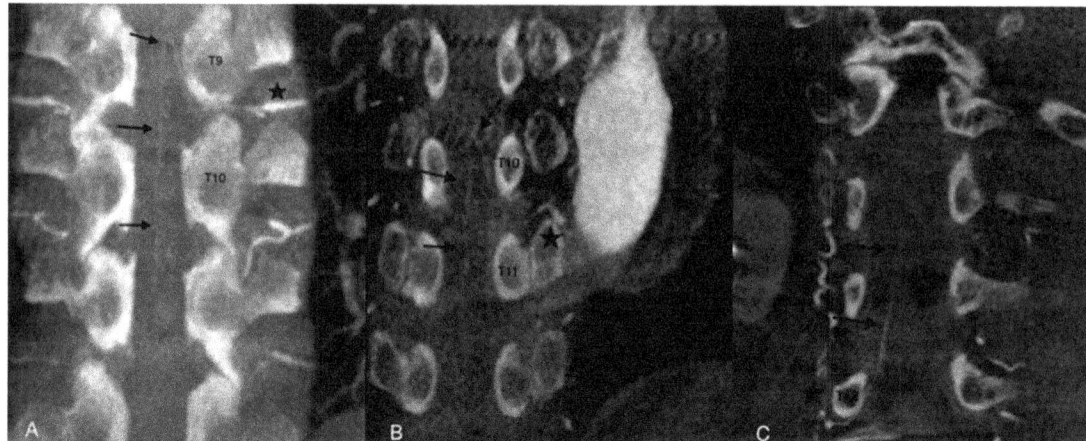

Figure 2. Examples of angio-CBCT reconstructions showing the Adamkiewicz artery (AA) (black arrows) in three different patients. The AA is seen running obliquely along the anterior surface of the spinal cord with a classic hairpin turn and connection to the anterior spinal artery (star). In cases (**A**,**B**), the feeding artery of the AA was clearly depicted. In case (**C**), complementary selective arteriography was performed.

If the feeding artery was not clearly visualized on angio-CBCT alone, selective DSA angiography catheterization of the arteries at the probable origin of the AA was performed. In this case, we used 3D road-mapping extracted from angio-CBCT, reconstructed in volume rendering reconstructions, with the localization of the intercostals and lumbar artery ostia to facilitate catheterization (Figure 3).

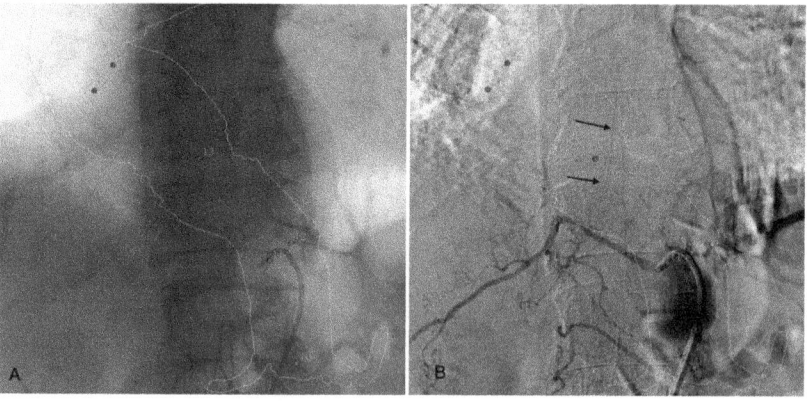

Figure 3. Three-dimensional road-mapping of the intercostal and lumbar artery ostia (red dots) and aortic wall mask (yellow lines), extracted from angio-CBCT acquisition (**A**). Selective angiography of a patent intercostal artery with visualization of the classic hairpin turns (black arrows) (**B**).

AA was considered not assessable on angio-CBCT and angio-CBCT negative if no artery meeting the AA definition was visible, even after 2 angio-CBCT procedures. In this situation, selective DSA angiography catheterization of the arteries was performed. The 3D road-map extracted from the angio-CBCT acquisition was also used, but in contrast to the previous situation, catheterization was not guided by AA detection, and all intercostal and lumbar arteries from the region were catheterized. Selective angiography of patent intercostal/lumbar arteries requires different types of catheters, and the choice of catheter was left at the discretion of the radiologist. A manual injection of 4 cc of contrast media iodixanol 320 (Visipaque, Gerbet, Aulnay-sous-Bois, France) was used for selective angiography. Selective DSA was considered successful when the feeding artery of the AA was located on the DSA. A procedure was considered unsuccessful if angio-CBCT and DSA failed to locate the feeding artery of the AA.

The location of the ostium of the intercostal or lumbar artery, which feeds the AA, was highlighted on the volume rendering reconstruction of angio-CBCT or on the preprocedural CT acquisition. These images were used during multidisciplinary discussions to define the surgical procedure.

2.3. Surgical Management and Neurological Follow-Up

Treatment decisions were standardized and validated in a multidisciplinary team including vascular surgeons, cardiologists, anesthesiologists, and radiologists. Concerning endovascular repair, if the AA arose near the stent graft ends, the preservation of the ostium was maintained by stent graft length reduction. If the AA arose in the aneurismal area and needed to be covered by TEVAR, preventive CSF drainage was performed. In the case of open surgical repair, surgical reimplantation of the AA was performed. All these procedure modifications based on AA localization were discussed and recorded during multidisciplinary team meetings. One month after aortic intervention, a follow-up examination recorded early neurological complications. All types of neurologic symptoms were recorded: spinal cord ischemia, paresthesia or motor disorders of the lower limb, and Parkinson's syndrome. The amount of iodine contrast injected, irradiation dose, fluoroscopy time, and procedure length were gathered. The continuous and categorical variables are described by the mean, standard deviation (SD) and range or median (Q1-median-Q3) and range, and n (%). The Mann Whitney U test was performed to evaluate both groups.

3. Results

A total of 21 patients were included in the study. Patient demographic and clinical characteristics are summarized in Table 1. All patients were able to benefit from the described diagnostic procedure with angio-CBCT. The average duration of the procedure was 48.7 ± 19.7 min for all 21 cases. In two cases, medullary arteriography was coupled to another intervention in the same operating time. The first was iliac stenting for aneurysmal exclusion, and the second was subclavian artery occlusion. Both interventions were performed in patients for whom angio-CBCT was positive and no extra DSA selective catheterization was necessary. The doses of contrast media and irradiation were combined in these two cases. No complications were noted during the procedure.

Table 1. Population characteristics (n = 21).

Variable	Patient Characteristics
Age, years (mean ± SD)	68 ± 11
Male, n (%)	17 (81)
BMI, kg/m^2 (mean ± SD)	27 ± 3.5
Hypertension, n (%)	17 (81)
Hyperlipidemia, n (%)	7 (33)
Diabetes, n (%)	2 (9)
Smoking, n (%)	14 (66)
Descending thoracic aorta pathology, n (%)	
Aneurysm	19 (90)
Dissection	2 (10)
Aortic diameter, mm (mean ± SD)	61.6 ± 8.1

AA was assessable on angio-CBCT in 15/21 (71%) cases. Among them, the feeding artery was undoubtedly visible in 5/15 patients (33%). For the remaining 10/15 patients (67%), DSA selective angiography was needed to confirm the feeding artery. The AA was not assessable on angio-CBCT in 6/21 patients (29%). Three-dimensional road-mapping-guided DSA angiography of all intercostals and lumbar arteries finally helped to visualize the AA and the feeding artery in 6/6 patients (100%). These six patients with negative angio-CBCT had bulky aneurysms with high diameters (64.6 ± 9.3 versus 60.33 ± 7.6; $p = 0.28$) causing major flow turbulence after iodine injection. Figure 4 summarizes the study flow-chart.

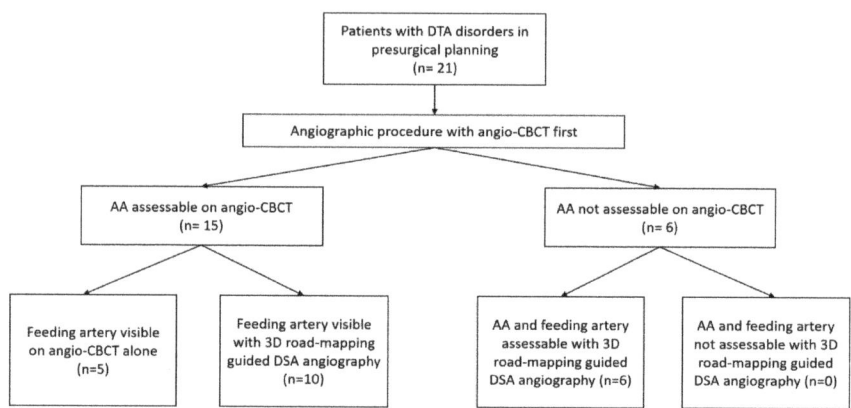

Figure 4. Study flow chart. DTA: descending thoracic aorta; AA: Adamkiewicz artery.

The median and interquartile irradiation dose was 25.5 (20.0–40.0) Gy/cm^2 for the positive angio-CBCT group and 70.4 (30.8–96.9) Gy/cm^2 for the negative angio-CBCT group ($p = 0.16$) (Table 2). There was no significant difference in fluoroscopy time or total procedure time depending on the angio-CBCT result (Table 2). The difference in iodine contrast dose was not statistically significant. In two cases, medullary arteriography was coupled to another intervention in the same operating time. The first was iliac stenting for aneurysmal exclusion, and the second was subclavian artery occlusion. Both interventions were performed in patients for whom angio-CBCT was positive and no extra DSA selective catheterization was necessary. The doses of contrast media and irradiation were combined in these two cases.

Table 2. Results of angiographies according to the visualization of the anterior spinal artery on the CBCT acquisition ($n = 21$). AA: Adamkiewicz artery.

	AA Assessable on CBCT ($n = 15$)	No AA Assessable on CBCT ($n = 6$)	p
Second angio-CBCT, n (%)	2 (13%)	6 (100%)	
Feeding artery visible on angio-CBCT, n (%)	5 (33)	x	
Feeding artery visible after selective guided DSA catheterization, n (%)	10 (67)	6 (100)	
Amount of iodine, mL (mean ± SD)	71.8 ± 38.7	90.0 ± 26.1	0.23
Fluoroscopy time, min (mean ± SD)	16.7 ± 10.8	13.1 ± 8.7	0.45
Length of the procedure, min (mean ± SD)	46.5 ± 17.2	47.9 ± 26.0	0.84
Irradiation, Gy/cm^2 (med (IQR))	25.5 (20.0–40.0)	70.4 (30.8–96.9)	0.41
Aortic aneurysm diameter, mm (mean ± SD)	60.33 ± 7.6	64.6 ± 9.3	0.28

The anterior spinal artery originated in 70% of cases from a left intercostal or lumbar artery and in 25% of cases from the 11th left intercostal artery. These data are presented in Table 3 [7].

Table 3. Distribution of the side and the level of the origin of the Adamkiewicz artery (AA) (n = 21).

	Right (n = 6)	Left (n = 15)
T7, n (%)	0 (0)	1 (5)
T9, n (%)	2 (10)	4 (20)
T10, n (%)	1 (5)	2 (10)
T11, n (%)	1 (5)	6 (25)
T12, n (%)	1 (5)	1 (5)
L1, n (%)	0 (0)	1 (5)
L3, n (%)	1 (5)	0 (0)

After presurgical planification, 16 out of 21 patients underwent aortic surgical repair (Table 4). Eleven patients were treated with endovascular surgical repair (TEVAR), and five were treated with open surgery. The identification of the AA artery led to eight modifications of the surgical strategy for the endovascular population: decision for stent graft length reduction in five (45.4%) of the patients to preserve the AA feeding artery ostium and/or CSF monitoring for seven patients (64%). In the open surgery group, bridging was chosen for three patients (60%) and/or CSF monitoring/drainage in two (40%) patients after the visualization of the AA feeding artery.

Table 4. Procedure modifications following presurgical identification of the AA for both endovascular and open surgery treatments and neurological complication follow-up (n = 16). CSF: cerebrospinal fluid; AA: Adamkiewicz artery.

	Endovascular (n = 11)	Open Surgery (n = 5)
Modification of the surgery, n (%)	8 (73%)	3 (60%)
- Stent graft length reduction, n (%)	5 (45%)	x
- Monitoring/CSF drainage, n (%)	7 (64%)	2 (40%)
- AA reimplantation, n (%)	x	3 (60%)
Neurologic complication, n (%)	0	1 (20%)

One month of follow-up revealed a unique severe neurologic complication described as a spinal cord injury with permanent paraplegia. The patient was selected for open surgery, and the feeding intercostal artery of the AA was reimplanted in association with CSF drainage. During surgery, the patient suffered circulatory arrest due to occlusion of the interventricular artery. The patient was resuscitated but exhibited permanent paraplegia in the recovery room.

4. Discussion

Angio-CBCT and selective DSA guided by 3D road-mapping allowed the location of the feeding artery of the AA in 100% of the patients included in the present study. Angio-CBCT decreases the need for selective catheterization. Kieffer et al. described neurological complications after selective catheterization of the spinal or intercostal artery [10,22]. These types of complications were not reported in our series, and their exact prevalence is difficult to evaluate with the use of up-to-date selective catheters. Three-dimensional road-mapping allowed the location of the patent ostium of the intercostal artery for selective catheterization. In our series, the addition of selective catheterization of the intercostal or lumbar artery did not significantly increase the procedure length, showing that the use of image 3D road-mapping and location of the patent artery might simplify image acquisition and AA location. The presence of an aneurysmal sack thrombus may promote ostial occlusion of the intercostal arteries arising from the aneurysm [23,24]. The precise surgical location of the artery that feeds the AA plays a role in planning the surgical strategy in our department. Matsuda reported that the estimated incidence of permanent and transient spinal cord injury was 3.7% in all TEVAR patients, 6.0% when part or all of the distal aorta was covered and 12.5% when the patent intercostal or lumbar artery that fed the AA was covered [25]. Preoperative identification of the feeding artery of the AA by selective spinal arteriography has been proposed by other groups [10,26–29]. Briefly, their procedure consisted of selective catheterization, usually by the femoral route, followed by the manual injection of contrast material for the imaging of intercostal and lumbar arteries until the arteries that supplied the anterior spinal artery were identified.

However, treatment of a DTA aneurysm might imply a voluntary occlusion of the feeding artery of the AA to avoid the risk of aortic rupture. Several methods have been developed to decrease the risk of spinal cord injury during treatment of a DTA aneurysm. Sequential treatment avoiding extensive covering of the intercostal artery and collateral of interest, such as the left subclavian artery or hypogastric artery, is recognized as an efficient method [30]. Preoperative coiling of the lumbar arteries is also described as a solution to reduce complications [31,32]. Curative treatment of spinal cord ischemia has been shown to be effective [4,29,33,34]. The goal of the treatment is to increase the medullary perfusion pressure and to increase the development of the collateral circulation. Banga et al. [35] increased the mean arterial blood pressure (>80–90 mmHg) and used cerebrospinal fluid drainage to increase the medullary perfusion pressure. Assessment of motor evoked potentials allows the monitoring of the blood supply to the spinal cord in real time during intervention and the adaptation of the arterial blood pressure to cerebrospinal fluid drainage. This setting has been shown to reduce postoperative complications [5,36]. In our clinical practice, all these methods are used and personally adapted according to the patient data. We thought that the precise location of the feeding artery of the AA could help us to better decide on neurological risk reduction techniques during surgery.

Recent innovations in CT or MR technology have made it possible to noninvasively identify the feeding artery of the AA. The detection rates for this artery have been reported to be 80–90% using CT or MR angiography [25–29,33] in patients with thoracic aneurysm or dissection. In fact, these noninvasive assessment methods are able to depict the morphologic hairpin turn configuration of the AA. However, the entire course of the AA should be identified by demonstrating continuity from the anterior spinal artery to the aorta via the AA to avoid misinterpretation of the arterial vascularization of the spinal cord. The rate for vascular continuity has been reported to be in the range of 25 to 60% for 16- or 64-detector row CT [12,14,15,17]. The difficulty in demonstrating continuity can be attributed to the small size of the artery and the proximity to the spine [37]. It is also important to emphasize that many studies have been conducted in different ethnic groups [10,23,28], whose physical characteristics differ from our population.

This study has some limitations, especially the small number of patients included. Angiography is invasive and requires radiation exposure, iodine chelate injection into the patient, and medical expertise and time. This was a proof-of-concept study, and we did not prove that the proposed method is able to decrease the occurrence of spinal cord injury.

5. Conclusions

These results suggest that the combined use of angio-CBCT and 3D road-mapping to guide the anatomical location of the feeding artery of the AA was feasible in all the patients included in our series. In our team's experience, precise knowledge of the arterial vascularization of the spinal cord allowed us to modify and personalize the treatment of DTA diseases.

Author Contributions: Conceptualization, A.J., P.-A.B., M.G., A.G. and A.B.; methodology, P.-A.B., A.G. and A.J.; validation, J.-F.H., M.D.M. and P.B.; formal analysis, P.-A.B.; investigation, P.-A.B., A.G. and A.B.; resources, M.D.M. and A.B.; data curation, A.G.; writing—original draft preparation, P.-A.B., A.G. and A.J.; writing—review and editing, A.B., J.-F.H., M.G., M.D.M., P.B. and F.T.; visualization, M.G.; supervision, A.J. All authors have read and agreed to the published version of the manuscript.

Funding: This research received no external funding.

Institutional Review Board Statement: Not applicable.

Informed Consent Statement: Informed consent was obtained from all subjects involved in the study.

Data Availability Statement: Not applicable.

Conflicts of Interest: The authors declare no conflict of interest.

References

1. Coselli, J.S.; Bozinovski, J.; Le Maire, S.A. Open Surgical Repair of 2286 Thoracoabdominal Aortic Aneurysms. *Ann. Thorac. Surg.* **2007**, *83*, S862–S864. [CrossRef]
2. Schepens, M.A.; Heijmen, R.H.; Ranschaert, W.; Sonker, U.; Morshuis, W.J. Thoracoabdominal Aortic Aneurysm Repair: Results of Conventional Open Surgery. *Eur. J. Vasc. Endovasc. Surg.* **2009**, *37*, 640–645. [CrossRef]
3. Gialdini, G.; Parikh, N.S.; Chatterjee, A.; Lerario, M.P.; Kamel, H.; Schneider, D.B.; Navi, B.B.; Murthy, S.B.; Iadecola, C.; Merkler, A.E. Rates of Spinal Cord Infarction After Repair of Aortic Aneurysm or Dissection. *Stroke* **2017**, *48*, 2073–2077. [CrossRef] [PubMed]
4. Ogino, H.; Sasaki, H.; Minatoya, K.; Matsuda, H.; Yamada, N.; Kitamura, S. Combined Use of Adamkiewicz Artery Demonstration and Motor-Evoked Potentials in Descending and Thoracoabdominal Repair. *Ann. Thorac. Surg.* **2006**, *82*, 592–596. [CrossRef] [PubMed]
5. Coselli, J.S.; LeMaire, S.A.; Köksoy, C.; Schmittling, Z.C.; Curling, P.E. Cerebrospinal Fluid Drainage Reduces Paraplegia after Thoracoabdominal Aortic Aneurysm Repair: Results of a Randomized Clinical Trial. *J. Vasc. Surg.* **2002**, *35*, 631–639. [CrossRef] [PubMed]
6. Lazorthes, G.; Gouaze, A.; Zadeh, J.O.; Santini, J.J.; Lazorthes, Y.; Burdin, P. Arterial Vascularization of the Spinal Cord. Recent Studies of the Anastomotic Substitution Pathways. *J. Neurosurg.* **1971**, *35*, 253–262. [CrossRef]
7. Alleyne, C.H.; Cawley, C.M.; Shengelaia, G.G.; Barrow, D.L. Microsurgical Anatomy of the Artery of Adamkiewicz and Its Segmental Artery. *J. Neurosurg.* **1998**, *89*, 791–795. [CrossRef]
8. Kamada, T.; Yoshioka, K.; Tanaka, R.; Makita, S.; Abiko, A.; Mukaida, M.; Ikai, A.; Okabayashi, H. Strategy for Thoracic Endovascular Aortic Repair Based on Collateral Circulation to the Artery of Adamkiewicz. *Surg. Today* **2016**, *46*, 1024–1030. [CrossRef]
9. Maier, S.; Shcherbakova, M.; Beyersdorf, F.; Benk, C.; Kari, F.A.; Siepe, M.; Czerny, M.; Rylski, B. Benefits and Risks of Prophylactic Cerebrospinal Fluid Catheter and Evoked Potential Monitoring in Symptomatic Spinal Cord Ischemia Low-Risk Thoracic Endovascular Aortic Repair. *Thorac. Cardiovasc. Surg.* **2019**, *67*, 379–384. [CrossRef]
10. Kieffer, E.; Fukui, S.; Chiras, J.; Koskas, F.; Bahnini, A.; Cormier, E. Spinal Cord Arteriography: A Safe Adjunct before Descending Thoracic or Thoracoabdominal Aortic Aneurysmectomy. *J. Vasc. Surg.* **2002**, *35*, 262–268. [CrossRef]
11. Yoshioka, K.; Niinuma, H.; Ohira, A.; Nasu, K.; Kawakami, T.; Sasaki, M.; Kawazoe, K. MR Angiography and CT Angiography of the Artery of Adamkiewicz: Noninvasive Preoperative Assessment of Thoracoabdominal Aortic Aneurysm. *Radiographics* **2003**, *23*, 1215–1225. [CrossRef]
12. Yoshioka, K.; Niinuma, H.; Ehara, S.; Nakajima, T.; Nakamura, M.; Kawazoe, K. MR Angiography and CT Angiography of the Artery of Adamkiewicz: State of the Art. *Radiographics* **2006**, *26*, S63–S73. [CrossRef]
13. Bley, T.A.; Duffek, C.C.; François, C.J.; Schiebler, M.L.; Acher, C.W.; Mell, M.; Grist, T.M.; Reeder, S.B. Presurgical Localization of the Artery of Adamkiewicz with Time-Resolved 3.0-T MR Angiography. *Radiology* **2010**, *255*, 873–881. [CrossRef]
14. Nishida, J.; Kitagawa, K.; Nagata, M.; Yamazaki, A.; Nagasawa, H.; Sakuma, H. Model-Based Iterative Reconstruction for Multi-Detector Row CT Assessment of the Adamkiewicz Artery. *Radiology* **2014**, *270*, 282–291. [CrossRef]
15. Yoshioka, K.; Tanaka, R.; Takagi, H.; Ueyama, Y.; Kikuchi, K.; Chiba, T.; Arakita, K.; Schuijf, J.D.; Saito, Y. Ultra-High-Resolution CT Angiography of the Artery of Adamkiewicz: A Feasibility Study. *Neuroradiology* **2018**, *60*, 109–115. [CrossRef]
16. Takagi, H.; Ota, H.; Natsuaki, Y.; Komori, Y.; Ito, K.; Saiki, Y.; Takase, K. Identifying the Adamkiewicz Artery Using 3-T Time-Resolved Magnetic Resonance Angiography: Its Role in Addition to Multidetector Computed Tomography Angiography. *Jpn. J. Radiol.* **2015**, *33*, 749–756. [CrossRef]
17. Shimoyama, S.; Nishii, T.; Watanabe, Y.; Kono, A.K.; Kagawa, K.; Takahashi, S.; Sugimura, K. Advantages of 70-KV CT Angiography for the Visualization of the Adamkiewicz Artery: Comparison with 120-KV Imaging. *AJNR Am. J. Neuroradiol.* **2017**, *38*, 2399–2405. [CrossRef]
18. Floridi, C.; Radaelli, A.; Abi-Jaoudeh, N.; Grass, M.; Grass, M.; Lin, M.; De Lin, M.; Chiaradia, M.; Geschwind, J.-F.; Kobeiter, H.; et al. C-Arm Cone-Beam Computed Tomography in Interventional Oncology: Technical Aspects and Clinical Applications. *Radiol. Med.* **2014**, *119*, 521–532. [CrossRef]
19. Hermie, L.; Dhondt, E.; Vanlangenhove, P.; De Waele, J.; Degroote, H.; Defreyne, L. Empiric Cone-Beam CT-Guided Embolization in Acute Lower Gastrointestinal Bleeding. *Eur. Radiol.* **2021**, *31*, 2161–2172. [CrossRef]
20. Peisen, F.; Maurer, M.; Grosse, U.; Nikolaou, K.; Syha, R.; Artzner, C.; Bitzer, M.; Horger, M.; Grözinger, G. Intraprocedural Cone-Beam CT with Parenchymal Blood Volume Assessment for Transarterial Chemoembolization Guidance: Impact on the Effectiveness of the Individual TACE Sessions Compared to DSA Guidance Alone. *Eur. J. Radiol.* **2021**, *140*, 109768. [CrossRef]

21. Honarmand, A.R.; Gemmete, J.J.; Hurley, M.C.; Shaibani, A.; Chaudhary, N.; Pandey, A.S.; Bendok, B.R.; Ansari, S.A. Adjunctive Value of Intra-Arterial Cone Beam CT Angiography Relative to DSA in the Evaluation of Cranial and Spinal Arteriovenous Fistulas. *J. Neurointerv. Surg.* **2015**, *7*, 517–523. [CrossRef]
22. Williams, G.M.; Roseborough, G.S.; Webb, T.H.; Perler, B.A.; Krosnick, T. Preoperative Selective Intercostal Angiography in Patients Undergoing Thoracoabdominal Aneurysm Repair. *J. Vasc. Surg.* **2004**, *39*, 314–321. [CrossRef]
23. Yogendranathan, N.; Herath, H.M.M.T.B.; Jayamali, W.D.; Matthias, A.T.; Pallewatte, A.; Kulatunga, A. A Case of Anterior Spinal Cord Syndrome in a Patient with Unruptured Thoracic Aortic Aneurysm with a Mural Thrombus. *BMC Cardiovasc. Disord* **2018**, *18*, 48. [CrossRef]
24. Aydin, A. Mechanisms and Prevention of Anterior Spinal Artery Syndrome Following Abdominal Aortic Surgery. *Angiol. Sosud. Khirurgiia* **2015**, *21*, 155–164.
25. Matsuda, H.; Fukuda, T.; Iritani, O.; Nakazawa, T.; Tanaka, H.; Sasaki, H.; Minatoya, K.; Ogino, H. Spinal Cord Injury Is Not Negligible after TEVAR for Lower Descending Aorta. *Eur. J. Vasc. Endovasc. Surg.* **2010**, *39*, 179–186. [CrossRef]
26. Heinemann, M.K.; Brassel, F.; Herzog, T.; Dresler, C.; Becker, H.; Borst, H.G. The Role of Spinal Angiography in Operations on the Thoracic Aorta: Myth or Reality? *Ann. Thorac. Surg.* **1998**, *65*, 346–351. [CrossRef]
27. Minatoya, K.; Karck, M.; Hagl, C.; Meyer, A.; Brassel, F.; Harringer, W.; Haverich, A. The Impact of Spinal Angiography on the Neurological Outcome after Surgery on the Descending Thoracic and Thoracoabdominal Aorta. *Ann. Thorac. Surg.* **2002**, *74*, S1870–S1872. [CrossRef]
28. Dias-Neto, M.; Reis, P.; Mendes, L.; Rodrigues, M.; Amaral, C.; Afonso, G.; Fernando Teixeira, J. Institutional Protocol for Prevention of TEVAR-Related Spinal Cord Ischemia—The First 9 Cases. *Rev. Port. Cir. Cardio-Torac. Vasc.* **2017**, *24*, 151.
29. Uchida, N. How to Prevent Spinal Cord Injury during Endovascular Repair of Thoracic Aortic Disease. *Gen. Thorac. Cardiovasc. Surg.* **2014**, *62*, 391–397. [CrossRef]
30. Bisdas, T.; Panuccio, G.; Sugimoto, M.; Torsello, G.; Austermann, M. Risk Factors for Spinal Cord Ischemia after Endovascular Repair of Thoracoabdominal Aortic Aneurysms. *J. Vasc. Surg.* **2015**, *61*, 1408–1416. [CrossRef]
31. Etz, C.D.; Debus, E.S.; Mohr, F.-W.; Kölbel, T. First-in-Man Endovascular Preconditioning of the Paraspinal Collateral Network by Segmental Artery Coil Embolization to Prevent Ischemic Spinal Cord Injury. *J. Thorac. Cardiovasc. Surg.* **2015**, *149*, 1074–1079. [CrossRef] [PubMed]
32. Geisbüsch, S.; Stefanovic, A.; Koruth, J.; Lin, H.; Morgello, S.; Weisz, D.; Griepp, R.; Di Luozzo, G. Endovascular Coil Embolization of Segmental Arteries Prevents Paraplegia After Subsequent TAAA Repair—An Experimental Model. *J. Thorac. Cardiovasc. Surg.* **2014**, *147*, 220–226. [CrossRef] [PubMed]
33. Epstein, N.E. Cerebrospinal Fluid Drains Reduce Risk of Spinal Cord Injury for Thoracic/Thoracoabdominal Aneurysm Surgery: A Review. *Surg. Neurol. Int.* **2018**, *9*, 48. [CrossRef] [PubMed]
34. Matsuda, H.; Ogino, H.; Fukuda, T.; Iritani, O.; Sato, S.; Iba, Y.; Tanaka, H.; Sasaki, H.; Minatoya, K.; Kobayashi, J.; et al. Multidisciplinary Approach to Prevent Spinal Cord Ischemia After Thoracic Endovascular Aneurysm Repair for Distal Descending Aorta. *Ann. Thorac. Surg.* **2010**, *90*, 561–565. [CrossRef]
35. Banga, P.V.; Oderich, G.S.; de Souza, L.R.; Hofer, J.; Gonzalez, M.L.C.; Pulido, J.N.; Cha, S.; Gloviczki, P. Neuromonitoring, Cerebrospinal Fluid Drainage, and Selective Use of Iliofemoral Conduits to Minimize Risk of Spinal Cord Injury During Complex Endovascular Aortic Repair. *J. Endovasc. Ther.* **2015**, *23*. [CrossRef]
36. Cinà, C.S.; Abouzahr, L.; Arena, G.O.; Laganà, A.; Devereaux, P.J.; Farrokhyar, F. Cerebrospinal Fluid Drainage to Prevent Paraplegia during Thoracic and Thoracoabdominal Aortic Aneurysm Surgery: A Systematic Review and Meta-Analysis. *J. Vasc. Surg.* **2004**, *40*, 36–44. [CrossRef] [PubMed]
37. Nishii, T.; Kono, A.K.; Nishio, M.; Negi, N.; Fujita, A.; Kohmura, E.; Sugimura, K. Bone-Subtracted Spinal CT Angiography Using Nonrigid Registration for Better Visualization of Arterial Feeders in Spinal Arteriovenous Fistulas. *AJNR Am. J. Neuroradiol.* **2015**, *36*, 2400–2406. [CrossRef]

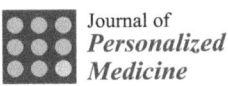

Article

Pelvic Venous Insufficiency: Input of Short Tau Inversion Recovery Sequence

Eva Jambon, Yann Le Bras, Gregoire Cazalas, Nicolas Grenier and Clement Marcelin *

Department of Radiology, Pellegrin Hospital, Place Amélie Raba Léon, 33076 Bordeaux, France
* Correspondence: clement.marcelin@gmail.com; Tel.: +33-65-914-4733; Fax: +33-557-82-16-50

Abstract: Objectives: To evaluate indirect criteria of pelvic venous insufficiency (PVI) of a short tau inversion recovery (STIR) sequence retrospectively compared with phlebographic findings. **Methods:** Between 2008 and 2018, 164 women who had received MRI and phlebography for pelvic congestion syndrome (60), varicose veins in the lower limbs (45), both (43), or other symptoms (16) were included. The presence of periuterine varicosities and perivaginal varicosities were compared to the findings of phlebography: grading of left ovarian vein reflux and presence of internal pudendal or obturator leak. **Results:** There was a correlation between the grading of LOV reflux on phlebography and the diameter of periuterine varicosities on STIR sequence (p = 0.008, rho = 0.206, CIrho [0.0549 to 0.349]). Periuterine varicosities had a positive predictive value of 93% for left ovarian reflux (95% CI [88.84% to 95.50%]). Obturator or internal pudendal leaks were found for 118 women (72%) and iliac insufficiency for 120 women (73%). **Conclusions:** Non-injected MRI offers a satisfactory exploration of PVI with STIR sequence. STIR sequences alone enabled the detection of left ovarian and iliac insufficiency.

Keywords: magnetic resonance imaging; pelvis; venous congestion; phlebography; varicose veins; venous insufficiency

1. Introduction

Pelvic venous insufficiency (PVI) is a pathology of premenopausal and multiparous women that is still poorly understood and frequently misdiagnosed [1]. Regularly responsible for pelvic congestion syndrome (PCS), combining chronic pelvic pain, dysmenorrhea, and dyspareunia, PVI induces recurrent varicose veins in the lower limbs (VVLL) and unsightly varicosities on the buttock, perineal, or vulvar [2–4]. These interrelated symptoms were recently grouped under the term "Pelvic Venous Disorders" [5]. The diversity of symptoms and the poor understanding of pathogenic mechanisms are major concerns. Although first described by Taylor in 1949, PCS frequency remains unknown [6,7]. The prevalence of retrograde flow in the ovarian veins has been estimated at 9.9% based on 273 angiographic studies including healthy female renal transplant donors, with 59% of them reporting chronic pelvic pain compatible with PCS and 77% reporting improvement after ovarian vein ligation [8,9]. A recent study on 2384 abdomino-pelvic computed tomography (CT) images found that 8% of premenopausal women had PCS with dilated left ovarian veins (LOV) [10].

Non-invasive investigations are recommended as an initial assessment for PVI, but phlebography remains the gold standard with a sensitivity and specificity of 91% and 89%, respectively [11–13]. However, phlebography is an invasive diagnostic technique, exposes the pelvis of women of childbearing age to irradiation, is costly, and is time-consuming [14,15]. Thanks to non-invasive diagnostic tools, pre-therapeutic phlebography could be facilitated [15].

CT is an effective technique for this indication but it is irradiating [16–20]. MRI is the imaging modality of choice for female pelvic exploration with an optimal exploration of internal genital organs [21] to eliminate differential diagnoses of chronic pain, in particular, endometriosis with similar symptoms [15,22].

Many women with PVI had an important diagnostic delay, sometimes for many years. A non-injected sequence could be added to MRI for "undetermined chronic pelvic pain" suitable for PVI.

Short-tau inversion recovery (STIR) sequence is an IR technique that nulls fat signal intensity based on T1 values. The STIR sequence uses an initial 180° RF pulse to invert spins in the longitudinal plane. After a short time delay (known as inversion time (TI)), this initial RF pulse is followed by a conventional spin-echo. To achieve fat suppression, a TI should be selected such that the longitudinal magnetization of the fat spins is zero when a subsequent 90° pulse is applied. The TI that will negate the signal from fat is equal to 0.69 times the Ti relaxation time of fat, provided that the selected TA is significantly greater than Ti. As Ti relaxation times are proportional to the applied magnetic field, the appropriate TI with a STIR for nulling the signal from fat must be adjusted for a given magnet strength. Even at a given magnetic field strength, the TI that maximally nulls the fat signal varies slightly from patient to patient, possibly because of differences in fat composition. STIR pulse sequences rely on the relatively short Ti relaxation time of adipose tissue to achieve fat suppression. This technique is quite different from the frequency-selective fat suppression technique, in which the signal from fat protons is selectively nulled on the basis of the intrinsic chemical shift differences between lipid and water protons. As STIR sequences will suppress the signal from any tissue or fluid that, like fat, has a short Ti relaxation time, this technique of fat suppression may be considered nonselective [23]. The STIR sequence allows unparalleled cartography of the pelvis. It is not yet evaluated despite its excellent tissue contrast and spatial resolution. PVI induces important varicosities visualized like hyperintense dilated tortuous structures around the uterus and vagina.

The aim of this study was to evaluate the indirect criteria of PVI of STIR sequences retrospectively compared with phlebographic findings.

2. Material and Methods

2.1. Patients

This was a single-centre, retrospective study performed in a regional University Hospital. Ethical approval was obtained by the Publication Group of the Ethics committee of the University Hospital (CE-GP-2019-20). Using radiology databases and medical records at our institution, from 2008 to 2018, we consecutively included all women who had MRI and phlebography for suspicion of PVI based on clinical features, defined as chronic pelvic pain (>6 months) with dysmenorrhea, dyspareunia, or post-coital pain, that typically increased at the end of the day and while standing. Other signs could be associated with dysuria, nocturia, or rectal symptoms. VVLL included were evaluated by US and pelvic leaks were identified. Unsightly varicosities on the buttock, perineal, or vulvar were described by the patients and clinically observed. A pelvic leak was defined as an abnormal communication between VVLL and pelvic veins. Exclusion criteria were other aetiologies of chronic pelvic pain (uterine fibroma, adenomyosis, or endometriosis).

2.2. Magnetic Resonance Imaging

Imaging was performed on a 1.5 Tesla instrument (Avanto, Siemens Healthcare, Forchheim, Germany) The duration of the examination was 30 to 40 min. After the acquisition of the scout images, 2-dimensional T2-weighted STIR BLADE sagittal and coronal images were acquired as the detailed scout images. The acquisition parameters for STIR images were as follows: TR, 4810 ms; TE, 82 ms; matrix, 256 × 256; slices, 30; slice thickness/gap, 4.5 mm/10% and imaging time, 3 min 22 s. Then, 2-dimensional T2-weighted STIR BLADE axial images were acquired. The acquisition parameters for axial STIR images were as follows: TR, 5771 ms; TE, 82 ms; matrix, 256 × 256; slices, 35; slice thickness/gap, 4.5 mm/10% and imaging time, 4 min 02 s. After, the other sequences were realized: axial T2 TRUFI, Axial T1 DIXON 3D VIBE, Angio Dynamic TWIST with coronal MIP reconstruction then 3D T1 VIBE. Dotarem© was injected at 3 mL/sec at the third dynamic for 2 mL/kg and flushed with 20 mL of NaCl.

A differential diagnosis or a type II or III venous compression, according to the classification of Greiner et al., had to be eliminated [24]. Indirect criteria of PVI of STIR in the 3 spatial planes with visualization of the top of the thighs were obtained to record the diameter of periuterine veins and the presence of perivaginal or external varicosities. A diameter > 5 mm was considered a periuterine varicosity, according to the Guidelines of the Society of Interventional Radiology [12]. The presence of paravaginal, perineal, vulvar varicosities or varicosities on the buttock was defined by abnormal dilated and tortuous veins. The presence of a hyposignal STIR sequence within pelvic veins was noted like "flow voids".

2.3. Phlebography

All procedures were undertaken on the same angiographic unit (Philips Medical Systems). Phlebography was performed by two investigators with experience in interventional radiology of 5 and 20 years before the embolization. A brachial or femoral venous approach was used, using a 4- or 5-French sheath. LRV was catheterized with a 4-French Cobra catheter and phlebography was performed. If a Nutcracker syndrome was suspected with clinical symptoms (haematuria, lumbar pain), a measurement of the vena cava and renal vein pressures was realized (Normal $\leq$ 3 mmHg) [24]. Then, LOV was catheterized and a phlebography with Valsalva manoeuvre was realized with automatic injection (Visipaque®: volume of 20 mL, rate of 10 mL/s). The internal iliac veins were catheterized with a Cobra catheter or a UAC catheter and were looking for incompetent collectors, leaks to the legs, and a May-Thurner syndrome with automatic injection (Visipaque®: volume of 20 mL, rate of 10 mL/s).

LOV insufficiency was defined by reflux towards the pelvis. LOV diameter was noticed and reflux was scored from 0 to 3 according to the description by Hiromura et al. [25]. In grade 1, retrograde flow remained in the LOV, not reaching the parauterine veins. In grade 2, the retrograde flow advanced into the ipsilateral parauterine veins and no further. In grade 3, the retrograde flow crossed the midline passing through the uterus from the left into the right parauterine plexus [25].

Iliac insufficiency was defined by reflux into its tributaries. A superior gluteal leak was visualized in front of the iliac wing, an inferior gluteal leak in front of the femoral head, an obturator leak passed over the obturator foramen and a pudendal leak followed the iliopubic rami. Irradiation data were not relevant because the embolization was performed on the same day.

2.4. Imaging Analysis

Images were reviewed in a blinded fashion by one radiologist with five years of experience and one radiologist with twenty years of experience. Inter-observer variability was evaluated for dilatation of iliac tributaries. In case of disagreement, a consensus reading was organized for a final decision. Only clinical patient information was available. To avoid any recognition bias, the studies were presented in random order. All imaging investigation data were assessed on a Picture Archiving and Communication system (PACS) station (Vue PACS; Carestream Health, Rochester, NY, USA).

2.5. Statistical Analysis

Statistical analysis was performed with Excel and MedCalc® software version 12.3 (Ostend, Belgium). Qualitative variables are expressed as raw numbers, proportions, and percentages. Quantitative variables are expressed as medians with 1st (Q1) and 3rd (Q3) quartiles and ranges.

The positive predictive value was calculated for every criterion. The correlation between reflux grading and periuterine varicosities was tested using Spearman's rank correlation. A *p*-value < 0.05 was considered statistically significant.

The inter-observer variability coefficient was calculated by the Kappa Cohen coefficient.

3. Results

3.1. Patients and Anatomical Analysis

Two hundred and twenty-five women had a phlebography for suspicion of PVI between 2008 and 2018 at our centre. One hundred and sixty-four women (median age: 39 years; Q1–Q3: 34–45) were included in the study (Table 1): 60 women for a PCS, 45 for VVLL, 43 for both, and 16 for other isolated symptoms (6 women with vulvar varicosities, 4 patients with perineal varicosities, 1 patient with varicosities on the buttock and 5 women suffering with lumbar pain and haematuria were included with suspicion of Nutcracker syndrome).

Table 1. Patients' characteristics. All quantitative variables are expressed in mean, SD, and range/median (Q1–Q3); all qualitative variables are expressed with raw numbers, proportions, and percentages.

	164
Age (years)	39 ± 9 (21–69)/39 (34–45)
Number of pregnancies	2 ± 1 (0–6)/2 (2–3)
PCS	60 (60/164; 36.59%)
VVLL	45 (45/164; 27.44%)
PCS + VVLL	43 (43/164; 26.22%)
Presence of external varicosities * Isolated	34 (34/164; 20.73%) 16 (16/164; 9.76%)
Dysuria	4 (4/164; 2.44%)

* Vulvar, perineal or on the buttock, isolated, or in association. N: Number of patients, PCS: pelvic congestion syndrome, VVLL: varicose veins of the lower limbs.

Referrals were made by vascular specialists in 62% of cases, vascular surgeons in 26%, and gynaecologists in 12%. The median time between MRI and phlebography was 41 days (28–65). One patient had an angioedema caused by a Gadolinium injection that required a short stay in intensive care.

Anatomical variability was found for 16 women (10%). Seven patients had LOV variability: six women with two LOV (4%) and one woman with three. There were five patients with LRV variability: one woman with two LRV, three with retroaortic LRV (2%), and one with circumaortic. There were three ROV draining into the right renal vein (2%).

3.2. STIR and Phlebographic Findings

On the STIR sequence, the median diameter of periuterine veins was 7 mm (6–8). One hundred and twenty-six women had periuterine varicosities with a diameter > 5 mm (77%). Ninety-eight patients had "flow voids" in their pelvic varicosities (60%).

One hundred and twenty-nine patients had perivaginal varicosities (79%), thirty-nine vulvar varicosities (24%), fifty-seven perineal varicosities (35%), and five varicosities on the buttock (3%).

One hundred and forty-four women had left ovarian reflux on phlebography (88%). Six reflux were grade 1 (4%), thirty-nine reflux were grade 2 (27%), and ninety-nine were grade 3 (69%).

There was a correlation between the grading of LOV reflux on phlebography and the diameter of periuterine varicosities on the STIR sequence ($p = 0.008$, rho = 0.206, CIrho [0.0549 to 0.349]). Periuterine varicosities had a positive predictive value of 93% for left ovarian reflux (95% CI [88.84% to 95.50%]).

Obturator or internal pudendal leaks were found for 118 women (72%) and iliac insufficiency for 120 women (73%) (Figure 1). Inter-observer agreement for iliac insufficiency was substantial (k = 0.72).

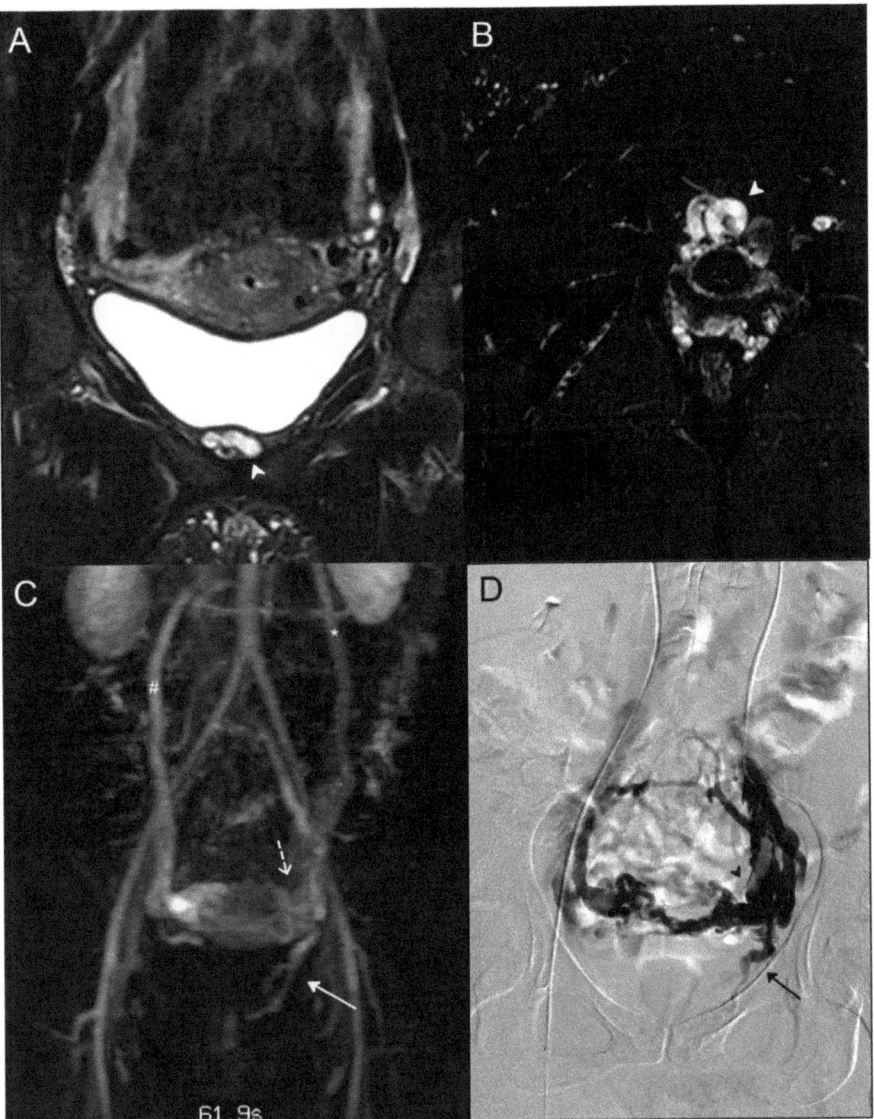

Figure 1. A 38-year-old woman who suffered from recurrent varicose veins in the lower limbs had magnetic resonance imaging (MRI) and a phlebography for suspicion of pelvic venous insufficiency. A/B: MRI coronal (**A**) and axial (**B**) T2 short inversion time inversion recovery (STIR) sequence: Dilated left internal pudendal vein *(white arrowhead)*. (**C**) Maximal intensity projection (MIP) coronal reconstruction of MRI angiography sequence: Voluminous periuterine varicose *(dotted arrow)*, reflux in the left internal pudendal vein *(white arrow)*, incompetent left ovarian vein (*), and vicarious right ovarian vein (#). (**D**) Phlebography: Confirmation of an incompetent left internal pudendal vein *(black arrow)*. Visualization of important periuterine varicose *(black arrowhead)*.

Perivaginal varicosities had a positive predictive value of 78% for obturator or internal pudendal leak (95% CI [64.41% to 78.68%]) (Figure 2). Perivaginal or external varicosities had a predictive value of 76% for iliac insufficiency (95% CI [72.51% to 79.71%]) (Table 2).

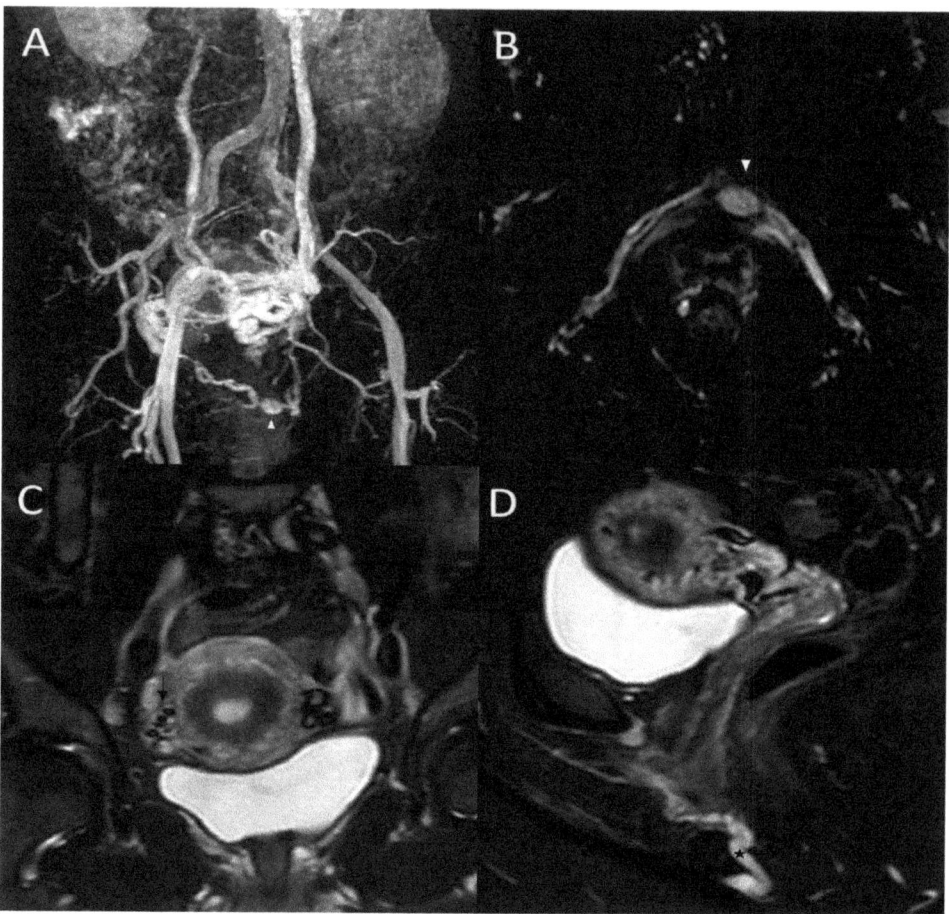

Figure 2. (**A**) 50-year-old woman who suffered from pelvic pain and vulvar varicosities had magnetic resonance imaging (MRI). Maximal intensity projection (MIP) coronal reconstruction of MRI angiography sequence: Voluminous left periuterine varicose with reflux in the internal pudendal veins *(white arrowhead)*, incompetent left ovarian vein, and vicarious right ovarian vein. (**B**) MRI axial T2 short inversion time inversion recovery (STIR) sequence: Dilated left internal pudendal vein with aneurysm *(white arrowhead)*. (**C**) MRI coronal T2 short inversion time inversion recovery (STIR) sequence: Flow voids in dilated pelvic varicose veins *(dark arrow)*. (**D**) MRI sagittal T2 short inversion time inversion recovery (STIR) sequence: Flow voids in dilated pelvic varicose veins *(dark arrow)* and dilated left internal pudendal vein (*).

Table 2. Diagnostic performance of the STIR sequence.

Criterion	Sensitivity	Specificity	PPV	NPV
Detection of leaks	0.92	0.77	0.93	0.73
Iliac insufficiency by detection of leaks	0.91	0.27	0.68	0.63
Left ovarian insufficiency by detection of Periuterine varicosities > 5 mm	0.82	0.53	0.93	0.26
Internal pudendal or obturator leak by detection of perivaginal varicosities	0.87	0.56	0.78	0.62

PPV: positive predictive value; NPV: negative predictive value.

4. Discussion

Based on 10 years of experience reported here, these data confirm that the STIR sequence is indirectly reliable to detect PVI. Detection of periuterine varicosities had a positive predictive value of 82% for LOV reflux. This result was according to the transvaginal US findings in the literature relating a sensitivity and specificity of 100% and 83–100%, respectively [26,27]. Pelvic US had many advantages: localization of pain at the passage of the probe and use of a Valsalva maneuver to objective reflux. US had the main disadvantage of being direct and operator-dependent. The STIR sequence allows for realistic cartography of pelvic varicosities for optimal anticipation and processing of the procedure of embolization. The iliac, ovarian, or mixt supply is visualized with the facility.

The presence of perivaginal varicosities had a 78% positive predictive value for obturator or pudendal leaks. The composite criterion containing peri-vaginal and external varicosities detected on the STIR sequence had a positive predicted value of 76% for iliac insufficiency.

In the literature, the evaluation of PVI was limited to direct reflux analysis [9,14,28,29]. Asciutto et al. evaluated dynamic MRI versus phlebography in 23 patients with PCS. The sensitivity and specificity of MRI were, respectively, 88% and 67% for ovarian veins, 100% and 38% for hypogastric veins, and 91% and 42% for periuterine varicosity [14]. Yang et al. compared the grading of reflux in the ovarian veins on dynamic MRI versus phlebography in 19 patients: the sensitivity, specificity, and diagnosis relevance of MRI were 66.7%, 100%, 78.9%, and 75%, 100%, 84.2% for the two observers, respectively [29]. Meneses et al. used a phase-contrast velocity mapping and found a sensitivity of 100% and specificity of 50%, based on nine patients with suspected PCS [30].

Perivaginal varicosities were responsible for deep dyspareunia and post-coital pains. Any radiologists could detect these varicosities with an endovaginal probe, with the copying of usual pains [31]. The sagittal STIR sequence allows complete visualization of peri-vaginal varicosities and these venous supplies. This criterion could be used to facilitate the phlebography and to search for internal pudendal or obturator incompetency even if the vein is valvulated.

External varicosities were visualized very well by the STIR sequence like a serpiginous dilated hypersignal vein in subcutaneous tissue. These veins were often in communication with varicose in the lower limbs. They could be treated directly by sclerotherapy with 2% polidocanol (Aetoxisclerol, Kreussler, Wiesbaden, Hessen, Germany) under ultrasound and X-ray guidance [32].

It is well known that PVI was a complex pathology and the ovarian vein reflux analysis is not sufficient. The dynamic MRI sequence does not allow for analyzing the iliac vein and afferents reflux [14]. STIR sequence allows a direct and indirect analysis of ovarian and iliac veins with a good spatial resolution.

Our study has some limitations, notably with recruitment, as all symptomatic patients had a final diagnosis of PVI. No patient had an MRI or phlebography that did not result in a PVI diagnosis. The retrospective review of imaging examinations could lead to the recognition of records. We have tried to minimize this bias by presenting the studies in random order.

In conclusion, non-injected MRI offers a satisfactory exploration of symptomatic PVI with the STIR sequence. Indirectly, the STIR sequence alone enabled the detection of left ovarian and iliac insufficiency.

Gynecological imaging included 3D T2 weight or sagittal T2 weight, however, these sequences provide detection of anomalies in pelvic organs, but the pelvic fat avoids correctly detecting varicose veins or they are likely sub-estimated.

The STIR sequence could be added as an option after a usual MRI protocol performed for unexplained pelvic pain. After detection of symptomatic pelvic varicosities without other etiology of pelvic pain on MRI, the patient should be addressed to an interventional radiologist.

Author Contributions: Conceptualization, E.J. and C.M.; methodology, E.J.; software, E.J.; validation, C.M., Y.L.B. and N.G.; formal analysis, E.J.; investigation, E.J.; data curation, E.J.; writing—original draft preparation, E.J.; writing—review and editing, E.J.; visualization, C.M. and G.C.; supervision, C.M.; project administration, C.M. All authors have read and agreed to the published version of the manuscript.

Funding: This research received no external funding.

Institutional Review Board Statement: Ethical approval was obtained by the Publication Group of the Ethics committee of the University Hospital (CE-GP-2019-20).

Informed Consent Statement: Not applicable.

Data Availability Statement: Not applicable.

Conflicts of Interest: The authors declare no conflict of interest.

Abbreviations

PVI	pelvic venous insufficiency
MRI	magnetic resonance imaging
LOV	left ovarian vein
LRV	left renal vein
STIR	short tau inversion recovery
ROV	right ovarian vein
PCS	pelvic congestion syndrome
VVLL	varicose veins in the lower limbs
CT	computed tomography
MIP	maximum intensity projection
PPV	positive predictive value
NPV	negative predictive value

References

1. Gültaşli, N.Z.; Kurt, A.; Ipek, A.; Gümüş, M.; Yazicioğlu, K.R.; Dilmen, G.; Taş, I. The relation between pelvic varicose veins, chronic pelvic pain and lower extremity venous insufficiency in women. *Diagn. Interv. Radiol.* **2006**, *12*, 34–38. [PubMed]
2. Phillips, D.; Deipolyi, A.R.; Hesketh, R.L.; Midia, M.; Oklu, R. Pelvic Congestion Syndrome: Etiology of Pain, Diagnosis, and Clinical Management. *J. Vasc. Interv. Radiol.* **2014**, *25*, 725–733. [CrossRef]
3. Greiner, M.; Gilling-Smith, G.L. Leg Varices Originating from the Pelvis: Diagnosis and Treatment. *Vascular* **2007**, *15*, 70–78. [CrossRef] [PubMed]
4. Bora, A.; Avcu, S.; Arslan, H.; Adali, E.; Bulut, M.D. The relation between pelvic varicose veins and lower extremity venous insufficiency in women with chronic pelvic pain. *JBR-BTR* **2012**, *95*, 215. [CrossRef] [PubMed]
5. Khilnani, N.M.; Meissner, M.H.; Learman, L.A.; Gibson, K.D.; Daniels, J.P.; Winokur, R.S.; Marvel, R.P.; Machan, L.; Venbrux, A.C.; Tu, F.F.; et al. Research Priorities in Pelvic Venous Disorders in Women: Recommendations from a Multidisciplinary Research Consensus Panel. *J. Vasc. Interv. Radiol.* **2019**, *30*, 781–789. [CrossRef]
6. Taylor, H.C. Vascular congestion and hyperemia; their effect on function and structure in the female reproductive organs; the clinical aspects of the congestion-fibrosis syndrome. *Am. J. Obstet. Gynecol.* **1949**, *57*, 637–653. [CrossRef]
7. Champaneria, R.; Shah, L.; Moss, J.; Gupta, J.K.; Birch, J.; Middleton, L.J.; Daniels, J.P. The relationship between pelvic vein incompetence and chronic pelvic pain in women: Systematic reviews of diagnosis and treatment effectiveness. *Health Technol. Assess.* **2016**, *20*, 1–108. [CrossRef]

8. Belenky, A.; Bartal, G.; Atar, E.; Cohen, M.; Bachar, G.N. Ovarian Varices in Healthy Female Kidney Donors: Incidence, Morbidity, and Clinical Outcome. *Am. J. Roentgenol.* **2002**, *179*, 625–627. [CrossRef]
9. Kim, C.Y.; Miller, M.J.; Merkle, E.M. Time-Resolved MR Angiography as a Useful Sequence for Assessment of Ovarian Vein Reflux. *Am. J. Roentgenol.* **2009**, *193*, W458–W463. [CrossRef]
10. Jurga-Karwacka, A.; Karwacki, G.M.; Schoetzau, A.; Zech, C.J.; Heinzelmann-Schwarz, V.; Schwab, F.D. A forgotten disease: Pelvic congestion syndrome as a cause of chronic lower abdominal pain. *PLoS ONE* **2019**, *14*, e0213834. [CrossRef]
11. Ganeshan, A.; Upponi, S.; Hon, L.-Q.; Uthappa, M.C.; Warakaulle, D.R.; Uberoi, R. Chronic Pelvic Pain due to Pelvic Congestion Syndrome: The Role of Diagnostic and Interventional Radiology. *Cardiovasc. Interv. Radiol.* **2007**, *30*, 1105–1111. [CrossRef]
12. Black, C.M.; Thorpe, K.; Venrbux, A.; Kim, H.S.; Millward, S.F.; Clark, T.W.; Kundu, S.; Martin, L.G.; Sacks, D.; York, J.; et al. Research Reporting Standards for Endovascular Treatment of Pelvic Venous Insufficiency. *J. Vasc. Interv. Radiol.* **2010**, *21*, 796–803. [CrossRef]
13. Beard, R.; Pearce, S.; Highman, J.; Reginald, P. Diagnosis of pelvic varicosities in women with chronic pelvic pain. *Lancet* **1984**, *2*, 946–949. [CrossRef]
14. Asciutto, G.; Mumme, A.; Marpe, B.; Köster, O.; Asciutto, K.; Geier, B. MR Venography in the Detection of Pelvic Venous Congestion. *Eur. J. Vasc. Endovasc. Surg.* **2008**, *36*, 491–496. [CrossRef]
15. Steenbeek, M.P.; van der Vleuten, C.J.; Kool, L.J.S.; Nieboer, T.E. Noninvasive diagnostic tools for pelvic congestion syndrome: A systematic review. *Acta Obstet. Gynecol. Scand.* **2018**, *97*, 776–786. [CrossRef]
16. Bookwalter, C.A.; VanBuren, W.M.; Neisen, M.J.; Bjarnason, H. Imaging Appearance and Nonsurgical Management of Pelvic Venous Congestion Syndrome. *RadioGraphics* **2019**, *39*, 596–608. [CrossRef]
17. Jin, K.N.; Lee, W.; Jae, H.J.; Yin, Y.H.; Chung, J.W.; Park, J.H. Venous reflux from the pelvis and vulvoperineal region as a possible cause of lower extremity varicose veins: Diagnosis with computed tomographic and ultrasonographic findings. *J. Comput. Assist. Tomogr.* **2009**, *33*, 763–769. [CrossRef]
18. Arnoldussen, C.W.K.P.; de Wolf, M.A.F.; Wittens, C.H.A. Diagnostic imaging of pelvic congestive syndrome. *Phlebology* **2015**, *30* (Suppl. S1), 67–72. [CrossRef]
19. Coakley, F.V.; Varghese, S.L.; Hricak, H. CT and MRI of Pelvic Varices in Women. *J. Comput. Assist. Tomogr.* **1999**, *23*, 429–434. [CrossRef]
20. Borghi, C.; Dell'Atti, L. Pelvic congestion syndrome: The current state of the literature. *Arch. Gynecol. Obstet.* **2015**, *293*, 291–301. [CrossRef]
21. Schwartz, L.B.; Panageas, E.; Lange, R.; Rizzo, J.; Comite, F.; McCarthy, S. Female pelvis: Impact of MR imaging on treatment decisions and net cost analysis. *Radiology* **1994**, *192*, 55–60. [CrossRef] [PubMed]
22. Juhan, V. Chronic pelvic pain: An imaging approach. *Diagn. Interv. Imaging* **2015**, *96*, 997–1007. [CrossRef] [PubMed]
23. Krinsky, G.; Rofsky, N.M.; Weinreb, J.C. Nonspecificity of short inversion time inversion recovery (STIR) as a technique of fat suppression: Pitfalls in image interpretation. *Am. J. Roentgenol.* **1996**, *166*, 523–526. [CrossRef] [PubMed]
24. Greiner, M.; Dadon, M.; Lemasle, P.; Cluzel, P. How Does the Pathophysiology Influence the Treatment of Pelvic Congestion Syndrome and is the Result Long-lasting? *Phlebology* **2012**, *27*, 58–64. [CrossRef] [PubMed]
25. Hiromura, T.; Nishioka, T.; Nishioka, S.; Ikeda, H.; Tomita, K. Reflux in the Left Ovarian Vein: Analysis of MDCT Findings in Asymptomatic Women. *Am. J. Roentgenol.* **2004**, *183*, 1411–1415. [CrossRef]
26. Giacchetto, C.; Cotroneo, G.B.; Marincolo, F.; Cammisuli, F.; Caruso, G.; Catizone, F. Ovarian varicocele: Ultrasonic and phlebographic evaluation. *J. Clin. Ultrasound* **1990**, *18*, 551–555. [CrossRef]
27. Park, S.J.; Lim, J.W.; Ko, Y.T.; Lee, D.H.; Yoon, Y.; Oh, J.H.; Lee, H.K.; Huh, C.Y. Diagnosis of Pelvic Congestion Syndrome Using Transabdominal and Transvaginal Sonography. *Am. J. Roentgenol.* **2004**, *182*, 683–688. [CrossRef]
28. Pandey, T.; Shaikh, R.; Viswamitra, S.; Jambhekar, K. Use of time resolved magnetic resonance imaging in the diagnosis of pelvic congestion syndrome. *J. Magn. Reson. Imaging* **2010**, *32*, 700–704. [CrossRef]
29. Yang, D.M.; Kim, H.C.; Nam, D.H.; Jahng, G.H.; Huh, C.Y.; Lim, J.W. Time-resolved MR angiography for detecting and grading ovarian venous reflux: Comparison with conventional venography. *Br. J. Radiol.* **2012**, *85*, e117–e122. [CrossRef]
30. Meneses, L.Q.; Uribe, S.; Tejos, C.; Andía, M.E.; Fava, M.; Irarrazaval, P. Using magnetic resonance phase-contrast velocity mapping for diagnosing pelvic congestion syndrome. *Phlebology* **2011**, *26*, 157–161. [CrossRef]
31. Valero, I.; Garcia-Jimenez, R.; Valdevieso, P.; Garcia-Mejido, J.A.; Gonzalez-Herráez, J.V.; Pelayo-Delgado, I.; Fernandez-Palacin, A.; Sainz-Bueno, J.A. Identification of Pelvic Congestion Syndrome Using Transvaginal Ultrasonography. A Useful Tool. *Tomography* **2022**, *8*, 89–99. [CrossRef]
32. Gavrilov, S.G. Vulvar varicosities: Diagnosis, treatment, and prevention. *Int. J. Women's Health* **2017**, *9*, 463–475. [CrossRef]

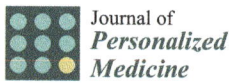

Article

Transarterial Embolization for Spontaneous Soft-Tissue Hematomas: Predictive Factors for Early Death

Rémi Grange [1,*], Lucile Grange [2], Clément Chevalier [1], Alexandre Mayaud [1], Loïc Villeneuve [1], Claire Boutet [1] and Sylvain Grange [1]

[1] Department of Radiology, University Hospital of Saint-Etienne, 42270 Saint-Priest-en-Jarez, France
[2] Department of Internal Medicine, University Hospital of Saint-Etienne, 42270 Saint-Priest-en-Jarez, France
* Correspondence: remgrange1@gmail.com; Tel.: +33-477-828-963

Abstract: Introduction: The aim of this retrospective monocentric study was to assess the safety and efficacy of spontaneous soft-tissue hematoma transarterial embolization (TAE) and to evaluate predictive factors for early mortality ($\leq$30 days) after TAE for spontaneous soft-tissue hematoma (SSTH). Materials and methods: Between January 2010 and March 2022, all patients referred to our hospital for spontaneous soft-tissue hematoma and treated by emergency TAE were reviewed. Inclusion criteria were patients: $\geq$18-year-old, with active bleeding shown on preoperative multidetector row computed tomography, with spontaneous soft-tissue hematoma, and treated by TAE. Exclusion criteria were patients with soft-tissue hematomas of traumatic, iatrogenic, or tumoral origin. Clinical, biological, and imaging records were reviewed. Imaging data included delimitation of hematoma volume and presence of fluid level. Univariate and multivariate analyses were performed to check for associations with early mortality. Results: Fifty-six patients were included. Median age was 75.5 [9–83] ([Q1–Q3]) years and 23 (41.1%) were males. Fifty-one patients (91.1%) received antiplatelet agent and/or anticoagulant therapy. All 56 patients had active bleeding shown on a preoperative CT scan. Thirty-seven (66.0%) hematomas involved the retroperitoneum. Median hemoglobin level was 7.6 [4.4–8.2] g/dL. Gelatine sponge was used in 32/56 (57.1%) procedures. Clinical success was obtained in 48/56 (85.7%) patients and early mortality occurred in 15/56 (26.8%) patients. In univariate and multivariate analysis, retroperitoneal location and volume of hematoma were associated with early mortality. Conclusion: Retroperitoneal location and volume of hematoma seem to be risk factors for early death in the context of TAE for spontaneous soft-tissue hematoma. Larger multicenter studies are necessary to identify others predictive factors for early mortality and to anticipate which patients may benefit from an interventional strategy with TAE.

Keywords: hematoma; soft-tissue; embolization; anticoagulant; bleeding

Citation: Grange, R.; Grange, L.; Chevalier, C.; Mayaud, A.; Villeneuve, L.; Boutet, C.; Grange, S. Transarterial Embolization for Spontaneous Soft-Tissue Hematomas: Predictive Factors for Early Death. *J. Pers. Med.* **2023**, *13*, 15. https://doi.org/10.3390/jpm13010015

Academic Editors: Julien Frandon and Taimur Saleem

Received: 12 October 2022
Revised: 13 December 2022
Accepted: 20 December 2022
Published: 22 December 2022

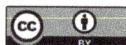

Copyright: © 2022 by the authors. Licensee MDPI, Basel, Switzerland. This article is an open access article distributed under the terms and conditions of the Creative Commons Attribution (CC BY) license (https://creativecommons.org/licenses/by/4.0/).

1. Introduction

Spontaneous soft-tissue hematoma (SSTH) is a relatively rare but potentially life-threatening condition [1]. The prevalence of SSTH is expected to increase due to the increasing use of anticoagulants among older patients and its diagnosis due to routine use of multidetector row computed tomography (MDCT) [2]. SSTH may cause pain, deglobulization, hemodynamic instability, and death [3]. SSTH may cause hospitalization or a clinically aggravating event in a hospitalized patient, especially in intensive-care units (ICUs) [4]. Its diagnosis may be delayed in the absence of apparent symptoms. There is no common consensus for appropriate SSTH management. Different options include conservative treatment or transarterial embolization (TAE). Surgical treatment [5] should be reserved as a last resort if TAE is unsuccessful. Moreover, depending on the clinical severity and history of the patient, preservation, discontinuation, or reversal of anticoagulant treatment should be discussed with the management team [6]. Preoperative MDCT plays a central role in locating the hematoma by assessing its volume and muscular relationships and by anticipating emergency TAE [7]. Nevertheless, the injection of contrast media may aggravate acute renal failure and require extracorporeal purification [8,9]. On the one hand, TAE is effective in stopping SSTH bleeding [10,11] but may generate or aggravate acute renal failure of multi-factorial origin in the aftermath of the acute bleed. On the other hand, active bleeding may stop spontaneously, especially in the absence of fascial rupture by intrinsic muscle compression. The clinical success rate of TAE for SSTH is estimated at 94.3% [3]. However, the mortality rate of these patients is high in 22.7% of the cases, with an early rebleeding rate of 9.4% [3]. Even if there is no standard of care for the diagnosis and treatment of SSTH, a management algorithm has been proposed [12]. Previous studies have focused on the occurrence of SSTH in patients admitted to intensive care [13], in patients treated with anticoagulants [6,14], and experiencing SARS-CoV-2 infection [15]. Moreover, studies on TAE in SSTH focused on a particular muscle [16] or a particular embolic agent [17,18]. Evaluating predictive factors for early mortality after TAE of SSTH has received little research attention: Barral et al. [7] showed that hematoma volume, retroperitoneal hematoma, and simplified acute physiology score II were independent predictors of early mortality after TAE. It is, therefore, essential to better understand the predictive factors of mortality to improve the selection of patients who may benefit from emergency TAE.

This retrospective monocentric study aimed to assess the safety and efficacy of spontaneous soft-tissue hematoma transarterial embolization and to evaluate predictive factors for early mortality after TAE for SSTH.

2. Methods

2.1. Study Population

Between January 2010 and March 2022, we reviewed clinical decisions and MDCT images for all patients referred to our hospital for SSTH treated by emergency TAE. The inclusion criteria were: patients (1) ≥18 years old, (2) with active bleeding shown on MDCT, (3) and treated by TAE. The exclusion criteria were: patients (1) <18 years old, (2) with soft-tissue hematomas of traumatic, (3) iatrogenic, or (4) tumoral origin, and (5) without preoperative MDCT angiography before TAE.

2.2. Patient Characteristics

We retrospectively reviewed medical records for old clinical history, including high blood pressure, diabetes mellitus, chronic renal failure, cardiovascular diseases, cirrhosis, performance status, antiaggregant and anticoagulant treatments, and indications to administer anticoagulant therapy. The recent clinical history included the presence and reasons for hospitalization at the time of diagnosis. Biological variables were collected at presentation, before TAE, including serum hemoglobin level, prothrombin time (PT), international normalized ratio (INR), and platelet count. The numbers of red blood cells, fresh frozen plasma, and platelets transfused were also reported. We considered transfusions performed within 24 h before and 48 h after the procedure. Hemoglobin drop was defined as the difference between the baseline hemoglobin level and hemoglobin level at the time of the procedure. Hemodynamic instability was defined as a decrease in blood pressure requiring the use of amines. Discontinuation, reversion of anticoagulant therapy, and the type of medication used to achieve reversion were reviewed.

2.3. Imaging and Procedure Data

All patients underwent an abdominal MDCT scan (SOMATOM SENSATION before September 2014 and SOMATOM, Siemens® AG, Medical solutions, Erlangen, Germany). Patients received ≥90 mL contrast medium (Xenetix 350, Guerbet®, Villepinte, France) with a flow rate ≥ 3 mL/s. Acquisitions without and with the injection of iodinated contrast medium at the arterial and portal phase were routinely performed in order to demonstrate active bleeding, defined by the contrast medium leaking during the arterial phase in MDCT images that grows during the portal phase. The location of and number of hematomas were recorded. Hematoma volume was evaluated by semi-automatic delimitation using the Carestream® software (Rochestern, NY, USA) by one experienced radiologist. In the case of multiple locations, the sum of the volume of all hematomas was calculated. The presence of a fluid level within the hematoma was also assessed.

All emergency TAEs were performed by 5 interventional radiologists with at least 3 years of experience in performing TAEs, after a collegial discussion between the interventional radiologist, the intensive-care physician, and the surgeon. After local anesthesia with 5% lidocaine, the right common femoral artery was accessed. First, global aortography was performed with a Pigtail 5F probe and a hydrophilic guidewire (Terumo, Tokyo, Japan). Then, a catheterization of the artery feeding the bleeding was performed with a Cobra 5F probe, and a 2.7F supraselective microcatheteter (Progreat, Terumo®, Tokyo, Japan) was used at the discretion of the interventional radiologist. TAEs were performed under fluoroscopic monitoring using micro coils (Interlock and IDC, Boston® Scientifics), N-butyl-2-cyanoacrylate (Glubran® GEM, Viareggio, Italy), gelatine sponge (Gelitaspon®), or microparticles (Embosphere®, Microspheres, BioSphere Medical, Rockland, MA, USA), depending on the location of the active bleeding, the intensity of the active bleeding, the presence of collateral arteries, the clinical severity, and the habits of the interventional radiologist. In the absence of active bleeding, an empirical TAE could be performed in case of hemodynamic instability based on the data from the preoperative MDCT. Complete fluoroscopic angiography controls were performed in order to confirm that bleeding had been successfully controlled. After the treatment, the introducer was sutured to the skin and removed the following day if there was no recurrence of bleeding. After TAE, all patients were monitored closely in the ICU for clinical signs and symptoms that were potentially suggestive of ischemic complication or recurrent bleeding until discharge or death.

2.4. Outcomes

These clinical findings were supplemented by laboratory studies. The long-term outcomes of the patients, specifically the incidence of rebleeding, mortality, and procedure-related complications, were determined by chart review. MDCT angiography following TAE was not routine practice in the hospital unit during this period. Technical success was defined as the stopping of active bleeding, based on the angiographic control findings. Clinical failure was defined as bleeding-related death or rebleeding that required repeat TAE during the 30-day follow-up period. In the case of suspected recurrent bleeding, MDCT with contrast injection was performed. Recurrent bleeding was defined by the presence of active bleeding on the follow-up MDCT after the TAE. Rebleeding was defined as early if it occurred within 30 days of TAE and as a late rebleeding event if it occurred after 30 days of TAE. Overall survival was calculated from the date of TAE until death from any cause. Complications of TAE were defined as ischemic complication in embolized territories, non-target embolization, or hematoma at the puncture site. Complications were defined as early when they occurred within the first 2 h following TAE and late complications at least 24 h after the procedure. Grades A and B were considered to be minor complications and grades C, D, E, and F were considered to be major complications according to the SIR classification [19].

2.5. Statistical Analysis

Data are presented either as absolute numbers with percentages for qualitative variables or as median (Q1–Q3) for quantitative variables. Univariable and multivariate analyses were conducted by using the Cox proportional hazard model to identify potential prognostic factors of survival and to estimate the adjusted odds ratio (OR) with 95% CI. R® software 3.6.2(R Foundation for Statistical Computing, Vienna, Austria) was used for this study. A Kaplan–Meier curve was created with Prism Graphpad® software 8.4.2 (GraphPad Software Inc., San Diego, CA, USA).

2.6. Ethical Considerations

This study was performed in accordance with the ethical standards of the Helsinki Declaration and was approved by the ethic committee of the University Hospital of Saint-Etienne.

3. Results

Between January 2010 and March 2022, 63 patients were referred to TAE for SSTH in our institute. Seven patients had angiography without TAE: six patients had negative angiography without TAE and one had a technical failure, resulting in a total of 56 patients treated with TAE.

3.1. Patient Characteristics

Patient characteristics are detailed in Table 1. Our study population included 56 patients. The median age was 75.5 (39–83) years and 23/56 (41.1%) were men. Among the population, 24/56 (42.8%) patients had a Performance Status ≥ 2. Regarding comorbidities, 27/56 (48.2%) patients had high blood pressure, 16/56 (33.9%) patients had diabetes, 32/56 (57.1%) patients had cardiovascular disease, 9/56 (16.1%) patients had chronic renal failure, 12/56 (21.4%) patients had a history of cancer, and 4/56 (7.1%) had cirrhosis. Before the occurrence of SSTH, 24/56 (42.9%) patients were already hospitalized. In 26/56 (46.4%) patients, no clinical symptoms except hypotension and/or blood loss were found. Of the 56, 5 (8.9%) patients received antiplatelet therapy, 39/56 (69.6%) patients received anticoagulation therapy, 7/56 (12.5%) received both antiplatelet and anticoagulation therapy, and 5/56 (8.9%) did not receive antiplatelet or anticoagulation therapy. The two main indications for antithrombotic therapy were cardiac arrhythmia in 27/51 (53.0%) patients and deep vein thrombosis in 10/51 (19.6%). Overdosage was found in 13/51 (25.5%) patients. All patients reported the discontinuation of antithrombotic therapy and 13/25 (25.5%) patients reported the reversion of anticoagulation. A clinical symptom was present in 30/56 (53.6%) patients, including abdominal pain (n = 26) and tumefaction (n = 4).

Table 1. Patient characteristics.

Variables	56
Age, years median [Q25–75]	75.5 [39–83]
Male n. (%)	23 (41.1)
Performance Status median [Q25–75]	1 [0–2]
Comorbidities n. (%)	
Diabete	16 (33.9)
HBP	27 (48.2)
Chronic renal failure	9 (16.1)
History of cancer	12 (21.4)
Cirrhosis	4 (7.1)
Antithrombotic therapy, n. (%)	**51 (91.1)**
Indication for antithrombotic therapy, n. (%)	
Atrial fibrillation	27 (53.0)
Deep venous thrombosis	10 (19.6)
Ischemic stroke	5 (9.8)
Cardiopathy	3 (5.9)
Mechanical valve prosthesis	2 (3.9)
Prophylaxy	2 (3.9)
Others	2 (3.9)
Hospitalized at the time of diagnosis n. (%)	24 (42.9)
Causes of hospitalization n. (%)	
Infection	7 (12.5)
Surgery	8 (14.3)

Table 1. Cont.

Variables	56
Cardiovascular disease	7 (12.5)
Infection and surgery	2 (3.6)
Hemodynamic instability n. (%)	30 (53.6)
Main symptom n. (%)	
Abdominal pain	26 (46.4)
Tumefaction	4 (7.2)
No clinical symptom	26 (46.4)

Concerning biological data, the median Hb was 7.6 (4.4–8.2) g/dL, the median drop of Hb was 3.45 (0.9–4.9) g/dL, and 41/56 (73.2%) patients received red blood cell (RBC) transfusion. The median INR was 1.45 (1–2.7) the median PT was 65 (8–75)% and the median platelet count was 180 (38–255) G/L. A total of 41 (71.9%) patients had red blood cell transfusion and the median red blood cell units transfused was 4 (1–7.5) per patients. A total of 25 (44.6%) patients had fresh frozen plasma and 7/56 (12.5%) patients had platelet transfusion. The median fresh frozen plasma and platelet units transfused was 3 (1–6) and 2 [2,3] per patient, respectively. Biological data are detailed in Table 2.

Table 2. Patient biological data.

Variables	56
Antithrombotic therapy n. (%)	51
Antiplatelet	5 (8.9)
Clopidogrel	2
Aspirin	3
Anticoagulant	39 (69.6)
LMWH	7
UFH	14
VKA	12
Apixaban	3
Rivaroxaban	2
Antiplatelet and Anticoagulation	7 (12.5)
VKA + Aspirin	1
UFH + Aspirin	6
No antithrombotic therapy	5 (8.9)
Discontinuation of anticoagulant therapy n. (%)	51 (100)
Overdosage n. (%)	13 (25.5)
Reversion of anticoagulant therapy n. (%)	13 (25.5)
Prothrombin complex concentrates	10 (19.6)
K Vitamin	9 (17.6)
Tranexamic Acid	5 (9.8)
Biology, median [Q25–75]	
INR	1.45 [1–2.7]
PT(%)	65 [8–75]
Platelet (G/L)	180 [38–255]
Hemoglobin (g/dL)	7.6 [4.4–8.2]
Drop of Hemoblogin (g/dL)	3.45 [0.9–4.9]
RBC Transfusion n. (%)	41 (71.9)
Number of RBC, median [Q25–75]	4 [1–7.5]
Fresh frozen plasma transfusion n. (%)	25 (44.6)
Number of fresh frozen plasma units, median [Q25–75]	3 [1–6]
Platelet transfusion n. (%)	7 (12.5)
Number of platelet units, median [Q25–75]	2 [2,3]

Abbreviations: INR: international normalized ratio, PT: prothrombin time test, UFH: Unfractionated heparin, LMWH: Low-molecular-weight Heparin.

3.2. Imaging and Procedure Data

On MDCT, the hematoma was located in the retroperitoneum in 37/56 (66.1%) patients, the rectus sheath in 13/56 (23.2%) patients, and the thigh muscle in 3/56 (5.4%) patients. Three patients (3.2%) had two SSTHs: one patient had psoas and thigh hematomas, one patient had rectus and thigh hematomas, and one patient had thigh and retroperitoneal hematomas. The median volume of SSTH was 1336 (135–1664) ml and 32/56 (57.1%) patients had a fluid level within the hematoma(s). Pre-procedure data are detailed in Table 2.

Angiographic active bleeding was detected in 50/56 (89.3%) patients, resulting in 6/56 (10.7%) patients being treated by empiric TAE. Procedures were performed using a gelatine sponge for 32/56 (57.2%) patients, microparticles for 11/56 (19.6%) patients; N-Butyl Cyanoacrylate (NBCA) for 4/56 (7.1%), with a combination of sponge and microparticles for 2/56 (3.6%) patients; a combination of gelatine sponge and NBCA in 1/56 (1.8%) patients; and a combination of coils, gelatine sponge, and particles for 1/56 (1.8%) patients (Figure 1).

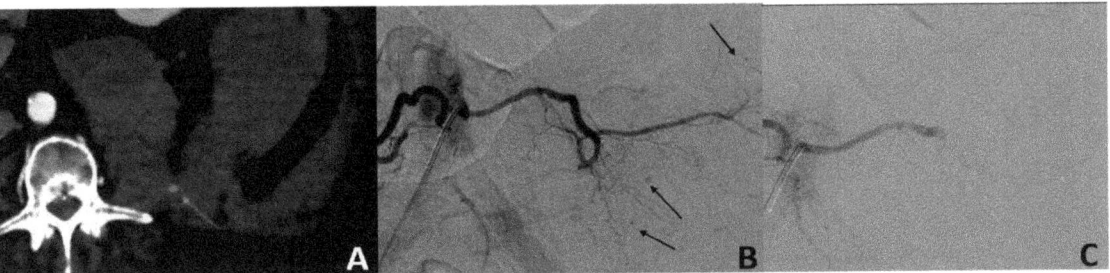

Figure 1. Isolated blood loss in a 74-year-old patient 2 days after cardiac surgery. (**A**) The MDCT scan showed active bleeding (blue arrow) from a large left retroperitoneal hematoma. (**B**) Angiography confirmed active multifocal bleeding from the left L5 lumbar artery (black arrows). (**C**) After embolization with NBCA, the control showed no opacification of the distal branches of the left L5 lumbar artery.

The main arteries embolized were: the lumbar artery in 30/56 (53.6%) patients, the inferior epigastric artery in 15/56 (26.8%) patients, and the ilio-lumbar artery in 14/56 (25.0%) patients. Multiple arteries were embolized in 8/56 (14.3%) patients. Two hematomas at the puncture site were reported (Grade A). Pre-procedure data are detailed in Table 3.

Table 3. Pre-procedure patient characteristics.

Variables	56
Preoperative CT n. (%)	
Active bleeding	56 (100)
Volume of hematoma median [Q25–75]	1336 [135–1664]
Fluid level	32 (57.14)
≥2 locations of hematoma	3 (5.4)
Location of hematoma n. (%)	
Retroperitoneum	37 (66.0)
Rectus sheath	13 (23.2)
Thigh	3 (5.4)
Psoas + Thigh	1 (1.8)
Rectus sheath + thigh	1 (1.8)
Rectus sheath + retroperitoneum	1 (1.8)

Table 3. Cont.

Variables	56
Angiographic data n. (%)	
Active bleeding	50 (89.3)
Empirical Embolization	6 (10.7)
Arteries Embolized n. (%)	
Lumbar	30 (53.6)
Ilio-lumbar	14 (25.0)
Epigastric inferior	15 (26.8)
Deep femoral	4 (7.1)
Number of embolized arteries n. (%)	
1	48 (85.7)
≥2	8 (14.3)
Embolic Agents n. (%)	
Gelatine sponge	32 (57.2)
Microparticles	11 (19.6)
Coils	5 (8.9)
NBCA	4 (7.1)
NBCA + gelatine sponge	1 (1.8)
Microparticle + gelatine sponge	2 (3.6)
Microparticle + gelatine sponge + coils	1 (1.8)
Time of procedure (min) median [Q25–75]	43 [16–60]

Abbreviations: NBCA: N-Butyl-Cyanoacrylate.

3.3. Outcomes and Prognostic Factors

Within 30 days, 8/56 (14.3%) patients had a recurrence of bleeding, all of whom were treated by repeat TAE. A flowchart of the patient outcomes is illustrated in Figure 2. One patient had a third TAE. During the follow-up period, 20/56 (35.7%) patients died. Of these, 15/56 (26.8%) deaths occurred ≤30 days and 5/56 (8.9%) deaths occurred >30 days after TAE (Figure 3). Of the patients who had a bleeding recurrence, 4/8 (50%) died ≤30 days. No surgical management or radiological drainage of the hematoma was performed. One patient with a retroperitoneal hematoma had partial ischemia of the kidney on arterial plication by extrinsic compression of the hematoma. The other patients did not present symptomatic compression of the surrounding organs. No related TAE-delayed complications were noticed. Figure 4 shows a Kaplan–Meier survival curve of the study population. Patient outcomes are detailed in Table 4.

Table 4. Patient outcomes.

Variables	56
Clinical Success n. (%)	48 (85.7)
Mortality during follow-up n. (%)	20 (35.7)
Day-30 mortality n. (%)	15 (26.8)
Day-3 mortality n. (%)	5 (8.9)
Per-operative Complications n. (%)	2 (3.6)
Post-Operative Complications n. (%)	0
Recurrence of Bleeding n. (%)	8 (14.3)
Early ≤ 30 days	8 (14.3)
Delayed > 30 days	0
Management of Early Rebleeding n. (%)	
Repeat TAE	8/8 (100)
Duration of follow-up (days) median [Q25–75]	31 [0–210]

Abbreviations: TAE: Transarterial embolization.

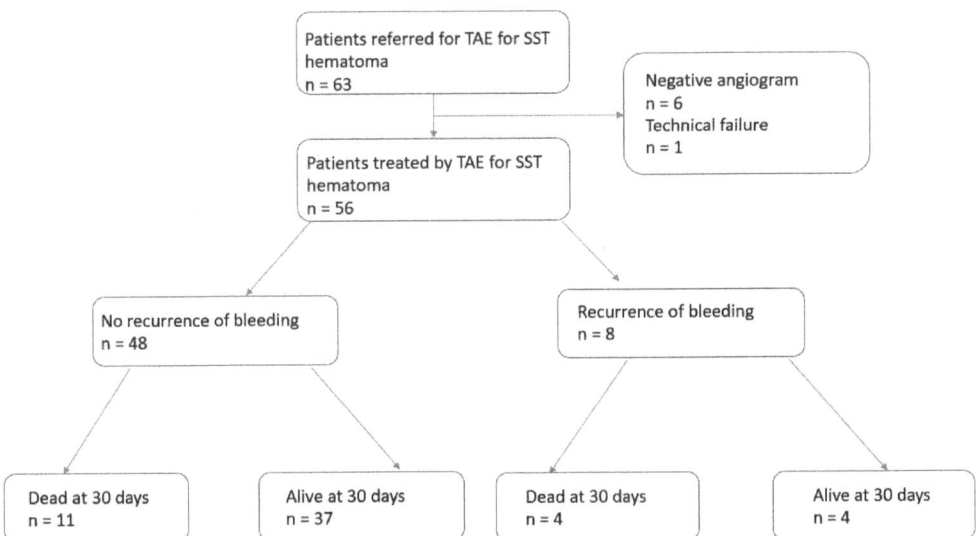

Figure 2. Flowchart of patient outcomes.

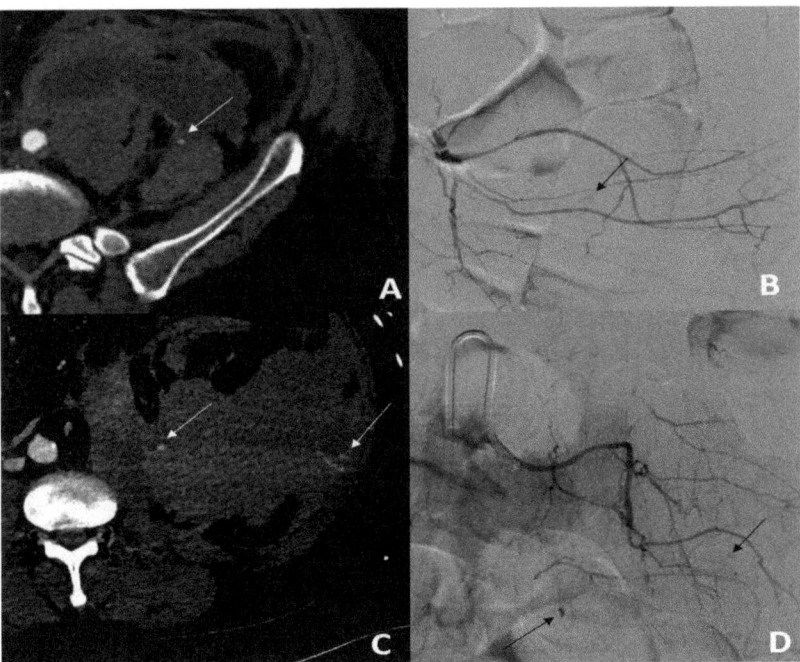

Figure 3. Back pain in a 45-year-old patient hospitalized for Sars-cov2 infection and pulmonary embolism. (A) The MDCT scan showed active bleeding (white arrow) from a large left retroperitoneal hematoma. (B) Angiography confirmed active unifocal bleeding (black arrow) from the left L5 lumbar artery, treated with gelatine sponge (C). On day 1, the patient presented with persistent blood loss. The MDCT scan showed a persistent hematoma with active bleeding (white arrows). (D) Angiography showed new multifocal active bleeding (black arrows) treated using 1 coil.

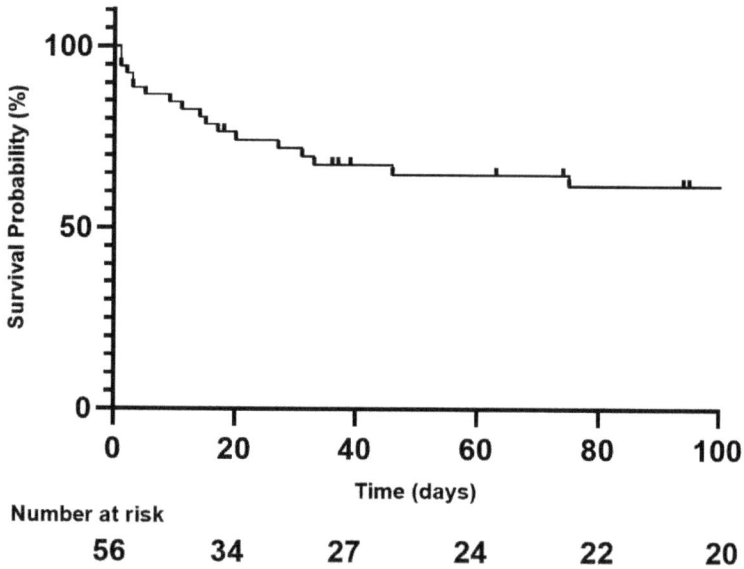

Figure 4. Kaplan–Meier curve of overall survival during the first 100 days following TAE.

Univariate and multivariate analyses are detailed in Table 5. There was no association between early death and age, sex, performance status, target artery, or the use of coils.

Table 5. Univariate and multivariate regression analysis for early death.

	Early Death ≤ 30 Days			
	Univariate Analysis		Multivariate Analysis	
Characteristics	OR	p Value	OR	p Value
Demographics data				
Age (years)	1.03 (0.98–1.10)	0.23	-	-
Male	1.36 (0.41–4.50)	0.61	-	-
HBP	1.40 (0.41–4.80)	0.59	-	-
Diabetes	2.22 (0.61–7.81)	0.23	-	-
Chronic renal failure	0.76 (0.13–4.19)	0.75	-	-
Active cancer	0.91 (0.16–5.17)	0.92	-	-
Antiplatelet therapy	0.66 (0.06–6.46)	0.72	-	-
Anticoagulant therapy	0.82 (0.23–2.93)	0.77	-	-
Hospitalization at diagnosis	1.23 (0.37–4.05)	0.72	-	-
Coagulation disorder				
INR	0.06 (0.76–1.46)	0.72	-	-
Hb < 7	1.31 (0.38–4.69)	0.67	-	-
MDCT Imaging data				
Retroperitoneum	4.65 (1.32–16.31)	0.016	4.08 (1.01–61.4)	0.047
Volume of hematoma (ml)	7.7 (1.86–31.92)	0.004	1.01 (1.00–1.02)	0.023
Fluid level on CT scan	0.81 (0.24–2.66)	0.727		
TAE data				
Blush at angiography	1.82 (0–∞)	0.99	-	-
Use of gelatine sponge	0.53 (0.61–1.78)	0.3	-	-
Lumbar artery	2.1 (0.61–7.22)	0.24	-	-
Number of embolized arteries	1.08 (0.23–5.04)	0.92	-	-

Abbreviations: HBP: High Blood Pressure, INR: international normalized ratio, MDCT: Multidetector Row Computed Tomography, TAE: Transarterial embolization, OR: odds ratio.

In univariate analysis, the retroperitoneal location (OR = 4.65 (1.32–13.31), p = 0.016) and the volume of hematoma (OR = 7.70 (1.86–31.92), p = 0.004) were associated with early mortality.

In multivariate analysis, the retroperitoneal location (OR = 4.08 (1.01–61.4), p = 0.047) and the volume of hematoma (OR = 1.01 (1.00–1.02), p = 0.023) were associated with early mortality.

4. Discussion

This retrospective study showed that emergency TAE of SSTH allows for the rapid control of bleeding, with high clinical success (85.7%), a relatively high early mortality rate (26.8%), and a significant rebleeding rate (14.3%). Moreover, it demonstrated an association between the hematoma volume, retroperitoneal location, and overall survival in multivariate analysis.

There are no official recommendations for managing patients treated with SSTH, especially those patients receiving thrombotic therapy. A review by Touma et al. [3] reported a high clinical success (93.1%), a moderate overall mortality rate (22.8%), and a significant recurrence rate (10.1%). This review showed that only 10 studies included >4 patients.

In line with previous studies, the present one showed a significant rate of early mortality rate (26.8%) within the first 30 days following TAE in patients treated for SSTH. That said, TAE was able to stop bleeding in all procedures. SSTH appears as a triggering event or may aggravate a precarious clinical situation in polypathological patients. Barral et al. [7] reported a 27% 30-day mortality rate following TAE for SSTH, despite high clinical success (83%). Our study found a gap between significant technical success (98.2%), clinical success (85.7%), and early mortality rate (26.8%). It is, therefore, essential to adopt an aggressive strategy in patients experiencing recurrences of bleeding and to monitor them closely for early recurrence.

We found that the retroperitoneal location and hematoma volume were associated with early mortality following TAE. Barral et al. [7] also found that retroperitoneal hematoma location was associated with mortality within 30 days. This can be explained by the higher rate of fascia rupture, resulting in a larger hematoma volume and a delayed symptomatology, leading to delayed medical management [7]. Volume measurement can be performed semi-automatically or with three measures within seconds on the pre-therapeutic CT scan and is a simple, quick way to argue for a therapeutic decision. The fluid level was not associated with early mortality in our study. Nakayama et al. [20] showed fluid level in 28/47 (60%) MDCT of patients with coagulopathy-related SSTH and an association between fluid level and active bleeding. However, the fluid level was only present in 32/56 (57.1%) patients with active bleeding in this study and was not associated with early mortality after TAE. Therefore, the relevance of its description in patients receiving preoperative MDCT angiography seems modest.

Almost all patients included in the study had anticoagulant and/or antiplatelet therapies at the time of TAE. This shows the important association between antithrombotic use and the occurrence of SSTH, which has already received attention in the published literature [3]. Barral et al. [7] and Popov et al. [12] recommended conservative treatment in patients with spontaneous soft-tissue bleeding, with active bleeding on CT and/or hemodynamic instability, and without fascia rupture. However, the withdrawal and reversal of anticoagulants are subject to the benefit–risk balance in patients with cardiovascular co-morbidities, particularly patients with cardiac rhythm disorders at risk of embolism. In our study, the reversal of anticoagulant is moderate (25.5%), highlighting the apprehension of reversing anticoagulants in patients with thrombogenic risk.

The present study showed a moderate rate of 14.3% of recurrent bleeding after TAE, which is in line with previous literature. Dohan et al. [21] showed rebleeding in 9/34 (26.4%) patients. This can be explained by the continued use of anticoagulants or by the delay in the reversion of anticoagulants. It is worth noting that all eight patients who presented with recurrent bleeding had clinical success during a repeat TAE. However, the early mortality rate in these patients is relatively high (50%), as was the case in Dohan et al.'s study [21], which showed 4/9 (44.4%) patients who experienced early death after presenting with a recurrence of bleeding after TAE.

MDCT angiography showed excellent sensitivity for detecting active bleeding of SSTH. There is no consensus on the pertinence of preoperative MDCT, which is not routinely performed. Vincenzo et al. [6] performed a systematic angiography in patients with persistent bleeding requiring iterative transfusions but not necessarily preoperative MDCT, which explains the large number of negative angiograms (25%) in their study. MDCT can limit the injection of contrast medium during TAE, to limit irradiation and to accelerate the TAE procedure by directly catheterizing the target artery. Contrary to Barral et al. [7], an MDCT angiogram was performed before TAE for all patients in the present study. However, we reserved iodine contrast injection for patients with hemodynamic instability and a glomerular filtration rate <30 mL/min or for patients with a glomerular filtration rate $\geq$30 mL/min in cases with a suspicion of active bleeding. The preoperative MDCT scan has a fundamental role in the choice of the target artery. In addition, it can avoid unnecessary angiography in patients without active bleeding. In fact, the sensitivity of MDCT is more effective at detecting active bleeding than angiography ($\geq$0.3 vs. 0.5 mL/min, respectively) [22,23]. The benefit–risk balance must be assessed, without underestimating the expected benefits of the injection of iodine contrast on patient management, especially since iodine-induced nephropathy has often been overestimated in studies [8].

Complications following TAE of SSTH are rare. Our study showed two puncture-site hematomas, without any ischemic muscle complications or worsening of pain that might suggest a muscle infarction, in line with the literature. However, cases of parietal muscle necrosis have been described with NBCA [24].

In our study, using a non-absorbable agent was not associated with a worse clinical prognosis than non-absorbable agents. This is in line with the literature, which does not find any influence of the embolizing agent on the prognosis [3]. However, given the low rate of ischemic complications [3] and the high risk of recurrence, a permanent embolizing agent should be prioritized to avoid any recurrence of bleeding on the embolized artery, in case the target artery can be selectively catheterized.

The present study has some limitations. It is a single-center retrospective study, with a limited number of patients; therefore, the results must be interpreted cautiously. All patients had pre-procedural MDCT, which does not reflect the habits of other hospitals and may lead to a selection bias. We studied only patients treated with TAE. The severity of the patients in this population does not reflect the population of patients followed for SSTH.

In conclusion, our study confirmed the safety and efficacy of TAE for SSTH. Nevertheless, early death remains high. The retroperitoneal location and hematoma volume seem to be risk factors for early death. Future multicenter studies are necessary to stratify the risk of early mortality and to anticipate which patients may benefit from an interventional strategy with TAE.

Author Contributions: Conceptualization R.G. and L.G.; Methodology, R.G. and L.G.; Software R.G. and L.G.; Validation, R.G. and L.G.; Formal analysis, R.G. and L.G.; Investigation, R.G.; Resources and data curation, R.G., L.G., C.C., A.M., L.V., C.B. and S.G.; Writing—Original draft preparation R.G.; Writing—review and editing R.G., L.G., C.C., A.M., L.V., C.B. and S.G.; Supervision S.G. and C.B. All authors have read and agreed to the published version of the manuscript.

Funding: This study was not supported by any funding.

Institutional Review Board Statement: This study was conducted in accordance with the Declaration of Helsinki and approved by the Institutional Review Board of the University Hospital of Saint-Etienne.

Informed Consent Statement: This study obtained IRB approval form the University of Saint-Etienne and informed consent was obtained.

Data Availability Statement: The data presented in this study are available on request from the corresponding author.

Acknowledgments: The authors thank Michael J. Deml for proofreading the manuscript.

Conflicts of Interest: The authors declare no conflict of interest.

Abbreviations

INR	International Normalized Ratio
MDCT	Multidetector row computed tomography
NBCA	N-butyl-2-cyanoacrylate
PC	Platelet count
PT	Prothrombin Time
RBC	Red Blood Cell
SSTH	Spontaneous soft-tissue hematoma
TAE	Transarterial Embolization

References

1. Decker, J.A.; Brill, L.M.; Orlowski, U.; Varga-Szemes, A.; Emrich, T.; Schoepf, U.J.; Schwarz, F.; Kröncke, T.J.; Scheurig-Münkler, C. Spontaneous Iliopsoas Muscle Hemorrhage–Predictors of Associated Mortality. *Acad. Radiol.* **2022**, *29*, 536–542. [CrossRef] [PubMed]
2. Neumayer, B.; Hassler, E.; Petrovic, A.; Widek, T.; Ogris, K.; Scheurer, E. Age determination of soft tissue hematomas: Hematoma Age Determination. *NMR Biomed.* **2014**, *27*, 1397–1402. [CrossRef]
3. Touma, L.; Cohen, S.; Cassinotto, C.; Reinhold, C.; Barkun, A.; Tran, V.T.; Banon, O.; Valenti, D.; Gallix, B.; Dohan, A. Transcatheter Arterial Embolization of Spontaneous Soft Tissue Hematomas: A Systematic Review. *Cardiovasc. Interv. Radiol.* **2019**, *42*, 335–343. [CrossRef]
4. Llitjos, J.F.; Daviaud, F.; Grimaldi, D.; Legriel, S.; Georges, J.L.; Guerot, E.; Bedos, J.P.; Fagon, J.Y.; Charpentier, J.; Mira, J.P. Ilio-psoas hematoma in the intensive care unit: A multicentric study. *Ann. Intensive Care* **2016**, *6*, 8. [CrossRef]
5. Nagraj, S.K.; Prashanti, E.; Aggarwal, H.; Lingappa, A.; Muthu, M.S.; Krishanappa, S.K.K.; Hassan, H. Interventions for treating post-extraction bleeding. *Cochrane Database Syst. Rev.* **2018**, *3*, CD011930.
6. Menditto, V.G.; Fulgenzi, F.; Lombardi, S.; Dimitriadou, A.; Mincarelli, C.; Rosati, M.; Candelari, R.; Pomponio, G.; Salvi, A.; Gabrielli, A. Management of spontaneous soft-tissue hemorrhage secondary to anticoagulant therapy: A cohort study. *Am. J. Emerg. Med.* **2018**, *36*, 2177–2181. [CrossRef] [PubMed]
7. Barral, M.; Pellerin, O.; Tran, V.T.; Gallix, B.; Boucher, L.M.; Valenti, D.; Sapoval, M.; Soyer, P.; Dohan, A. Predictors of Mortality from Spontaneous Soft-Tissue Hematomas in a Large Multicenter Cohort Who Underwent Percutaneous Transarterial Embolization. *Radiology* **2019**, *291*, 250–258. [CrossRef]
8. Luk, L.; Steinman, J.; Newhouse, J.H. Intravenous Contrast-Induced Nephropathy—The Rise and Fall of a Threatening Idea. *Adv. Chronic Kidney Dis.* **2017**, *24*, 169–175. [CrossRef]
9. van der Molen, A.J.; Reimer, P.; Dekkers, I.A.; Bongartz, G.; Bellin, M.F.; Bertolotto, M.; Clement, O.; Heinz-Peer, G.; Stacul, F.; Webb, J.A.; et al. Post-contrast acute kidney injury—Part 1: Definition, clinical features, incidence, role of contrast medium and risk factors: Recommendations for updated ESUR Contrast Medium Safety Committee guidelines. *Eur. Radiol.* **2018**, *28*, 2845–2855. [CrossRef]
10. Sharafuddin, M.J.; Andresen, K.J.; Sun, S.; Lang, E.; Stecker, M.S.; Wibbenmeyer, L.A. Spontaneous extraperitoneal hemorrhage with hemodynamic collapse in patients undergoing anticoagulation: Management with selective arterial embolization. *J. Vasc. Interv. Radiol.* **2001**, *12*, 1231–1234. [CrossRef]
11. Klausenitz, C.; Kuehn, J.P.; Noeckler, K.; Radosa, C.G.; Hoffmann, R.T.; Teichgraeber, U.; Mensel, B. Efficacy of transarterial embolisation in patients with life-threatening spontaneous retroperitoneal haematoma. *Clin. Radiol.* **2021**, *76*, 157.e11–157.e18. [CrossRef] [PubMed]
12. Popov, M.; Sotiriadis, C.; Gay, F.; Jouannic, A.-M.; Lachenal, Y.; Hajdu, S.D.; Doenz, F.; Qanadli, S.D. Spontaneous Intramuscular Hematomas of the Abdomen and Pelvis: A New Multilevel Algorithm to Direct Transarterial Embolization and Patient Management. *Cardiovasc. Interv. Radiol.* **2017**, *40*, 537–545. [CrossRef]
13. Artzner, T.; Clere-Jehl, R.; Schenck, M.; Greget, M.; Merdji, H.; De Marini, P.; Tuzin, N.; Helms, J.; Meziani, F. Spontaneous ilio-psoas hematomas complicating intensive care unit hospitalizations. *PLoS ONE* **2019**, *14*, e0211680. [CrossRef]
14. Basile, A.; Medina, J.G.; Mundo, E.; Medina, V.G.; Leal, R. Transcatheter arterial embolization of concurrent spontaneous hematomas of the rectus sheath and psoas muscle in patients undergoing anticoagulation. *Cardiovasc. Interv. Radiol.* **2004**, *27*, 659–662. [CrossRef] [PubMed]
15. Teta, M.; Drabkin, M.J. Fatal retroperitoneal hematoma associated with Covid-19 prophylactic anticoagulation protocol. *Radiol. Case Rep.* **2021**, *16*, 1618–1621. [CrossRef] [PubMed]

16. Qanadli, S.D.; El Hajjam, M.; Mignon, F.; Bruckert, F.; Chagnon, S.; Lacombe, P. Life-threatening spontaneous psoas haematoma treated by transcatheter arterial embolization. *Eur. Radiol.* **1999**, *9*, 1231–1234. [CrossRef] [PubMed]
17. Patidar, Y.; Srinivasan, S.V.; Singh, J.; Patel, R.K.; Chandel, K.; Mukund, A.; Sharma, M.K.; Sarin, S.K. Clinical Outcomes of Transcatheter Arterial Embolization Using N-butyl-2-cyanoacrylate (NBCA) in Cirrhotic Patients. *J. Clin. Exp. Hepatol.* **2022**, *12*, 353–361. [CrossRef] [PubMed]
18. Yoo, D.H.; Jae, H.J.; Kim, H.-C.; Chung, J.W.; Park, J.H. Transcatheter arterial embolization of intramuscular active hemorrhage with N-butyl cyanoacrylate. *Cardiovasc. Interv. Radiol.* **2012**, *35*, 292–298. [CrossRef]
19. Khalilzadeh, O.; Baerlocher, M.O.; Shyn, P.B.; Connolly, B.L.; Devane, A.M.; Morris, C.S.; Cohen, A.M.; Midia, M.; Thornton, R.H.; Gross, K.; et al. Proposal of a New Adverse Event Classification by the Society of Interventional Radiology Standards of Practice Committee. *J. Vasc. Interv. Radiol.* **2017**, *28*, 1432–1437.e3. [CrossRef]
20. Nakayama, M.; Kato, K.; Yoshioka, K.; Sato, H. Coagulopathy-related soft tissue hematoma: A comparison between computed tomography findings and clinical severity. *Acta Radiol. Open* **2020**, *9*, 2058460120923266. [CrossRef]
21. Dohan, A.; Sapoval, M.; Chousterman, B.G.; di Primio, M.; Guerot, E.; Pellerin, O. Spontaneous Soft-Tissue Hemorrhage in Anticoagulated Patients: Safety and Efficacy of Embolization. *Am. J. Roentgenol.* **2015**, *204*, 1303–1310. [CrossRef] [PubMed]
22. Geffroy, Y.; Rodallec, M.H.; Boulay-Coletta, I.; Jullès, M.-C.; Ridereau-Zins, C.; Zins, M. Multidetector CT angiography in acute gastrointestinal bleeding: Why, when, and how. *Radiographics* **2011**, *31*, E35–E46. [CrossRef] [PubMed]
23. Chua, A.E.; Ridley, L.J. Diagnostic accuracy of CT angiography in acute gastrointestinal bleeding. *J. Med. Imaging Radiat. Oncol.* **2008**, *52*, 333–338. [CrossRef] [PubMed]
24. Djaber, S.; Bohelay, G.; Moussa, N.; Déan, C.; del Giudicce, C.; Sapoval, M.; Dohan, A.; Pellerin, O. Cutaneous necrosis after embolization of spontaneous soft-tissue hematoma of the abdominal wall. *Diagn. Interv. Imaging* **2018**, *99*, 831–833. [CrossRef]

Disclaimer/Publisher's Note: The statements, opinions and data contained in all publications are solely those of the individual author(s) and contributor(s) and not of MDPI and/or the editor(s). MDPI and/or the editor(s) disclaim responsibility for any injury to people or property resulting from any ideas, methods, instructions or products referred to in the content.

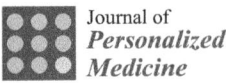

Article

Treatment of Acute Mesenteric Ischemia: Individual Challenges for Interventional Radiologists and Abdominal Surgeons

Arne Estler [1,*], Eva Estler [2], You-Shan Feng [3], Ferdinand Seith [1], Maximilian Wießmeier [2], Rami Archid [4], Konstantin Nikolaou [1], Gerd Grözinger [1] and Christoph Artzner [1]

[1] Diagnostic and Interventional Radiology, University Hospital Tuebingen, 72076 Tübingen, Germany
[2] Faculty of Medicine, University of Tuebingen, 72074 Tübingen, Germany
[3] Institute for Clinical Epidemiology and Applied Biometrics, Medical University of Tübingen, 72076 Tübingen, Germany
[4] Department of General & Transplant Surgery, University Hospital Tuebingen, 72076 Tübingen, Germany
* Correspondence: arne.estler@med.uni-tuebingen.de; Tel.: +49-707-1298-5453

Abstract: Background: Acute mesenteric ischemia (AMI) is a life-threatening condition resulting from occlusion of the mesenteric arterial vessels. AMI requires immediate treatment with revascularization of the occluded vessels. Purpose: to evaluate the technical success, clinical outcomes and survival of patients receiving endovascular treatment for AMI followed by surgery. Material and Methods: A search of our institution's database for AMI revealed 149 potential patients between 08/2016 and 08/2021, of which 91 were excluded due to incomplete clinical data, insufficient imaging or missing follow-up laparoscopy. The final cohort included 58 consecutive patients [(median age 73.5 years [range: 43–96 years], 55% female), median BMI 26.2 kg/m^2 (range:16.0–39.2 kg/m^2)]. Periinterventional imaging regarding the cause of AMI (acute-embolic or acute-on-chronic) was evaluated by two radiologists in consensus. The extent of AMI and the degree of technical success was graded according to a modified TICI (Thrombolysis in Cerebral Infarction scale) score (TICI-AMI) classification (0: no perfusion; 1: minimal; 2a < 50% filling; 2b > 50%; 2c: near complete or slow; 3: complete). Lab data and clinical data were collected, including the results of follow-up laparoscopy. Non-parametric statistics were used. Results: All interventions were considered technically successful. The most common causes of AMI were emboli (51.7%) and acute-on-chronic thrombotic occlusions (37.9%). Initial imaging showed a TICI-AMI score of 0, 1 or 2a in 87.9% ($n = 51$) of patients. Post-therapeutic TICI-AMI scores improved significantly with 87.9% of patients grade 2b and better. Median lactate levels reduced from 2.7 (IQR 2.0–3.7) mg/dL (1–18) to 1.45 (IQR 0.99–1.90). Intestinal ischemia was documented in 79.1% of cases with resection of the infarcted intestinal loops. In total, 22/58 (37.9%) patients died during the first 30 days after intervention and surgery. According to CIRSE criteria, we did not observe any SAE scores of grade 2 or higher. Conclusions: AMI is a serious disease with high lethality within the first 30 days despite optimal treatment. However, interventional revascularization before surgery with resection of the infarcted bowel can save two out of three of critically ill patients.

Keywords: acute mesenteric ischemia; revascularization; laparoscopy

Citation: Estler, A.; Estler, E.; Feng, Y.-S.; Seith, F.; Wießmeier, M.; Archid, R.; Nikolaou, K.; Grözinger, G.; Artzner, C. Treatment of Acute Mesenteric Ischemia: Individual Challenges for Interventional Radiologists and Abdominal Surgeons. *J. Pers. Med.* **2023**, *13*, 55. https://doi.org/10.3390/jpm13010055

Academic Editor: Julien Frandon

Received: 11 November 2022
Revised: 23 December 2022
Accepted: 24 December 2022
Published: 27 December 2022

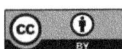

Copyright: © 2022 by the authors. Licensee MDPI, Basel, Switzerland. This article is an open access article distributed under the terms and conditions of the Creative Commons Attribution (CC BY) license (https://creativecommons.org/licenses/by/4.0/).

1. Introduction

Mesenteric ischemia is most often defined as a complex of symptoms resulting from acute or chronic occlusion of the mesenteric vessels that supply the intestines. Occlusion initially leads to cellular damage, tissue death due to ischemia and later to secondary inflammatory changes [1]. In untreated cases, mesenteric ischemia leads to life-threatening intestinal necrosis. Although the incidence of mesenteric ischemia is relatively low (0.09–0.2% of all acute surgical hospital admissions), it should always be excluded as a differential diagnosis because mortality is reported in the literature to be as high as 50–80% [2–5]. However, early diagnosis of mesenteric ischemia can significantly reduce mortality. Acute mesenteric ischemia (AMI) can have a variety of causes: it may be non-occlusive (NOMI) or occlusive and caused by either arterial embolism (50%), arterial thrombosis (15–25%) or mesenteric venous thrombosis (5–15%) [6,7].

A mesenteric embolus may originate from the left atrium in cardiac arrhythmias or in global heart failure with a poor ejection fraction. Less frequently, such emboli originate from an arteriosclerotic aorta. These emboli typically attach to the narrowest part of the vessel, making the superior mesenteric artery (SMA) a predestined site in addition to its shallow angle of origin from the aorta and its relatively large lumen [8]. In particular, the area 3–10 cm downstream of the SMA is particularly vulnerable to occlusions (>20% of emboli), which supplies the main portion of the ileum.

Mesenteric arterial thrombosis is almost always associated with pre-existing chronic atherosclerosis. The vast majority of these patients have a history of symptomatic chronic mesenteric ischemia, such as postprandial pain and weight loss [8]. Because mesenteric thrombosis of the SMA most commonly has an underlying calcified plaque, the truncus is usually also involved [9]. However, SMA thrombosis may also occur in the setting of vasculitis, dissection or aneurysm.

Once the diagnosis of acute mesenteric ischemia is made by contrast-enhanced computed tomography, therapy should be initiated immediately. This includes the immediate administration of fluids and broad-spectrum antibiotics, endovascular revascularization and subsequent diagnostic laparoscopy, especially in patients with signs of peritonism [10]. In selected cases, surgical embolectomy may also be the procedure of choice.

To date, limited data is available for this therapeutic regimen. Hence, the aim of this study was to evaluate patient outcomes after interventional revascularization of the SMA, considering the degree and time of ischemia, as well as the technical success of revascularization.

2. Material and Methods

This study was conducted retrospectively at a single center and was IRB approved. Electronic medical records from our primary medical centre were screened in order to identify patients who presented with the signs and symptoms of AMI due to occlusion of the SMA between August 2016 and August 2021. We included consecutive patients with either arterial thrombosis, arterial embolism or venous thrombosis. We excluded patients with AMI with (A) non-occlusive mesenteric ischemia, (B) incomplete clinical data, (C) insufficient imaging or (D) missing follow-up laparoscopy (see flow chart Figure 1). Other data collected from the electronic medical records were: age at intervention, sex, weight, height, access location and tool, type of thrombectomy or embolectomy, additional procedures such as percutaneous transluminal angioplasty (PTA) or stents, reports of previous abdominal surgery, lab work including lactate and partial thromboplastin time (PTT), medication (e.g., amount of intraprocedural heparin or post-procedure anticoagulation) and pre-existing medical conditions, such as coronary artery disease, hypertension, diabetes and atrial fibrillation. Survival data were assessed after 30 days and 12 months.

All patients presenting to our clinic with clinical signs of AMI underwent contrast-enhanced CT for primary evaluation. All CT scans were performed on a second or third-generation CT scanner (Siemens Somatom Force or Somatom AS+, Siemens Healthineers, Erlangen, Germany). Iodinated contrast medium (Imeron 400, Bracco Imaging Deutschland GmbH) was administered at a dosage of 1.5 mL/kg and at a rate of 3.5 mL/s in every patient. Image acquisition was performed in native, arterial and portal venous contrast medium phases, respectively. Patients with imaging findings suggestive of acute mesenteric ischemia were immediately discussed by an interdisciplinary team of radiologists and abdominal surgeons and were included in the in-house treatment scheme of AMI.

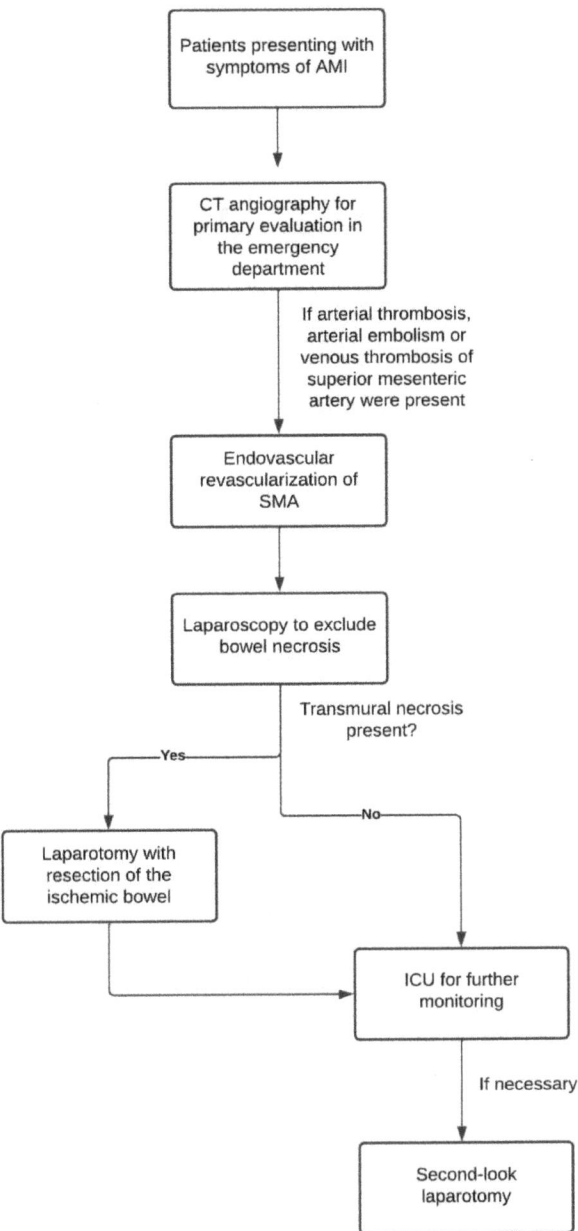

Figure 1. In-house procedure of treatment in patients presenting with AMI.

2.1. Endovascular Procedure

The patients were immediately transferred to the interventional radiology angiography suite. All patients were treated either under general anesthesia or sedation. After sterile draping, arterial access was made via the left brachial artery or the right common femoral artery. The access site was chosen at the judgment of the executing interventionalist, considering the steepness of the SMA origin. Accordingly, the access sheaths were either a wire-reinforced 6 French 60 cm sheath (Terumo) from the arm or a 6F 45 cm renal double curved (Terumo) configured sheath from the groin. The occluded vessels were probed via 4F angiography catheters in a multipurpose configuration cranially or in C2 or S1 form caudally (Cook). Angiograms were acquired before recanalization. A 0.018-inch wire (Command 18, Abbott) was used for the initial crossing of the occlusion. Depending on the aetiology of the occlusion, an interventional treatment regime was set. Thrombectomy was performed with hydrodynamic thrombectomy, including power pulse spray lysis with 10 mg of alteplase (AngioJet n = 21), rotational thrombectomy (Rotarex 6F n = 2) or aspiration thrombectomy with a 6F guide catheter (VistaBrite 6F n = 28). Additional short-term lysis with a 10 mg alteplase bolus was given in n = 36 cases. Stenting or PTA of the underlying stenoses was performed as necessary. The interventional success of recanalization was finally confirmed by angiography. The transbrachially inserted sheaths were removed after successful PTA. The transfemoral accesses sheaths were often changed to short 6F sheaths and remained in place until after surgery. The resected bowel parts were documented and included in the further evaluation of this study.

2.2. Surgery

All patients were taken to the operating room following intervention and underwent diagnostic laparoscopy. In cases with ischemic bowel loops, resection adapted to the extent of irreversible ischemia was performed. Patients with bowel loops with possible reversible ischemic damage underwent second-look laparoscopy after 24 h for definitive care.

2.3. Anticoagulation

In cases with remaining embolic occlusions, patients received therapeutic full heparinization with a target PTT of 50 to 70 s. After final surgical treatment, the patients were loaded with aspirin (500 mg) and clopidogrel (300 mg) orally. All patients were recommended dual antiplatelet therapy with 100 mg of aspirin and 75 mg of clopidogrel daily for four weeks. This was followed by single platelet inhibition with aspirin (100 mg). All patients with a cardiogenic cause for an embolic event were subsequently treated with an appropriate plasmatic anticoagulant.

2.4. Outcome Assessment

The extent of AMI and the degree of technical success was graded according to a modified TICI-AMI (Thrombolysis in Cerebral Infarction scale) classification (0: no perfusion; 1: minimal; 2a: < 50% filling; 2b: > 50%; 2c: near complete or slow; 3: complete) [11]. Other important parameters evaluated were the time from symptom onset to angiography and the time from angiography to surgical evaluation of the necrotic bowel loops. Furthermore, a correlation between the outcome and multiple parameters, including the TICI score, were established.

2.5. Statistical Analysis

Statistical evaluation was performed using SPSS Statistics 27 (IBM, Armonk, NY, USA) and GraphPad (GraphPad Prism version 9.0.0 for Windows, GraphPad Software, San Diego, CA, USA, www.graphpad.com accessed on 5 November 2008). In the descriptive statistics, continuous values fulfilling a normal distribution were reported as mean values including standard deviations. Ordinal data were reported as medians with the 10th to 90th percentiles in parentheses. The data were tested for normal distribution using the Shapiro–Wilk test. p-values of α < 0.05 were considered statistically significant.

3. Results

A total of 58 patients (55% females) (median age 73.5 years [range: 43 to 96 years], 59% female, median BMI 26.2 kg/m^2 [range: 16.0 to 39.2 kg/m^2]) were included in this study.

The patients' characteristics are summarized in Table 1.

Table 1. Patient characteristics at the time of mesenteric ischemia. All the values are given as median ± standard deviation. BMI: body mass index.

Age (mean years ± SD)	71.8 ± 14.4
BMI (mean kg/m^2 ± SD)	25.8 ± 5.3
Sex (m/f)	32 females (55.2%) 26 males (44.8%)
Coronary heart disease present?	n = 25 (43.1%)
Hypertension present?	n = 33 (56.9%)
Diabetes present?	n = 11 (19.0%)
Atrial fibrillation present?	n = 21 (36.2%)
Chronic peripheral arterial occlusive disease present?	n = 15 (25.9%)
Dialysis present?	n = 9 (15.5%)

Of the 58 patients enrolled, 100% had acute occlusion with acute symptoms. The predominant access site was brachial in 30 patients (51.7%) and femoral in 28 patients (48.3%), and the maximum sheath size was 6F in the vast majority of patients (87.9%). Other sheath sizes were 4F (n = 1, 1.7%), 5F (n = 3, 5.2%) and 7F (n = 2, 3.4%). The amount of heparin administered varied between 2500 units (3.4%), 5000 units (60.3%), 7500 units (5.2%) and 10,000 units (1.7%). A total of 17 patients (29.3%) received heparin via a perfusor during the intervention. Abdominal 3-phase CT angiography was conducted in 100% of cases. The extent of bowel ischemia was classified in the CT scan; the vast majority of patients had <50% initial (pre-interventional) filling of the mesenteric branches (89.6%). Pre-existing AMS stenosis was present in 74.1% of patients and a larger proportion of patients had embolic occlusion (51.7%), followed by mesenteric (arterial) thrombosis (37.9%). Mesenteric occlusion was often treated by a combined procedure of different recanalization methods, with aspiration thrombectomy in 48.3% of patients, systemic lysis in 55.2% of patients and hydrodynamic thrombectomy in 26.2% of patients. The mean time between the onset of symptoms to intervention was 222 min (Table 2). The TICI-AMI score before recanalization confirmed the CT results, with a large proportion of patients with <50% initially contrasted mesenteric vessels. After the intervention, the TICI AMI improved in total (Table 3).

Table 2. Details of Intervention.

Access Vessel	
• Brachial	n = 31 (53.4%)
• Femoral	n = 27 (46.6%)
Sheath size	
• 4 French	n = 1 (1.7%)
• 5 French	n = 3 (5.2%)
• 6 French	n = 52 (89.6%)
• 7 French	n = 2 (3.4%)
Complications	
• Access site	n = 0 (0%)
• Mesenteric arteries	n = 0 (0%)
Administered Heparin during procedure	
• 2500 i.u.	n = 2 (3.4%)
• 5000 i.u.	n = 25 (60.3%)
• 7500 i.u.	n = 3 (5.2%)
• 10,000 i.u.	n = 1 (1.7%)
• Continuous therapeutic heparinization	n = 17 (29.3%)
Pre-interventional imaging	
• Abdominal CT Angiography	n = 58 (100%)

Table 2. *Cont.*

Extent of bowel ischemia on CT	
• 0: no peripheral perfusion	n = 22 (37.9%)
• 1: minimal	n = 4 (6.9%)
• 2a: <50% filling	n = 26 (44.8%)
• 2b: >50% filling	n = 4 (6.9%)
• 2c: near complete	n = 0 (0%)
• 3: complete	n = 0 (0%)
Pre-existing AMS stenosis	
• Yes	n = 43 (74.1%)
• No	n = 15 (25.9%)
Type of occlusion	
• Embolus	n = 30 (51.7%)
• Thrombosis	n = 22 (37.9%)
• Dissection	n = 4 (6.9%)
• Vasculitis	n = 2 (3.4%)
Time onset of symptoms to intervention (mean min ± SD)	222 min ± 166 min
Method(s) of recanalization	
• Primary stent	n = 16 (27.6%)
• Hydrodynamic thrombectomy	n = 21 (36.2%)
• Rotational thrombectomy	n = 2 (3.4%)
• Aspiration thrombectomy	n = 28 (48.3%)
• Lysis	n = 32 (55.2%)
Additional	
• Balloon angioplasty	n = 31 (53.4%)
• Stent	n = 14 (24.1%)

Table 3. Change in TICI AMI before and after recanalization.

TICI AMI before recanalization	
• 0: no peripheral perfusion	n = 2 (3.4%)
• 1: minimal	n = 24 (41.4%)
• 2a: < 50% filling	n = 25 (43.1%)
• 2b: > 50% filling	n = 6 (10.3%)
• 2c: near complete or slow	n = 1 (1.7%)
• 3: complete	n = 0 (0%)
TICI AMI after recanalization	
• 0: no peripheral perfusion	n = 0 (0%)
• 1: minimal	n = 4 (6.9%)
• 2a: < 50% filling	n = 3 (5.2%)
• 2b: > 50% filling	n = 17 (29.3%)
• 2c: near complete of slow	n = 19 (32.8%)
• 3: complete	n = 15 (25.9%)

In laparoscopy following the intervention, intestinal ischemia was present in 55.2% of patients; a mean of 110 cm of ileum was resected (Table 4). Three patients even received a complete colectomy in combination with partial ileum resection.

After intervention, serum lactate level dropped statistically significantly from a mean value of 4.26 mmol/L initially to 1.8 mmol/L after 24 h ($p < 0.001$) (Figure 2).

There were statistically significant differences in the laboratory values of lactate and PTT in relation to the arrival value at the hospital or at the onset of symptoms, and also in relation to the course of laboratory values during the first 24 h (Figures 3 and 4). The patients who died within the first 12 months after symptom onset had significantly higher lactate and PTT initially and after 12 h (both $p < 0.05$).

Table 4. Results of surgical follow up after intervention.

Time interval between end of intervention and start of laparoscopy (mean min ± SD)	71 min ± 42 min
Bowel ischemia in laparoscopy • Yes • No	n = 32 (55.2%) n = 26 (44.8%)
Extend of bowel resection • Ileum • Right hemicolectomy • Total colectomy	Mean about 110 cm n = 5 n = 3

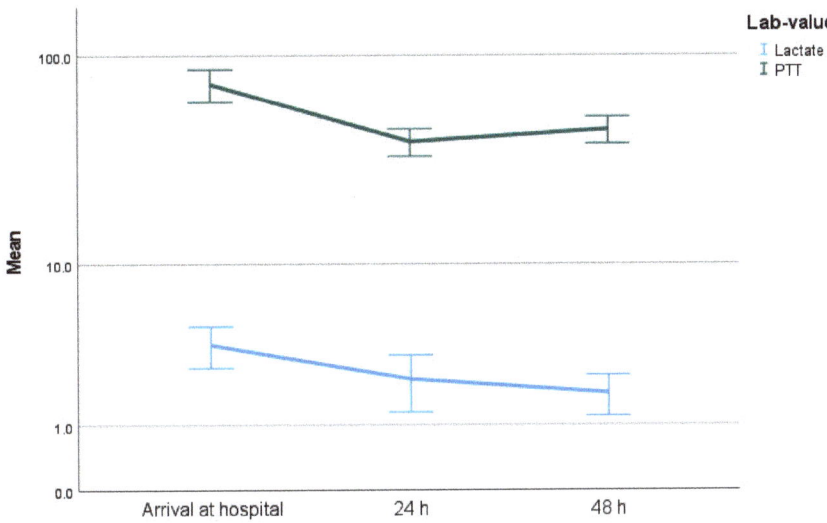

Figure 2. Significant decrease in serum lactate levels ($p < 0.001$) and in serum PTT ($p < 0.001$).

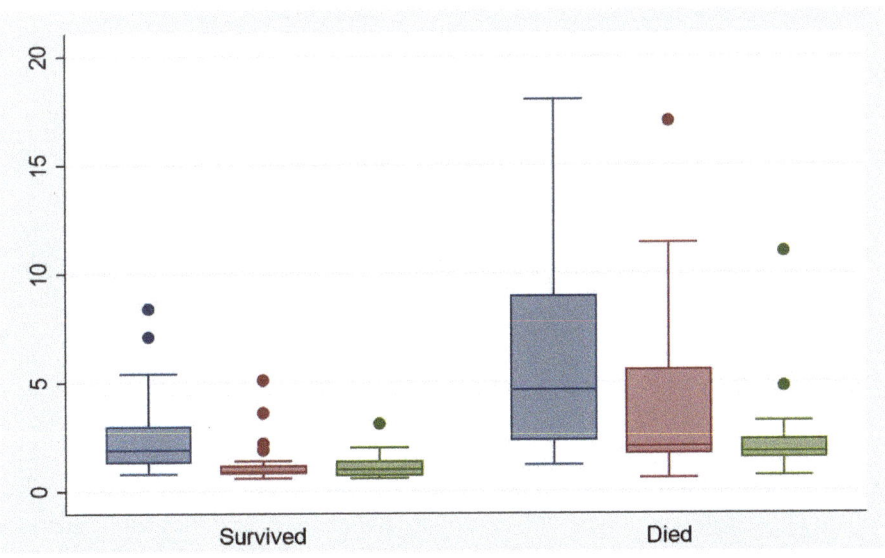

Figure 3. Serum lactate levels on arrival at hospital (blue), after 12 h (red) and after 24 h (green).

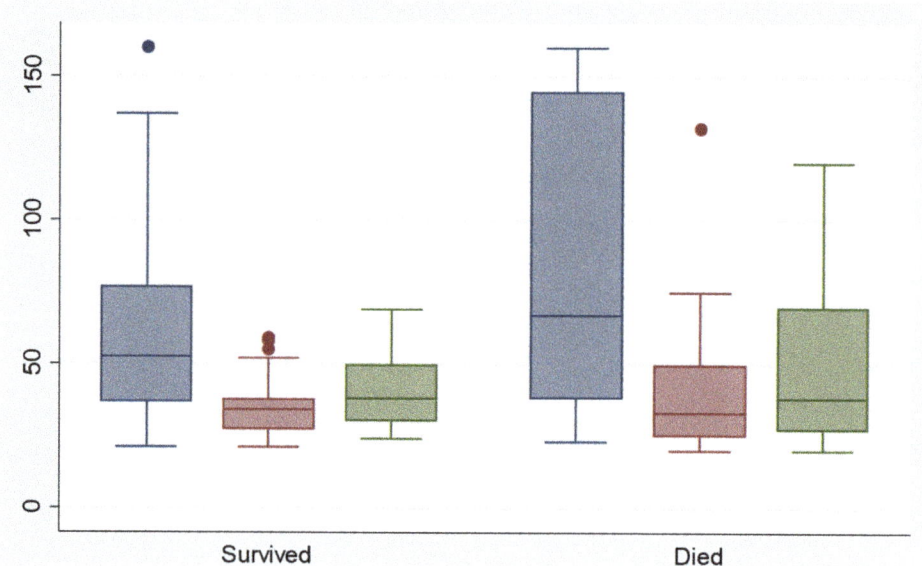

Figure 4. Serum PTT levels during angiography (blue), 12 h after angiography (red) and 24 h after angiography (green).

Kaplan–Meier estimates showed a 50% mortality within 6.9 months, whereas 25% mortality was already achieved at 0.67 months (Figure 5).

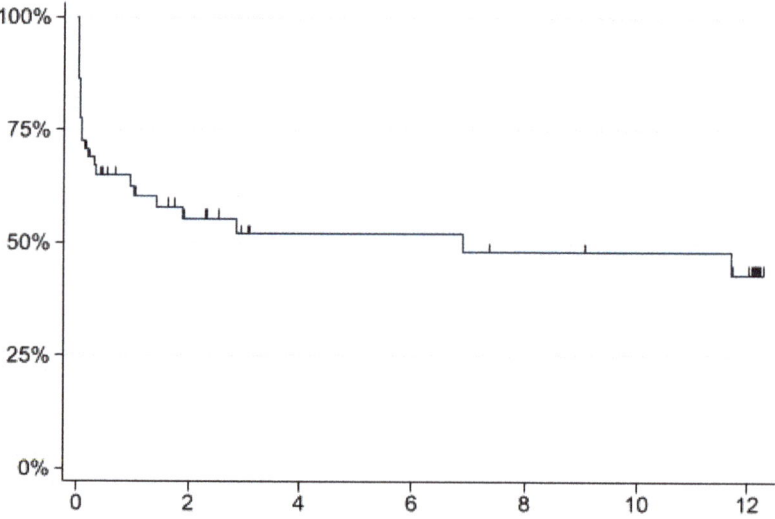

Figure 5. Kaplan–Meier mortality curve; x-axis: months; y-axis: probability of survival.

In our cohort, we did not find statistically significant correlations between the aetiology of mesenteric ischemia and patient death using the log-rank test (Chi^2 = 2.52, p = 0.28). However, we found a statistically significant correlation with respect to the extent of intestinal ischemia (see Figure 6 Chi = 12.25, p = 0.006). There were other factors that did not have a statistically significant effect on death (see Table 5).

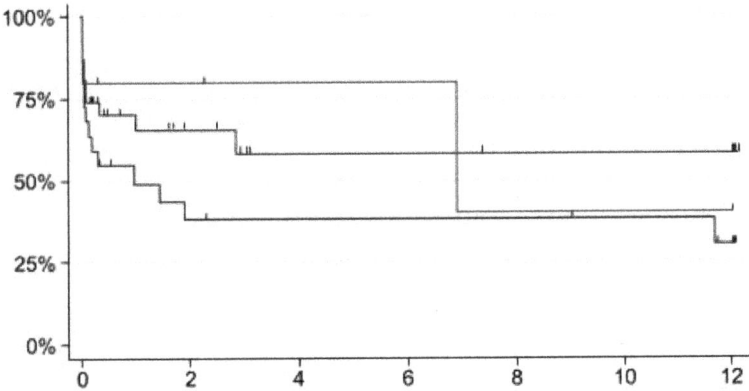

Figure 6. Kaplan–Meier estimate of the aetiology of mesenteric ischemia and patient death. The green line represents dissection, the blue line represents embolus and the red line represents thrombosis. Chi^2 = 12.25, p = 0.006; x-axis: months; y-axis: probability of survival.

Table 5. Log-rank test between several clinical parameters and death. All parameters were obtained as part of the treatment regimen for mesenteric ischemia.

Death	Chi^2	p-Value
Aetiology of mesenteric ischemia	2.52	0.28
Extent of intestinal ischemia	12.25	0.006
Resection of colon	1.37	0.24
Patient history of coronary heart disease	0.76	0.09
Patient history of hypertension	0.51	0.43
Patient history of diabetes	0.38	0.54
Patient history of atrial fibrillation	0.49	0.48
Patient history of chronic peripheral occlusive disease	0.6	0.44
Patient history of dialysis	0.55	0.46

There was no statistically significant association between the aetiology of ischemia and overall survival during the first 12 months (p = 0.28, see Figure 6). Although all three aetiologies showed high initial mortality, mesenteric thrombosis showed a slightly increased mortality compared with embolism.

An interesting side-fact resulting from our data was that resection of the ileum clearly correlated with survival; patients who had a portion of ileum resected had a 2.3-fold increased risk of death (p = 0.02). Furthermore, time from symptom onset statistically significantly correlated with patient mortality (p = 0.043), whereas patients with a shorter time period had a significantly longer survival (Table 6).

Table 6. Multivariate analysis of "time from symptom onset", "resection of ileum" and "survival" of patients.

Correlation	Time from Symptom Onset	Survival	Resection of Ileum
Time from symptom onset	x	r = −0.220, p = 0.043	r = −0.047, p = 0.73
Survival	r = −0.220, p = 0.043	x	r = 0.316, p = 0.01
Resection of ileum	r = −0.047, p = 0.73	r = 0.316, p = 0.01	x

4. Discussion

Acute mesenteric ischemia is a life-threatening condition that requires immediate treatment. Acute thrombosis of the ostia of the superior mesenteric artery has been described to be associated with the worst prognosis, since the affected patient population is mostly of advanced age with concomitant atherosclerosis and pre-existing stenosis of the ostium [4,12,13]. In this retrospective analysis, 74.1% of patients had a pre-existing stenosis of the ostium of the SMA. This, in the case of acute occlusion, usually involves a larger part of the bowel, in contrast to the purely arterial embolus, which might usually be located more distally in the vascular tree. Especially problematic in the context of mesenteric ischemia are elderly patients with atrial fibrillation who develop an embolic occlusion. In contrast to patients with chronic stenosis, these patients do not (yet) have any bypass circuits. There was no statistically significant correlation between death and aetiology of mesenteric ischemia ($p = 0.28$).

It is widely recognized that time is critical in the treatment of AMI. Therefore, the restoration of blood supply to the bowel is the first priority in these patients in order to avoid the occurrence of irreversible necrosis of the bowel wall. Nevertheless, the results of delayed diagnosis or treatment in predicting mortality after AMI are controversial in the literature [14,15], and current data suggest that ischemic changes are reversible in the first 6 h, although this is in contrast to ischemic stroke. Furthermore, current guidelines do not provide precise information on the correct timing for revascularization. In our cohort, a mean time between the onset of symptoms and revascularization of 222 min (=less than 4 h) could be achieved, which lead to improved survival compared to the existing literature. In our cohort, there was a statistically significant difference in terms of patient survival and the time from symptom onset to intervention.

Regarding the poor prognosis of patients with AMI and the fact that time plays a crucial role in the prevention of intestinal necrosis and survival [16], it would be useful to identify factors that can predict the outcome of patients after revascularization in order to improve treatment.

Several studies have suggested that elevated serum lactate levels, which result from anaerobic glycolysis, are associated with irreversible transmural necrosis [17,18] and a worse outcome [19,20]. Our results indicate a clear distinction between the laboratory parameters of lactate and PTT with respect to the subgroups "dead within 12 months" and "alive after 12 months" (both $p < 0.05$). This distinction is associated with the extent of mesenteric ischemia, as patients with extensive ischemia are also more likely to have a shorter survival time.

These factors could be indicators for poor outcomes and alternative treatment options as open surgery or hybrid retrograde open mesenteric stenting could be considered in these patients, whereas retrograde stenting requires dedicated preparation, but has shown promising results [21].

Another important predictor of the outcome for patients with mesenteric ischemia is the presence of pre-existing co-morbidities. In our cohort, 50 out of 58 patients had various pre-existing co-morbidities, of which 25 had CHD, 33 had hypertension, 11 had diabetes, 21 had cardiac arrhythmias, 15 suffered from chronic peripheral arterial occlusive disease and 9 patients were undergoing dialysis. None of these proved to be reliable in predicting the patients' outcome, which is consistent with the literature [12].

The limitations of this study include its retrospective nature and limited cohort size, as it was performed at a single centre and only in patients with clinically significant occlusion of the SMA, whereas patients with occlusion of the celiac trunk were excluded. In addition, all the patients were treated under emergency conditions by different interventionalists and there was no standardized follow-up.

In conclusion, the 30-day mortality rate in patients with AMI (independent of aetiology) remains high despite emergency endovascular revascularization/stenting of the SMA. In the absence of statistically reliable prognostic factors for clinical outcomes in this patient population that could potentially be used to guide patient management toward alternative treatments, we recommend immediate endovascular revascularization followed by surgical screening for ischemic bowel parts in all patients.

Author Contributions: Data curation, E.E. and M.W.; Writing—original draft, A.E.; Writing—review & editing, F.S., R.A., K.N., G.G. and C.A.; Visualization, Y.-S.F. All authors have read and agreed to the published version of the manuscript.

Funding: We acknowledge support by Open Access Publishing Fund of University of Tübingen.

Institutional Review Board Statement: The study was conducted in accordance with the Declaration of Helsinki, and approved by the Institutional Ethics Committee of the University of Tübingen (182/2021BO2, 8 April 2021).

Informed Consent Statement: Patient consent was waived since mortality is relatively very high in this clinical picture and is associated with a poor prognosis even with successful revascularization.

Conflicts of Interest: The authors declare no conflict of interest.

References

1. Patel, A.; Kaleya, R.N.; Sammartano, R.J. Pathophysiology of mesenteric ischemia. *Surg. Clin. N. Am.* **1992**, *72*, 31–41. [CrossRef] [PubMed]
2. Chang, R.-W.; Chang, J.-B.; Longo, W.-E. Update in management of mesenteric ischemia. *World J. Gastroenterol.* **2006**, *12*, 3243–3247. [CrossRef] [PubMed]
3. Horton, K.M.; Fishman, E.K. Multidetector CT angiography in the diagnosis of mesenteric ischemia. *Radiol. Clin. N. Am.* **2007**, *45*, 275–288. [CrossRef]
4. Schoots, I.G.; Koffeman, G.I.; Legemate, D.A.; Levi, M.; Van Gulik, T.M. Systematic review of survival after acute mesenteric ischaemia according to disease aetiology. *Br. J. Surg.* **2004**, *91*, 17–27. [CrossRef] [PubMed]
5. Beaulieu, R.J.; Arnaoutakis, K.D.; Abularrage, C.J.; Efron, D.T.; Schneider, E.; Black, J.H., III. Comparison of open and endovascular treatment of acute mesenteric ischemia. *J. Vasc. Surg.* **2014**, *59*, 159–164. [CrossRef] [PubMed]
6. Acosta, S. Mesenteric Ischemia. *Curr. Opin. Crit. Care* **2015**, *21*, 171–178. Available online: https://journals.lww.com/co-criticalcare/Fulltext/2015/04000/Mesenteric_ischemia.12.aspx (accessed on 21 April 2015). [CrossRef]
7. Clair, D.G.; Beach, J.M. Mesenteric Ischemia. *N. Engl. J. Med.* **2016**, *374*, 959–968. [CrossRef]
8. Kundan, M.; Chebrolu, H.; Muniswamppa, C.; Kumar, N.; Chintamani, C.; Varma, V. Outcomes of Management of Patients with Acute Mesenteric Ischemia: A Prospective Study. *Niger. J. Surg. Off. Publ. Niger. Surg. Res. Soc.* **2021**, *27*, 16–21. [CrossRef] [PubMed]
9. Kärkkäinen, J.M.; Acosta, S. Acute mesenteric ischemia (part I)—Incidence, etiologies, and how to improve early diagnosis. *Best Pract. Res. Clin. Gastroenterol.* **2017**, *31*, 15–25. [CrossRef]
10. Bala, M.; Kashuk, J.; Moore, E.E.; Kluger, Y.; Biffl, W.; Gomes, C.A.; Ben-Ishay, O.; Rubinstein, C.; Balogh, Z.J.; Civil, I.; et al. Acute mesenteric ischemia: Guidelines of the World Society of Emergency Surgery. *World J. Emerg. Surg. WJES* **2017**, *12*, 38. [CrossRef]
11. Zaidat, O.O.; Yoo, A.J.; Khatri, P.; Tomsick, T.A.; von Kummer, R.; Saver, J.L.; Marks, M.P.; Prabhakaran, S.; Kallmes, D.F.; Fitzsimmons, B.-F.M. Recommendations on angiographic revascularization grading standards for acute ischemic stroke: A consensus statement. *Stroke* **2013**, *44*, 2650–2663. [CrossRef]
12. Pedersoli, F.; Schönau, K.; Schulze-Hagen, M.; Keil, S.; Isfort, P.; Gombert, A.; Alizai, P.H.; Kuhl, C.K.; Bruners, P.; Zimmermann, M.; et al. Endovascular Revascularization with Stent Implantation in Patients with Acute Mesenteric Ischemia due to Acute Arterial Thrombosis: Clinical Outcome and Predictive Factors. *Cardiovasc. Interv. Radiol.* **2021**, *44*, 1030–1038. [CrossRef]
13. Kanasaki, S.; Furukawa, A.; Fumoto, K.; Hamanaka, Y.; Ota, S.; Hirose, T.; Inoue, A.; Shirakawa, T.; Nguyen, L.D.H.; Tulyeubai, S. Acute Mesenteric Ischemia: Multidetector CT Findings and Endovascular Management. *Radiogr. A Rev. Publ. Radiol. Soc. N. Am.* **2018**, *38*, 945–961. [CrossRef]
14. Wadman, M.; Syk, I.; Elmståhl, S. Survival after operations for ischaemic bowel disease. *Eur. J. Surg. Acta Chir.* **2000**, *166*, 872–877. [CrossRef]
15. Block, T.A.; Acosta, S.; Björck, M. Endovascular and open surgery for acute occlusion of the superior mesenteric artery. *J. Vasc. Surg.* **2010**, *52*, 959–966. [CrossRef] [PubMed]
16. Klar, E.; Rahmanian, P.B.; Bücker, A.; Hauenstein, K.; Jauch, K.W.; Luther, B. Acute mesenteric ischemia: A vascular emergency. *Dtsch. Arztebl. Int.* **2012**, *109*, 249–256. [PubMed]
17. Emile, S.H. Predictive Factors for Intestinal Transmural Necrosis in Patients with Acute Mesenteric Ischemia. *World J. Surg.* **2018**, *42*, 2364–2372. [CrossRef]
18. Canfora, A.; Ferronetti, A.; Marte, G.; di Maio, V.; Mauriello, C.; Maida, P.; Bottino, V.; Aprea, G.; Amato, B. Predictive Factors of Intestinal Necrosis in Acute Mesenteric Ischemia. *Open Med. (Wars. Pol.)* **2019**, *14*, 883–889. [CrossRef]
19. Caluwaerts, M.; Castanares-Zapatero, D.; Laterre, P.-F.; Hantson, P. Prognostic factors of acute mesenteric ischemia in ICU patients. *BMC Gastroenterol.* **2019**, *19*, 80. [CrossRef] [PubMed]

20. Grotelüschen, R.; Bergmann, W.; Welte, M.N.; Reeh, M.; Izbicki, J.R.; Bachmann, K. What predicts the outcome in patients with intestinal ischemia? A single center experience. *J. Visc. Surg.* **2019**, *156*, 405–411. [CrossRef]
21. Oderich, G.S.; Macedo, R.; Stone, D.H.; Woo, E.Y.; Panneton, J.M.; Resch, T.; Dias, N.V.; Sonesson, B.; Schermerhorn, M.L.; Lee, J.T.; et al. Multicenter study of retrograde open mesenteric artery stenting through laparotomy for treatment of acute and chronic mesenteric ischemia. *J. Vasc. Surg.* **2018**, *68*, 470–480.e1. [CrossRef] [PubMed]

Disclaimer/Publisher's Note: The statements, opinions and data contained in all publications are solely those of the individual author(s) and contributor(s) and not of MDPI and/or the editor(s). MDPI and/or the editor(s) disclaim responsibility for any injury to people or property resulting from any ideas, methods, instructions or products referred to in the content.

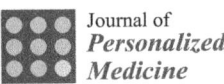

Journal of Personalized Medicine

Article

Stenting in Brain Hemodynamic Injury of Carotid Origin Caused by Type A Aortic Dissection: Local Experience and Systematic Literature Review

Jean-François Aita [1,2,3], Thibault Agripnidis [1,2,3], Benoit Testud [4], Pierre-Antoine Barral [4], Alexis Jacquier [4], Anthony Reyre [1], Ammar Alnuaimi [4], Nadine Girard [1], Farouk Tradi [2,3,4], Paul Habert [2,3,4], Vlad Gariboldi [5], Frederic Collart [5], Axel Bartoli [4] and Jean-François Hak [1,2,3,*]

1 Department of Neuroradiology, APHM La Timone, 13005 Marseille, France
2 LIIE, Aix Marseille University, 13007 Marseille, France
3 CERIMED, Aix Marseille University, 13007 Marseille, France
4 Department of Medical Imaging, APHM La Timone, 13005 Marseille, France
5 Department of Cardiac Surgery, La Timone Hospital, La Timone Hospital 264, Rue Saint Pierre, 13005 Marseille, France
* Correspondence: jean-francois.hak@ap-hm.fr

Abstract: In this study, we report our local experience of type A aortic dissections in patients with cerebral malperfusion treated with carotid stenting before or after aortic surgery, and present a systematic literature review on these patients treated either with carotid stenting (CS) before or after aortic surgery (AS) or with aortic and carotid surgery alone (ACS). We report on patients treated in our center with carotid stenting for brain hemodynamic injury of carotid origin caused by type A dissection since 2018, and a systematic review was conducted in PubMed for articles published from 1990 to 2021. Out of 5307 articles, 19 articles could be included with a total of 80 patients analyzed: 9 from our center, 29 patients from case reports, and 51 patients from two retrospective cohorts. In total, 8 patients were treated by stenting first, 72 by surgery first, and 7 by stenting after surgery. The mean age; initial NIHSS score; time from symptom onset to treatment; post-treatment clinical improvement; post-treatment clinical worsening; mortality rate; follow-up duration; and follow-up mRS were, respectively, for each group (local cohort, CS before AS, ACS, CS after AS): 71.2 ± 5.3 yo, 65.5 ± 11.0 yo; 65.3 ± 13.1 yo, 68.7 ± 5.8 yo; 4 ± 8.4, 11.3 ± 8.5, 14.3 ± 8.0, 0; 11.8 ± 14.3 h, 21 ± 39.3 h, 13.6 ± 17.8 h, 13 ± 17.2 h; 56%, 71%, 86%, 57%; 11%, 28%, 0%, 14%; 25%, 12.3%, 14%, 33%; 5.25 ± 2.9 months, 54 months, 6.8 ± 3.8 months, 14 ± 14.4 months; 1 ± 1; 0.25 ± 0.5, 1.3 ± 0.8, 0.68 ± 0.6. Preoperative carotid stenting for hemodynamic cerebral malperfusion by true lumen compression appears to be feasible, and could be effective and safe, although there is still a lack of evidence due to the absence of comparative statistical analysis. The literature, albeit growing, is still limited, and prospective comparative studies are needed.

Keywords: aortic; dissection; brain; malperfusion; carotid; stenting; surgery

1. Introduction

Type A aortic dissection (AAD) is a diagnostic and therapeutic emergency, always needing an urgent surgical repair.

Left untreated, mortality is 1–2% per hour, 25% the first day, 50% in 48 h and 75% in two weeks. Incidence is estimated at 3–6 people per 100,000 people per year [1].

Complications are related to extension of the dissection; retrograde extension to the aortic ring can lead to acute aortic insufficiency and to an intra-pericardial effusion, with cardiac tamponade, accounting for 70% of acute mortality. False lumen aneurysmal evolution may be complicated by aortic rupture [2].

Extension to visceral arteries, complicating 20–30% of AAD, may be responsible for a malperfusion syndrome in downstream organs, including cerebral ischemia.

"Radiographic" malperfusion (evidence of an organ's vascular compromise) should be distinguished from "clinical" malperfusion or "malperfusion syndrome", characterized by clinical symptoms, indicating ischemia of downstream organs: the latter carries a much worse prognosis [3].

Reperfusion can cause an increase in intracranial pressure. The brain, very sensitive to ischemia, is susceptible to reperfusion-related edema or hemorrhagic infarction and its complications. The longer the time to reperfusion, the more complications that may occur, thus minimizing the time to reperfusion is therefore essential [3].

Strokes are the major neurological complication, affecting up to one-third of AAD patients, occurring either initially or postoperatively; Zhao et al. reported an incidence of 36.7% of ischemic lesions on diffusion magnetic resonance imaging (MRI) [4]. Stroke is an independent risk factor for early and mid-term mortality [5].

Strokes complicating AAD are of ischemic type, most often multifactorial, due to:

— An extension of the dissection to the supra-aortic branches, with carotid or vertebral occlusion, by compression of the true lumen, or thrombo-embolic mechanism arising from the false lumen;
— Often coexisting with systemic hypotension, resulting in decreased cerebral perfusion [4,6].

Cerebral malperfusion (CM), to be distinguished from ischemic stroke, complicates 11% of AAD [3,7]. In the study by Geirsson et al., its presence in the preoperative period increased in-hospital mortality from 9.5 to 50%, the risk of postoperative stroke from 4.5 to 46.7%, the occurrence of coma from 4.5 to 40%, and confusion from 29.6 to 73.3% [8].

Extension of dissection to the common carotid arteries (CCA) has an incidence of 30%. It is associated with a significant increase in preoperative neurological deficits (23%, compared to 3% without extension) [9,10]. The right CCA is most frequently affected, in conjunction with the brachiocephalic artery [11].

Appearance of new deficits postoperatively may result from the increase in preoperative malperfusion, intraoperative hypoperfusion, or a perioperative embolic event [12]. A transient deficit may be observed in association with reperfusion edema.

Aortic and carotid surgery is the standard treatment in case of cerebral malperfusion.

Amr et al. noted that isolated hypoperfusion should not be a contraindication for surgery, regardless of its severity [13].

If CM occurs, the aim of surgery is to restore cerebral perfusion to minimize the risk of long-term complications. The usual attitude is to replace the arch and repair the dissected common carotid artery, hoping that repair of the dissection will correct the malperfusion [10].

There is no definitive recommendation regarding the place of carotid stenting (CS) in case of CM complicating an AAD extended to the carotid arteries [14].

Several authors have reported stenting management of the dissected carotid artery before surgery for downstream CM, but data in the literature remain limited.

Carotid angioplasty can be performed more rapidly than surgery, under local anesthesia. The goal is to cover the entire dissected portions with stents, allowing obliteration of the false lumen and re-expansion of the true lumen.

On the other hand, the benefit of CS in the aftermath of aortic surgery (AS) has also been reported, because of residual dissection with true lumen stenosis, resulting in symptomatic cerebral hypoperfusion.

Postoperative malperfusion syndrome is an independent predictor of early mortality according to the multicenter study by Czerny et al. [7,10]. Similarly, asymptomatic residual radiological malperfusion after surgical repair, has been associated with long-term neurological sequelae, with a fourfold relative risk of transient ischemic attack or stroke [3].

Our objective is to report our local experience of AAD patients with CM treated with CS before or after AS and to perform a systematic literature review of AAD patients with CM treated either with CS before or after AS or with aortic and carotid surgery alone (ACS).

2. Materials and Methods

2.1. Ethics

For the cohort study, as this was a non-interventional retrospective study of routinely acquired data, written informed consent for this study was not necessary. The manuscript was prepared following the Preferred Reporting Items for Systematic-Reviews and Meta-Analyses (PRISMA) guidelines.

2.2. Local Center Patients' Selection

We conducted a retrospective search in our center's PACS database, from January 2018 to June 2022.

The inclusion criteria were: (1) adult patients, aged 18 years old or more, (2) with uni- or bilateral carotid dissection, following acute type A aortic dissection, without intracranial vessel occlusion, (3) associated with brain hypoperfusion in the territory of the dissected vessels, attested by either hypoperfusion proved with perfusion–CT or perfusion–MRI sequence, or typical junctional stroke pattern on diffusion MRI sequence, (4) patients who underwent CS before or after AS.

Patients with carotid or large intracranial vessel occlusion due to an embolic mechanism, or who were managed conservatively or with thrombolysis were excluded.

2.3. Literature Review

A systematic review of the literature was performed in the PubMed database separately by two authors (J-FA and TA). The keyword associations used were "Aortic dissection AND Carotid stenting", "Aortic dissection AND carotid angioplasty", "aortic dissection AND carotid plasty", "Aortic dissection AND stroke", "Acute disease AND aneurysm, dissecting AND cerebrovascular disorders". All articles dating from 1990 to the research date (February 2022) were included for screening.

The inclusion and exclusion criteria for selecting the articles were the same.

Titles and abstracts were screened. Studies meeting prespecified inclusion criteria were reviewed in full. PRISMA guidelines were strictly adhered. Two authors completed the quality assessment and evaluation of bias according to specific guidelines.

We evaluated the outcome of these patients in terms of mortality, residual disability, and intra- and post-procedural complications.

Risk of bias was assessed according to the Joanna Briggs Institute Critical Appraisal tools for case reports, and to the Cochrane Collaboration tool for cohort studies (details in online Supplementary Tables S1 and S2).

2.4. Data Extraction and Expression of Results

Baseline characteristics were displayed as absolute number (percentage) or mean (SD) or median (interquartile range [IQR], e.g., 25th–75th quantiles).

Extracted data included bibliographic information, type of paper, stated aim, topic/focus of systematic review, study/review methodology, description of reported involvement, baseline characteristics and results about treatment and outcome.

3. Results

3.1. Local Center Patients' Selection (n = 9)

In total, nine patients were included in the study: four who underwent CS before AS, and five following AS, all of them because of neurologic deficits, attributed to a hemodynamic brain hypoperfusion. The characteristics of these patients are detailed in Table 1.

Table 1. Local patients characteristics.

Patient	1	2	3	4	5	6	7	8	9
Treatment	Carotid stenting before aortic surgery				Carotid stenting after aortic surgery				
Age	71	71	72	72	78	64	71	74	62
Sex	M	M	M	M	F	M	F	F	F
Arterial hypertension	yes	No	yes	yes	yes	yes	yes	no	yes
Current smoking	No	No	Yes	No	No	Yes	No	No	yes
Pre-stroke MRS	0	0	0	0	0	0	0	0	0
NIHSS on presentation	21	NA	10	0	NA	0	0	0	0
ASPECTS score	7	10	8	9	10	10	8	NA	NA
Supra-aortic branch involved	RCCA and ICA, LCCA and ICA	RCCA and ICA	RCCA and ICA	RCCA	RCCA	LCCA	RCCA	RCCA and ICA, LCCA	RCCA
Per-procedure complications	No	No	No	No	Yes (common carotid intra-stent thrombosis treated by aspiration, A2 distal emboli)	No	No	Yes M2 (sylvian emboli)	Yes (distal emboli)
New lesion on post-procedure MRI	No	No	No	Yes	No	No	No	Yes (junctionnal infarct)	Yes (diffuse distal ischemic lesions)
New neurological deficit post-procedure	No	No	No	No	No	Yes (transient majoration due to reperfusion oedema)	No	No	No
Post-procedure neurologic deficit regression	Partial	Partial	Partial	Yes	No Neurologic degradation (day 8)	Partial	Partial	No Cardiac arrest (day 4)	NA
Survived	Yes	No Mesenteric ischemia (day 2)	Yes	Yes		Yes	Yes		NA
MRS at discharge	2	-	4	NA	-	1	4	-	NA
MRS after 90 days	1	-	3	1	-	1	1	-	NA
Sent permeability at follow-up	Yes	Yes	Yes	Yes	Yes	Yes	Yes	Yes	NA

The nine patients managed in our center had a median age of 72 years (IQR 67.5–75.5), with a male predominance.

All patients had an mRS score of 0 before dissection. The median ASPECTS score was 9 (IQR 8–10) (n = 3). Following CS, the neurological deficit partially regressed in 66.7% of the patients. An increase in neurological deficit occurred in 11% for various reasons detailed in Table 1. During carotid stenting, three patients presented with distal emboli, e.g., a distal A2 embolus without endovascular rescue, a sylvian M2 embolus treated by thrombectomy; multiple distal emboli were not accessible by thrombectomy.

Following CS, three patients (33%) presented new ischemic lesion: a junctional infarct and a sylvian punctiform spot, distal diffuse ischemic lesions. Of these three patients, one patient presented with clinical worsening. All surviving patients had good stent permeability at follow-up.

3.2. Literature Review (n = 73)

A total of 5307 articles were identified. After exclusion based on the abstract, 703 articles were retained for detailed review. Finally, 19 articles matched all the criteria, 17 case reports, and 2 retrospective series were included. None of the studies were prospective; see flowchart of the included studies (Figure 1). The characteristics of included studies are shown in Table 2.

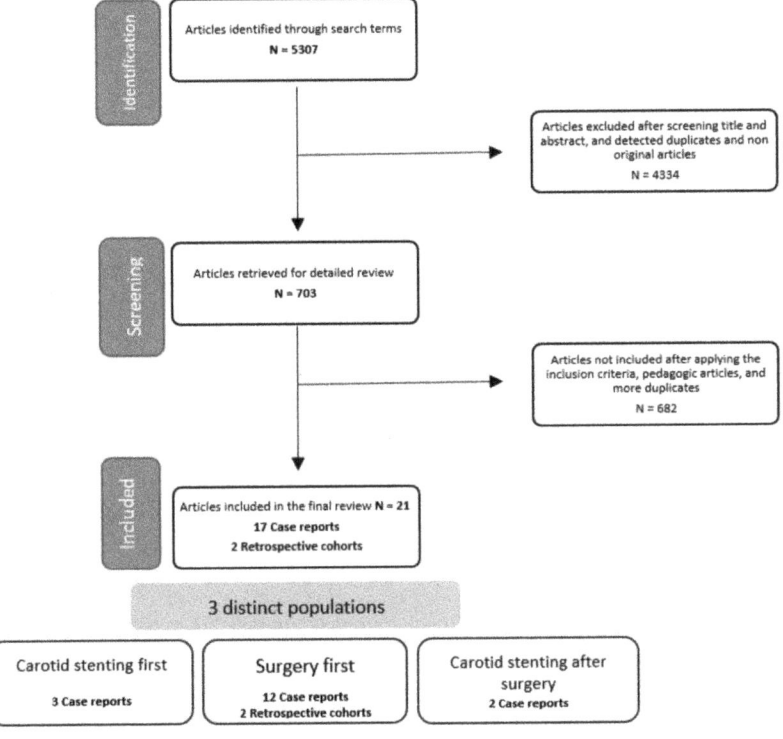

Figure 1. Flowchart of included studies.

Patients had a median age of 64.5 years (IQR 57–70) for the case reports [11,13–28], and 60.5 years and 68 years in the cohorts [12,17]; 52% were female. A history of arterial hypertension (AH) was found in 83% of the cases.

All patients had an mRS score of 0 before dissection. The mean initial NIHSS score (all items combined) was 13.6 ± 11.2. The median time from symptom onset to treatment was 6 h (IQR 3.5–15).

Table 2. Summary of included studies.

Study	Year	Study Type	Number of Patients Included	First Treatment
Schönholz et al. [15]	2008	Case report	1	Surgery
Chahine et al. [16]	2018	Case report	2	Surgery
Morihara et al. [17]	2016	Case report	1	Surgery
Matsumoto et al. [18]	2016	Case report	2	Surgery
Amr et al. [13]	2016	Case report	2	Surgery
Hong et al. [19]	2005	Case report	1	Surgery
Karawabuki et al. [20]	2006	Case report	1	Surgery
Kim et al. [29]	2006	Case report	1	Surgery
Ueyama et al. [22]	2007	Case report	1	Surgery
Roseborough et al. [11]	2006	Case report	1	Surgery then stenting
Sakaguchi et al. [23]	2005	Case report	1	Surgery
Usui et al. [24]	2021	Case report	1	Surgery
Fukuhara et al. [25]	2021	Case report	1	Surgery
Funakoshi et al. [26]	2020	Case report	2	Stenting then surgery
Heran et al. [27]	2019	Case report	1	Stenting then surgery
Popovic et al. [14]	2016	Case report	1	Stenting then surgery
Casana et al. [28]	2011	Case report	1	Surgery then stenting
Fichadaya et al. [12]	2022	Cohort	10	Surgery
Morimoto et al. [30]	2011	Cohort	41	Surgery

3.3. Aortic and Carotid Surgery (ACS) Group (n = 72)

The mean age of the group was 65.5 ± 11.0 years; 53% were female.

The median initial NIHSS score was 16 (IQR 5–19) for the case reports and 8 for the Morimoto et al. cohort [31]. The mean NIHSS for all articles was 11.3 ± 8.5. The median time from symptom onset to treatment for the case reports was 5.5 h (IQR 3–12), and the mean time for all articles was 21 ± 39.3 h.

One patient died during surgery [15] of an uncontrollable hemorrhage complication. No other intraoperative complications were reported.

A new persistent neurological deficit occurred for 28% of the operated patients. A new ischemic lesion on postoperative DWI–MRI occurred for 49% of the patients.

Overall, 13% of the patients (15/53) died during hospitalization (mRS 6). For the other patients, the median mRS score was 3 (IQR 2–3) at discharge, and 0 (IQR 0–0.5) at last follow-up. The mean follow-up time was 53.4 months.

Individual patient data for this group are available in Supplementary Table S3A.

3.4. Carotid Stenting (CS) before Aortic Surgery (AS) Group (n = 8)

The mean age of the group was 65.3 ± 13.1 years; 25% were female. A history of AH was found in 66% of cases. All patients had an mRS score of 0 before dissection.

The median initial NIHSS score was 14 (IQR 11–21). The mean NIHSS was 14.3 ± 8.0. The median time from symptom onset to treatment was 5.5 h (IQR 3–18), with a mean duration of 13.6 ± 17.8 h.

No deaths during CS or surgery occurred. No patient had any intra-CS or intra-operative complication. Partial regression of neurological deficits was achieved in six patients (86%). The median post-CS NIHSS was 4 (n = 3 patients).

A new ischemic lesion on post-CS imaging occurred in 2 patients.

One patient died before aortic surgery, at day 2, of mesenteric ischemia; 1 patient did not undergo surgery because of a history of Bentall surgery. The other patients received aortic replacement afterwards.

None of the operated patients presented new neurological deficits or new ischemic lesions on postoperative imaging.

One patient died postoperatively during hospitalization from mediastinitis on day 35 [16]. For the other patients, the median mRS score was 2 at discharge, and 1 at follow-up. The mean follow-up time was 6.8 ± 3.6 months. All stents were patented at follow-up.

An example of one of our treated patients is shown in Figure 2.

Individual patient data for this group are available in Supplementary Table S3B.

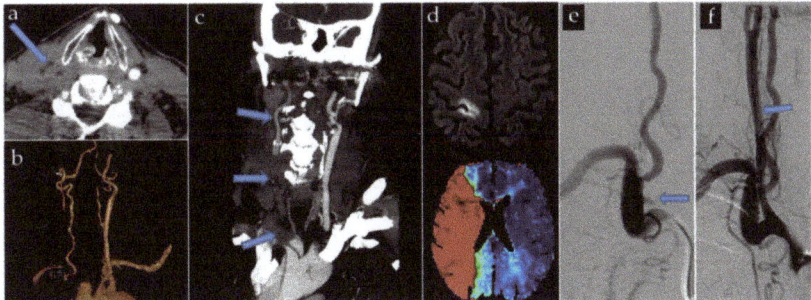

Figure 2. Local cohort case of a 72-year-old, who suffered a brutal left hemicorporal deficit. CT scan showed an AAD extended to the LCCA, with a subocclusive compression of the true lumen (**a–c**). Initial MRI showed a significant mismatch between the limited cytotoxic lesion of the rolandic area, and the hypoperfusion of the entire sylvian territory (**d**). Preoperative angioplasty was decided (**e**) The initial occlusion is shown. Stenting allowed to re-expand the true lumen, with coverage of the entire carotid dissection (**f**). The patient underwent aortic surgery 6 h later, without complications, and recovered gradually after. Post-surgical MRI (not shown) found no new cytotoxic lesion, and showed complete resolution of the hypoperfusion.

3.5. Carotid Stenting (CS) after Aortic Surgery (AS) Group (n = 7)

The mean age of the group was 68.7 ± 5.8 years; 71% were female. A history of AH was found in 66% of cases.

All patients had an mRS score of 0 before dissection.

The initial NIHSS score of all patients was 0. The median time from symptom onset to surgery was 6 h (IQR 6–8), with a mean duration of 13 ± 17.2 h.

All patients presented a new neurological deficit postoperatively, with six of the seven patients presenting new lesions and a hypoperfused cerebral territory on imaging, justifying management by stenting.

The median surgery to stenting time was 3 h (IQR 1–14). During the procedure, three patients presented distal emboli despite the use of an FilterWire EZ (Boston Scientific, Marlborough, MA, USA) distal protection filter in all cases:

- A 78 yo patient presented with a distal A2 embolus, too distant to be accessible by thrombectomy. Three 9 × 30 mm Carotid Wallstents were used, covering the entirety of the brachiocephalic trunk and right common carotid artery. After deployment of the first two Carotid Wallstents, an intra-stent thrombosis occurred, and was immediately and successfully treated by aspiration, and was not recurrent. Antiplatelet treatment was started the next day.

- A 74 yo patient presented a sylvian M2 embolus at the end of the procedure, successfully treated by thrombectomy immediately after stenting with three Carotid Wallstent (7 × 40 mm, 9 × 50 mm and 5 × 30 mm) and a Smart Control 14 × 40 mm. Antiplatelet treatment and preventive low molecular weight Heparin were started the next day.
- A 62 yo patient presented multiple distal emboli not accessible to thrombectomy. Antiplatelet treatment and curative low molecular weight Heparin were started 12 h post-procedure.

On postoperative imaging, the last two patients presented, respectively, a junctional infarct and distal embolic lesions.

Partial regression of neurological deficits was obtained in four patients (57%).

Only one patient presented a neurological worsening in the post-stenting period, related to reperfusion edema, which rapidly completely resolved.

One patient was still hospitalized at the time of writing, a few days after stenting, and the outcome could not be studied.

Two patients died during hospitalization. In the surviving patients, the median mRS score was 2 at discharge and 1 at follow-up.

Individual patient data for this group are available in Supplementary Table S3C.

4. Discussion

Regarding the patients from our local cohort (n = 9), the mean age was 71.2 ± 5.3 years, with a male predominance, a history of AH was found in 78%. The median ASPECTS score was 9 (IQR 8–10). Following CS, neurological deficits partially regressed in 0.67% (2/3) of the patients and remained stable in 0.33 (1/3) of the cases. During CS, three patients presented procedural complications: multiple distal emboli, an A2 emboli, and a homolateral sylvian M2 emboli, the latter being successfully treated by thrombectomy. The first patient had an immediate intra-stent thrombosis, successfully treated by aspiration. All surviving patients had good stent permeability at follow-up.

Experience in carotid stenting in the context of stroke derives from three situations: thrombectomy in thromboembolic stroke, urgent carotid repair in a traumatic setting, and isolated carotid artery stenosis or dissections (in rare cases).

The meta-analysis of Fabre et al. in the context of primitive carotid dissections, reported a technical success rate of 99.1% in 201 patients, with rare complications, including one embolic stroke, two subarachnoid hemorrhages, a transient vasospasm in two patients.

During follow-up, only 3.3% of patients developed intimal hyperplasia or intrastent stenosis; 2.1% had recurrent TIA in the territory of the stented vessels [32].

In the context of AAD extended to the carotid arteries, a limited number of case reports have been published in the literature, with stenting *before* [14,26,27], *during* [31,33,34], or *after* [11,21,28,34–38] aortic surgical repair: in all reported cases, technical success was achieved, with complete exclusion of false lumen, and stent patency at follow-up. All patients showed improvement or complete resolution of neurological symptoms. Only one case of death is reported, unrelated, from mediastinitis.

Recently, Mukherjee et al. reported three patients treated by retrograde carotid stenting after aortic repair, with residual stenosing carotid or brachial artery dissections. Venous stents (Boston Scientific VICI) were chosen because of their greater radial strength than the stents normally used, with the goal of a better obliteration of the false lumen [34].

Carotid angioplasty can be performed more rapidly than surgery, under local anesthesia.

Funakoshi et al. summarized the various challenges of performing carotid angioplasty-stenting preoperatively [26]:

(1) The need for double antiplatelet therapy in the immediate post-procedure period, which may lead to postpone the urgent aortic replacement surgery, which can only be carried out under mono-antiaggregation. (2) A risk of post-procedure reperfusion edema. A prior perfusion imaging (CT or MRI) allows to evaluate this risk. (3) The technical difficulty of catheterizing the true lumen. (4) Restriction of future surgical options: when stents cover the origin of aortic branches total arch replacement is impossible. Both patients

in the article were treated with hemi-arch replacement for this reason. (5) The risk of per-procedure distal emboli. However, according to a meta-analysis by Fabre et al., the risk of distal emboli is low for the treatment of dissections: for patients who benefited from a stenting treatment of primary internal carotid dissections, only 1 out of 201 treated patients presented an embolic stroke [32].

After the procedure, most patients are put on double antiplatelet therapy for 1–6 months, then on permanent single antiaggregant [32].

A summary of the benefits and drawbacks of the procedure is presented in Table 3.

Table 3. Comparison of benefits and drawbacks.

Carotid Stenting First	Aortic and Carotid Surgery First
Benefits	
Local anesthesia	Faster repair of ascending aorta
Faster installation (15 min of installation on table)	Correction of systemic hypotension
Treatment of distal internal carotid artery dissections	
Complete exclusion of the false lumen	
Drawbacks	
Double antiaggregation post-procedure: postponed surgery	Longer preparation
Difficulty in catheterizing the true lumen	General anesthesia
Restriction of surgical options: impossibility of total arch replacement when stents cover the origin of supra-aortic branches	Risk of intraoperative hypoperfusion under cardiopulmonary bypass
Risk of distal embolization per procedure	Risk of residual dissection and/or cerebral malperfusion if distal repair is impossible

The study by Fukuhara et al. found a significant difference in morbidity and mortality with ICA vs. CCA occlusion: every one of the ICA patients developed rapid cerebral edema with herniation, and died during hospitalization, whereas 79% of patients with occlusion limited to CCAs (uni- or bilateral) survived, and only one patient developed cerebral edema. These results suggest that occlusion of an ICA may be a marker at risk for cerebral edema and herniation [25].

The residual dissection of postoperative supra-aortic branches is associated with long-term neurological complications [11]. The prospective study by Neri et al., which followed 42 of these patients for a median of 3.17 years, found an incidence of neurological events of 30.9%, including stroke in 18 patients, with a relative risk of 3.99, all of which occurred in the territory of the initial dissected artery [39].

To the best of our knowledge, our study is the first aiming to synthesize the literature on carotid stenting for hemodynamic injury in the context of AAD.

Our study has many limitations. The included articles were mostly case reports, a source of important biases, notably publication bias. The patients' selection from our center was retrospective, non-randomized, and monocentric. Due to the small number of patients included, statistics comparing the different groups could not be performed. All the articles studied did not evaluate the long-term outcome of patients and did not allow us to obtain any hindsight on mortality or recurrence of symptoms in the long term.

5. Conclusions

Preoperative carotid stenting for hemodynamic CM by true lumen compression appears to be feasible, and could be effective and safe, although there is still a lack of evidence, due to the absence of comparative statistical analysis. The literature, albeit growing, is still limited, and prospective comparative studies are needed.

Supplementary Materials: The following supporting information can be downloaded at: https://www.mdpi.com/article/10.3390/jpm13010058/s1, Table S1: Risk of bias of each case report study according to the The Joanna Briggs Institute Critical Appraisal tools; Table S2: Risk of bias of each individual non-randomised study according to the Cochrane Collaboration tool; Table S3A: Individual patients data from the patients treated by aortic and carotid surgery; Table S3B: Individual patients data from the patients treated by carotid stenting before aortic surgery; Table S3C: Individual patients data from the patients treated by carotid stenting after aortic surgery.

Author Contributions: Conceptualization, J.-F.H. and J.-F.A.; methodology, J.-F.H.; software, J.-F.H.; validation, J.-F.A., T.A., B.T., P.-A.B., A.J., A.R., N.G., F.T., P.H., V.G., F.C., A.B. and J.-F.H.; formal analysis, J.-F.H. and J.-F.A.; investigation, A.A., J.-F.A., T.A., B.T., P.-A.B., A.J., A.R., N.G., F.T., P.H., V.G., F.C., A.B. and J.-F.H.; resources, J.-F.H. and J.-F.A.; data curation, J.-F.A., T.A., B.T., P.-A.B., A.J., A.R., N.G., F.T., P.H., V.G., F.C., A.B. and J.-F.H.; writing—original draft preparation J.-F.A.; writing—review and editing, J.-F.H.; visualization, J.-F.H. and J.-F.A. supervision, J.-F.H.; project administration, A.J., J.-F.H. and J.-F.A. All authors have read and agreed to the published version of the manuscript.

Funding: This research received no external funding.

Institutional Review Board Statement: The study was conducted according to the guidelines of the Declaration of Helsinki and approved by the Ethics Committee of the CERIM (IRB: CRM-2209-303).

Informed Consent Statement: Patient consent was waived due to the fact that the study was a non-interventional retrospective study of routinely acquired data.

Data Availability Statement: The data presented in this study are available on request from the corresponding author.

Conflicts of Interest: The authors declare no conflict of interest.

References

1. Sukockienė, E.; Laučkaitė, K.; Jankauskas, A.; Mickevičienė, D.; Jurkevičienė, G.; Vaitkus, A.; Stankevičius, E.; Petrikonis, K.; Rastenytė, D. Crucial role of carotid ultrasound for the rapid diagnosis of hyperacute aortic dissection complicated by cerebral infarction: A case report and literature review. *Medicina* 2016, 52, 378–388. [CrossRef] [PubMed]
2. Sullivan, P.R.; Wolfson, A.B.; Leckey, R.D.; Burke, J.L. Diagnosis of acute thoracic aortic dissection in the emergency department. *Am. J. Emerg. Med.* 2000, 18, 46–50. [CrossRef] [PubMed]
3. Goldberg, J.B.; Lansman, S.L.; Kai, M.; Tang, G.H.L.; Malekan, R.; Spielvogel, D. Malperfusion in Type A Dissection: Consider Reperfusion First. *Semin. Thorac. Cardiovasc. Surg.* 2017, 29, 181–185. [CrossRef] [PubMed]
4. Zhao, H.; Ma, W.; Wen, D.; Duan, W.; Zheng, M. Computed tomography angiography findings predict the risk factors for preoperative acute ischaemic stroke in patients with acute type A aortic dissection. *Eur. J. Cardio-Thorac. Surg.* 2020, 57, 912–919. [CrossRef]
5. Chemtob, R.A.; Fuglsang, S.; Geirsson, A.; Ahlsson, A.; Olsson, C.; Gunn, J.; Ahmad, K.; Hansson, E.C.; Pan, E.; O Arnadottir, L.; et al. Stroke in acute type A aortic dissection: The Nordic Consortium for Acute Type A Aortic Dissection (NORCAAD). *Eur. J. Cardio-Thorac. Surg.* 2020, 58, 1027–1034. [CrossRef]
6. Okita, Y.; Okada, K. Treatment strategies for malperfusion syndrome secondary to acute aortic dissection. *J. Card Surg.* 2021, 36, 1745–1752. [CrossRef]
7. Czerny, M.; Schoenhoff, F.; Etz, C.; Englberger, L.; Khaladj, N.; Zierer, A.; Weigang, E.; Hoffmann, I.; Blettner, M.; Carrel, T.P. The Impact of Pre-Operative Malperfusion on Outcome in Acute Type A Aortic Dissection. *J. Am. Coll. Cardiol.* 2015, 65, 2628–2635. [CrossRef]
8. Geirsson, A.; Szeto, W.Y.; Pochettino, A.; McGarvey, M.L.; Keane, M.G.; Woo, Y.J.; Augoustides, J.G.; Bavaria, J.E. Significance of malperfusion syndromes prior to contemporary surgical repair for acute type A dissection: Outcomes and need for additional revascularizations. *Eur. J. Cardio-Thorac. Surg.* 2007, 32, 255–262. [CrossRef]
9. Kreibich, M.; Desai, N.D.; Bavaria, J.E.; Szeto, W.Y.; Vallabhajosyula, P.; Beyersdorf, F.; Czerny, M.; Siepe, M.; Rylski, B.; Itagaki, R.; et al. Common carotid artery true lumen flow impairment in patients with type A aortic dissection. *Eur. J. Cardio-Thorac. Surg.* 2021, 59, 490–496. [CrossRef]
10. Munir, W.; Chong, J.H.; Harky, A.; Bashir, M.; Adams, B. Type A aortic dissection: Involvement of carotid artery and impact on cerebral malperfusion. *Asian Cardiovasc Thorac Ann.* 2021, 29, 635–642. [CrossRef]
11. Roseborough, G.S.; Murphy, K.P.; Barker, P.B.; Sussman, M. Correction of symptomatic cerebral malperfusion due to acute type I aortic dissection by transcarotid stenting of the innominate and carotid arteries. *J. Vasc. Surg.* 2006, 44, 1091–1096. [CrossRef] [PubMed]

12. Fichadiya, A.; Menon, B.K.; Gregory, A.J.; Teleg, E.; Appoo, J.J. Neuroanatomy and severity of stroke in patients with type A aortic dissection. *J. Card. Surg.* **2022**, *37*, 339–347. [CrossRef] [PubMed]
13. Amr, G.; Boulouis, G.; Bricout, N.; Modine, T.; Fayad, G.; Aguettaz, P.; Koussa, M. Stroke Presentation of Acute Type A Aortic Dissection with 100% Perfusion-Weighted Imaging–Diffusion-Weighted Imaging Mismatch: A Call for Urgent Action. *J. Stroke Cerebrovasc. Dis.* **2016**, *25*, 1280–1283. [CrossRef] [PubMed]
14. Popovic, R.; Radovinovic-Tasic, S.; Rusovic, S.; Lepic, T.; Ilic, R.; Raicevic, R.; Obradovic, D. Urgent carotid stenting before cardiac surgery in a young male patient with acute ischemic stroke caused by aortic and carotid dissection. *VSP* **2016**, *73*, 674–678. [CrossRef]
15. Schönholz, C.; Ikonomidis, J.S.; Hannegan, C.; Mendaro, E. Bailout Percutaneous External Shunt to Restore Carotid Flow in a Patient With Acute Type A Aortic Dissection and Carotid Occlusion. *J. Endovasc. Ther.* **2008**, *15*, 639–642. [CrossRef]
16. Chahine, J.; Thapa, B.; Gajulapalli, R.D.; Kadri, A. Acute Aortic Dissection Presenting with a Headache: An Easily Missed Life-threatening Emergency. *Cureus* **2018**, *10*, e3531. [CrossRef]
17. Morihara, R.; Yamashita, T.; Deguchi, K.; Tsunoda, K.; Manabe, Y.; Takahashi, Y.; Yunoki, T.; Sato, K.; Nakano, Y.; Kono, S.; et al. Successful Delayed Aortic Surgery for a Patient with Ischemic Stroke Secondary to Aortic Dissection. *Int. Med.* **2017**, *56*, 2343–2346. [CrossRef]
18. Matsumoto, H.; Yoshida, Y.; Hirata, Y. Usefulness of cervical magnetic resonance imaging for detecting type A acute aortic dissection with acute stroke symptoms. *Magn. Reson. Imaging* **2016**, *34*, 902–907. [CrossRef] [PubMed]
19. Hong, K.-S.; Park, S.-Y.; Whang, S.-I.; Seo, S.-Y.; Lee, D.-H.; Kim, H.-J.; Cho, J.-Y.; Cho, Y.-J.; Jang, W.-I.; Kim, C.Y. Intravenous Recombinant Tissue Plasminogen Activator Thrombolysis in a Patient with Acute Ischemic Stroke Secondary to Aortic Dissection. *J. Clin. Neurol.* **2009**, *5*, 49. [CrossRef]
20. Kawarabuki, K.; Sakakibara, T.; Hirai, M.; Shirasu, M.; Kohara, I.; Tanaka, H.; Oyamada, M.; Takamatsu, T.; Murayama, Y.; Yamaki, T. Acute Aortic Dissection Presenting as a Neurologic Disorder. *J. Stroke Cerebrovasc. Dis.* **2006**, *15*, 26–29. [CrossRef]
21. Kim, S.H.; Song, S.; Kim, S.-P.; Lee, J.; Lee, H.C.; Kim, E.S. Hybrid technique to correct cerebral malperfusion following repair of a type a aortic dissection. *Korean J. Thorac. Cardiovasc. Surg.* **2014**, *47*, 163–166. [CrossRef] [PubMed]
22. Ueyama, K.; Otaki, K.; Koyama, M.; Kamiyama, H. Urgent simultaneous revascularization of the carotid artery and ascending aortic replacement for type A acute aortic dissection with cerebral malperfusion. *Gen. Thorac. Cardiovasc. Surg.* **2007**, *55*, 284–286. [CrossRef] [PubMed]
23. Sakaguchi, G.; Komiya, T.; Tamura, N.; Obata, S.; Masuyama, S.; Kimura, C.; Kobayashi, T. Cerebral malperfusion in acute type A dissection: Direct innominate artery cannulation. *J. Thorac. Cardiovasc. Surg.* **2005**, *129*, 1190–1191. [CrossRef] [PubMed]
24. Usui, T.; Suzuki, K.; Niinami, H.; Sakai, S. Aortic dissection diagnosed on stroke computed tomography protocol: A case report. *J. Med. Case Rep.* **2021**, *15*, 299. [CrossRef] [PubMed]
25. Fukuhara, S.; Norton, E.L.; Chaudhary, N.; Burris, N.; Shiomi, S.; Kim, K.M.; Patel, H.J.; Deeb, G.M.; Yang, B. Type A Aortic Dissection With Cerebral Malperfusion: New Insights. *Ann. Thorac. Surg.* **2021**, *112*, 501–509. [CrossRef] [PubMed]
26. Funakoshi, Y.; Imamura, H.; Tokunaga, Y.; Murakami, Y.; Tani, S.; Adachi, H.; Ohara, N.; Kono, T.; Fukumitsu, R.; Sunohara, T.; et al. Carotid artery stenting before surgery for carotid artery occlusion associated with acute type A aortic dissection: Two case reports. *Interv. Neuroradiol.* **2020**, *26*, 814–820. [CrossRef]
27. Heran, M.K.S.; Balaji, N.; Cook, R.C. Novel Percutaneous Treatment of Cerebral Malperfusion Before Surgery for Acute Type A Dissection. *Ann. Thorac. Surg.* **2019**, *108*, e15–e17. [CrossRef]
28. Casana, R.; Tolva, V.; Majnardi, A.R.; Bianchi, P.G.; Addobati, L.; Bertoni, G.B.; Cireni, L.V.; Silani, V. Endovascular Management of Symptomatic Cerebral Malperfusion Due to Carotid Dissection After Type A Aortic Dissection Repair. *Vasc Endovasc. Surg.* **2011**, *45*, 641–645. [CrossRef]
29. Sik Kim, Y.; Chernyshev, O.Y.; Alexandrov, A.V. Nonpulsatile Cerebral Perfusion in Patient With Acute Neurological Deficits. *Stroke* **2006**, *37*, 1562–1564. [CrossRef]
30. Morimoto, N.; Okada, K.; Okita, Y. Lack of neurologic improvement after aortic repair for acute type A aortic dissection complicated by cerebral malperfusion: Predictors and association with survival. *J. Thorac. Cardiovasc. Surg.* **2011**, *142*, 1540–1544. [CrossRef]
31. Igarashi, T.; Takahashi, S.; Takase, S.; Yokoyama, H. Intraoperative thrombectomy for occluded carotid arteries in patients with acute aortic dissection: Report of two cases. *Surg. Today* **2014**, *44*, 1177–1179. [CrossRef]
32. Fabre, O.; Guesnier, L.; Renaut, C.; Gautier, L.; Geronimi, H.; Jasaitis, L.; Strauch, K. Prise en charge actuelle des dissections aortiques de type A. Traitement chirurgical et traitement des syndromes de malperfusion. *Ann. De Cardiol. Et D'angéiologie* **2005**, *54*, 332–338. [CrossRef] [PubMed]
33. Lentini, S.; Tancredi, F.; Benedetto, F.; Gaeta, R. Type A aortic dissection involving the carotid arteries: Carotid stenting during open aortic arch surgery. *Interact Cardiovasc. Thorac. Surg.* **2009**, *8*, 157–159. [CrossRef] [PubMed]
34. Mukherjee, D.; Lewis, E.; Spinosa, D.; Tang, D.; Ryan, L. Retrograde Carotid Stenting Using Newly Released Venous Stent for Cerebral Malperfusion in Type A Aortic Dissection. *J. Endovasc.* **2022**, *29*, 444–450. [CrossRef] [PubMed]
35. Gao, P.; Wang, Y.; Chen, Y.; Jiao, L. Open retrograde endovascular stenting for left common carotid artery dissection secondary to surgical repair of acute aortic dissection: A case report and review of the literature. *Ann. Vasc Surg.* **2015**, *29*, e11–e15. [CrossRef]
36. Tsai, K.-T.; Shen, T.-C. Challenging carotid intervention after total arch rerouting and hybrid zone 0 elephant trunk repair for a complicated type A aortic dissection. *J. Endovasc.* **2014**, *21*, 306–311. [CrossRef]

37. Cardaioli, P.; Rigatelli, G.; Giordan, M.; Faggian, G.; Chinaglia, M.; Roncon, L. Multiple carotid stenting for extended thoracic aorta dissection after initial aortic surgical repair. *Cardiovasc. Revasc. Med.* **2007**, *8*, 213–215. [CrossRef]
38. Pavkov, I.; Horner, S.; Klein, G.E.; Niederkorn, K. Percutaneous transluminal angioplasty with stenting in extended supra-aortic artery dissection. *Croat. Med. J.* **2004**, *45*, 217–219.
39. Neri, E.; Sani, G.; Massetti, M.; Frati, G.; Buklas, D.; Tassi, R.; Giubbolini, M.; Benvenuti, A.; Sassi, C. Residual dissection of the brachiocephalic arteries: Significance, management, and long-term outcome. *J. Thorac. Cardiovasc. Surg.* **2004**, *128*, 303–312. [CrossRef]

Disclaimer/Publisher's Note: The statements, opinions and data contained in all publications are solely those of the individual author(s) and contributor(s) and not of MDPI and/or the editor(s). MDPI and/or the editor(s) disclaim responsibility for any injury to people or property resulting from any ideas, methods, instructions or products referred to in the content.

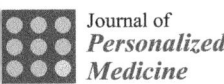

Article

Prostate Artery Embolization: Challenges, Tips, Tricks, and Perspectives

Benjamin Moulin *, Massimiliano Di Primio, Olivier Vignaux, Jean Luc Sarrazin, Georgios Angelopoulos and Antoine Hakime

Diagnostic and Interventional Radiology, American Hospital of Paris, 92200 Neuilly sur Seine, France
* Correspondence: b.moulin00@gmail.com

Abstract: Prostatic artery embolization (PAE) consists of blocking the arteries supplying the prostate to treat benign prostate hypertrophia (BPH). Its effectiveness on both urinary symptoms and flowmetric parameters has now been amply demonstrated by around a hundred studies, including several randomized trials. The main advantage of this procedure is the very low rate of urinary and sexual sequelae, including ejaculatory, with an excellent tolerance profile. The arterial anatomy is a key element for the realization of PAE. Its knowledge makes it possible to anticipate obstacles and prevent potential complications related to nontarget embolization. Nontarget embolization can occur with a small intraprostatic shunt or reflux and has no consequences except some local inflammation symptoms that resolve in a couple of days. Nevertheless, some situations with large arterial shunts arising from the prostatic artery must be recognized (accessory rectal, bladder, or pudendal branches), and must imperatively be protected before embolization, at the risk of exposing oneself to otherwise ischemic complications that are more severe, such as bladder necrosis and skin or mucosal necrosis. This article offers a step-by-step review of the various anatomical and technical key points to ensure technical and clinical success, while avoiding the occurrence of adverse events.

Keywords: prostate adenoma; benign prostate hypertrophia; embolization; prostate artery embolization; minigù mally invasive

Citation: Moulin, B.; Di Primio, M.; Vignaux, O.; Sarrazin, J.L.; Angelopoulos, G.; Hakime, A. Prostate Artery Embolization: Challenges, Tips, Tricks, and Perspectives. *J. Pers. Med.* 2023, 13, 87. https://doi.org/10.3390/jpm13010087

Academic Editors: Julien Frandon and Liang Cheng

Received: 22 November 2022
Revised: 13 December 2022
Accepted: 27 December 2022
Published: 29 December 2022

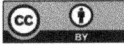

Copyright: © 2022 by the authors. Licensee MDPI, Basel, Switzerland. This article is an open access article distributed under the terms and conditions of the Creative Commons Attribution (CC BY) license (https://creativecommons.org/licenses/by/4.0/).

1. Introduction

A lower urinary tract symptom (LUTS) is a very common condition with significant socio-economic importance to the public health system. Benign prostatic hyperplasia (BPH) is the first etiology of a LUTS in men, with an incidence of 50% among men in the fifth decade [1]. The treatment is usually based on a conservative approach, pharmacological therapy, and surgical procedures. Trans-urethral resection of the prostate (TURP) is the standard therapy for the management of benign prostate enlargement (BPE), after the failure of medical therapy. Nevertheless, TURP is associated with relevant morbidity, including retrograde ejaculation and incontinence (early or permanent), and may present an adverse event such as infection, bleeding, and urethral stricture [2,3]. In this context, minimally invasive therapeutics emerged in the last decade, trying to ensure patients lower adverse event rates. Among them, prostate artery embolization (PAE) was first described in 2000 and consists of endovascular embolization of the prostate arteries with small, calibrated particles, which leads to an interruption of blood supply and then to prostate tissue necrosis and atrophy. This procedure offers advantages compared to surgery, such as the possibility to perform embolization under local anesthesia, without a Foley catheter or endourethral instrument insertion [4]. Additionally, PAE pretends to preserve sexual and urinary function in almost all cases, which seems essential given the expectations of patients [5]. On another hand, PAE remains less studied than TURP or other surgical technics, such as laser ablation. The purpose of this paper is to review the technical aspect and current perspective of PAE. Based on the experience and literature review, the authors provided a step-by-step approach with the first part of the manuscript focusing on technical aspects and challenges during embolization, and the second part reviewing the current evidence and controversies of this procedure.

2. Tips and Tricks to Perform Prostate Artery Embolization (PAE)

2.1. Perform an Arterial Mapping: Preoperative Computerized Tomography (CT) Angiogram or Intraoperative Cone-Beam CT (CBCT)

Cross-sectional imaging with vascular opacification is necessary before embolization for good anatomical understanding, the search for pitfalls, and the planning of the intervention. This imaging can be a CT angiogram performed prior to intervention (at the time of the pre-intervention assessment) or a CBCT angiogram performed at the beginning of the procedure. There are no clear guidelines on this topic. We suggest favoring the CT, given that it enables the easiest approach (radial or femoral) to be chosen before the intervention, and that it avoids injection of iodinated contrast media at the time of the procedure. Indeed, the accumulation of contrast in the bladder can prove to be problematic due to the discomfort encountered and the risk of urinary retention (teams using CBCT can have recourse to the placement of a penis sheath, or more rarely, an indwelling catheter, which from our point of view, is too invasive and thus we are in favor of performing arterial mapping by a pre-operative CT angiogram).

2.2. Manage Aortoiliac Anatomy

Aortoiliac imaging analysis is important for choosing the easier approach. In classical situations, radial or femoral roads can be performed without differences, depending on operator experience and preferences. For atheromatous patients, which commonly present with very sinuous vessels, aortoiliac catheterism can be very complicated in particular crossover maneuvers or ipsilateral iliac catheterization. Similarly, an important iliac bifurcation angulation can be conducted to a difficult homo-lateral internal iliac catheterization and can request a second ipsilateral femoral puncture.

A radial approach should be considered in the following situations:

- Tortuous common iliac arteries (Figure 1);
- Aortic or iliac bifurcation forming a very acute angle.

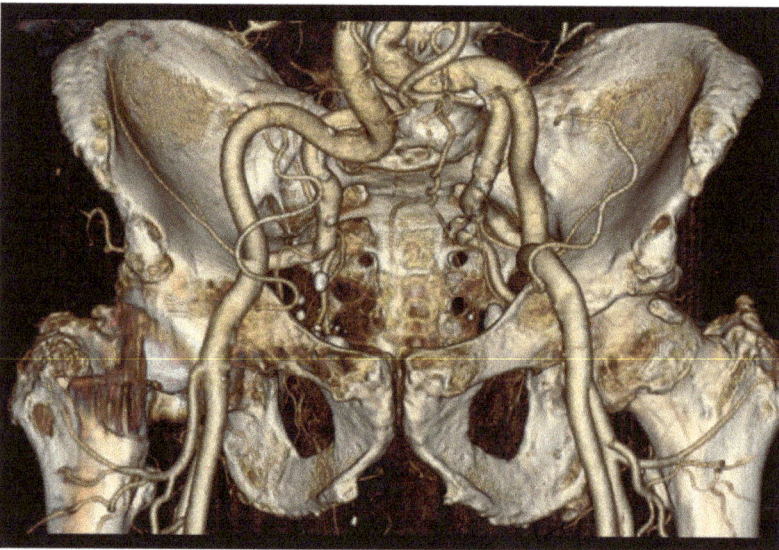

Figure 1. A CT scan with a 3D reconstruction showing very tortuous iliac arteries and very acute right internal/external iliac angulation. Upper radial access was privileged in the first intention.

2.3. Identify the Origin of the Prostatic Artery

Many studies have been published on the anatomy of the prostatic arteries. The most used classification is the one described by De Assis et al. (Figure 2), which classifies the anatomy into five types, depending on the origin of the prostatic artery (type I, II, III, and IV). Type V (5.6%) is a combination of situations that do not correspond to types 1 to 4 and correspond to prostatic arteries arising from a trifurcation of the anterior trunk of the internal iliac artery, gluteal artery, accessory pudendal artery, or epigastric artery.

Type 1: common trunk with the superior vesical artery =28.7%

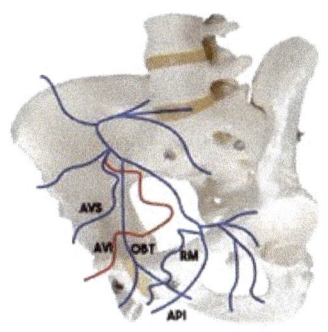

Type 2: anterior division of the Internal iliac artery =14.7%

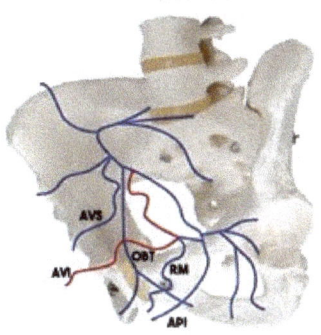

Type 3: obturator artery =14.7%

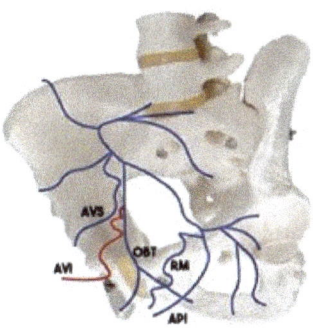

Type 4: internal pudendal artery : =14.7%

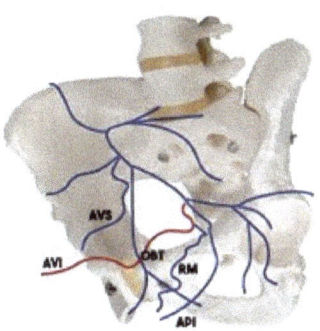

Figure 2. Prostatic artery origin description, from de Assis [6].

When no prostatic artery is found in the territory of the internal iliac, one should always consider looking for a possible origin from the external iliac via an accessory obturator artery (1.8% of patients [7]) or via the epigastric artery (the so-called "corona mortis artery"). Additionally, in the cases of occlusion of the prostatic artery and, in particular, of the central artery, the flow is usually supplied by collaterality, by a frequency in the distality of the internal pudendal artery (Figure 3), the peripheral or contralateral prostatic artery, and the obturator artery.

2.4. Manage the Prostatic Artery Catheterism

For an operator accustomed to endovascular navigation, catheterization of the prostatic artery is usually easy, once its origin has been identified. However, certain situations can make this catheterism very delicate. The risk factors making this catheterization potentially difficult have previously been reported [8]:

- Atheroma and sinuous arteries (increasing with age);
- Type 1 prostatic artery, with tight angulation between the anterior trunk of the internal iliac and the inferior bladder artery (this situation also sometimes occurs with the internal pudendal artery on type 4).

Here are some examples, as well as some tips to remedy them.

2.4.1. When the Internal Iliac Arteries Are Tortuous or When the Catheter Is Unstable

This situation can be solved

- with the use of a longer sheath (45 centimeters for example), when a femoral approach is intended;
- with the "buddy-wire technic" [9]: the use of an increased sheath caliber (7 french) and the positioning of a guidewire parallel to the catheter, to increase the stability of this one;
- and with a radial approach [10], which can be considered to overcome the loss of stability inherent in the cross-over.

2.4.2. When the Prostatic Artery Arises with a Very Acute Angulation

Pre-formed micro-catheters with significant terminal angulation can be used [9] (terminal angulation can also be personally shaped with steam). Torqueable microcatheters are also available [11]. The end of the microguide can also be modified (double curvature) to allow the strong angulation to pass. Torque microcatheters are also available. Additionally, the extremity of the microguide can also be shaped with a double curve.

- Use a rigid torque catheter with a tight distal curve to directly catheterize the artery without a microcatheter. This type of catheter should be handled with care, as it is very rigid and can easily lead to dissection of the prostatic artery.

2.5. Know the Intra-Prostatic Anatomy, Detect and Protect the Shunt and Collaterals

The prostatic artery is divided into two branches (Figure 4), the superior or anteromedial artery which supplies the central prostate (often called the central artery for convenience), and the inferior or posteromedial artery, which supplies the peripheral prostate (also called the capsular or peripheral artery). In about 8% of cases [5], the two branches of the prostatic artery have an independent birth. It is then necessary to specifically identify the central branch which will be the target of the embolization.

The origin of the inferior vesical, vesicular, and middle rectal branches, when present, is generally upstream of the central/peripheral prostatic artery bifurcation. A lot of connections have been described between the prostatic artery and other pelvic arteries. The most frequent are collateral with inferior vesical, middle rectal, and internal pudendal arteries.

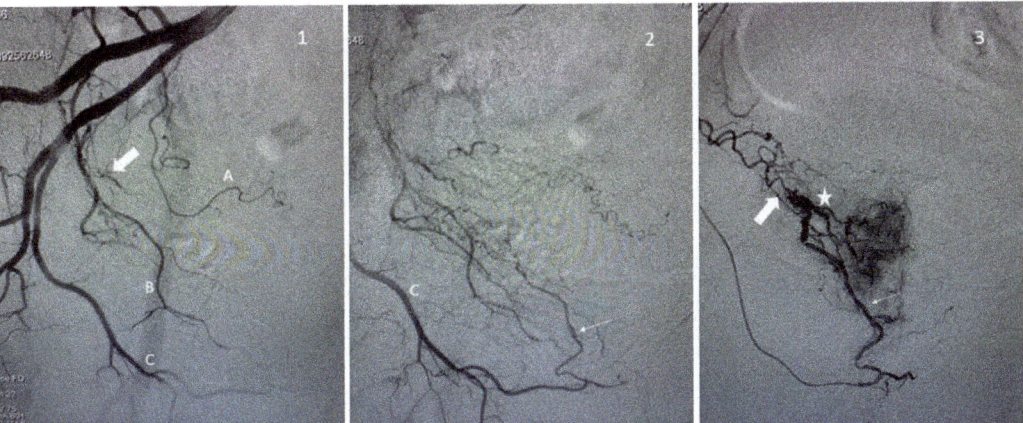

Figure 3. Examples of prostate artery occlusion and revascularization of the prostate via a distal pudendal/prostatic apical shunt. **Image 1**: Internal iliac angiography demonstrating a vesical inferior artery (A), an obturator artery (B), and an internal pudendal artery (C). Note the occluded prostatic artery (arrow). **Image 2**: Supraselective angiography of the internal pudendal artery (C) showing a connexion with the prostatic artery via an apical shunt (thin arrow). **Image 3**: Retrograde catheterism of the prostatic artery (thin arrow) and opacification demonstrating opacification of the prostatic central branch (star) and confirming occlusion of a proximal prostatic artery (large arrow).

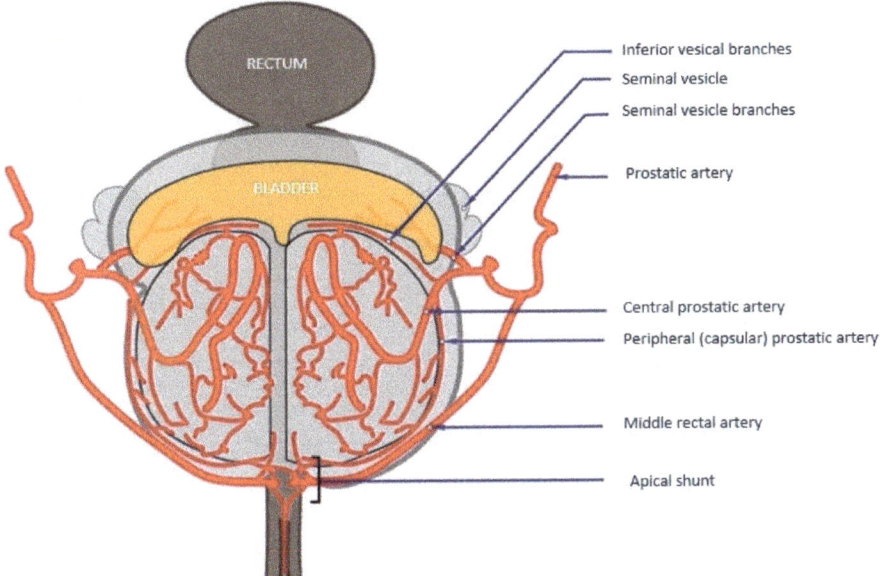

Figure 4. Vascular intra-prostatic anatomy (initial description by Picel) [12].

2.5.1. Middle Rectal and Inferior Vesical Collaterals

Collateral to the rectum (Figure 5, middle rectal branch, 14%) or bladder (inferior bladder arteries, 11%) are frequent situations [13]. If the prostatic branches can be catheterized supraselectively, these can be embolized directly. If supraselective embolization is not feasible, the middle rectal or lower bladder branch must be occluded using a microcoil, which redirects the flow to the prostatic artery.

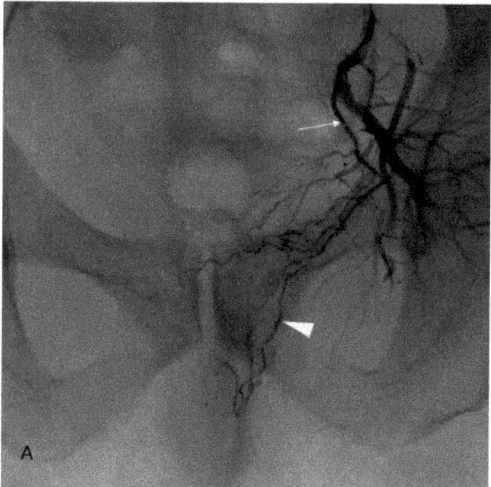 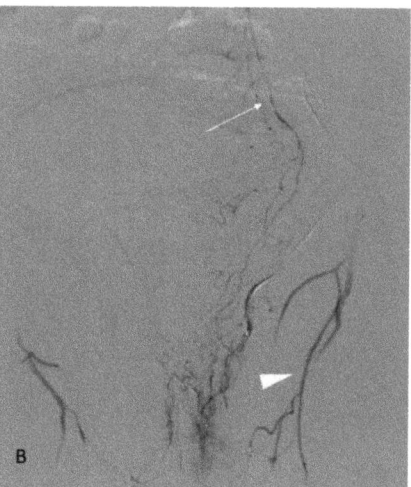

Figure 5. Prostate artery connection with the middle rectal artery. Image (**A**): Iliac angiography demonstrating a vesico-prostatic trunk (arrow) with collateral in the direction of the rectum (arrowhead). Image (**B**): Supraselective angiography in the middle rectal artery confirming the opacification of the rectum and connection with the superior rectal artery (arrow) arising from the inferior mesenteric artery. Note another shunt with the obturator artery (arrowhead).

2.5.2. Internal Pudendal Artery Collateral

Collaterals are frequently found with the internal pudendal arteries. These are clearly visible for a trained operator on supraselective DSA performed in the prostatic arteries, but can also be seen on preoperative or CBCT scans when the prostatic arteries are enhanced.

Two situations should be distinguished (Figure 6):

- **The post-capsular collaterals**, which are usually found at the apex, are opacified during DSA with a flow rate usually superior to 0.5 cc/s. These collaterals disappear with the decrease in the injection rate. In these cases, embolization can be performed without risk but must be performed at a low flow rate;
- **The pre-capsular collaterals**, which are true intra-prostatic arterial connections (usually described as the "accessory pudendal artery" (aPA)). In some extreme situations, there is no real prostatic artery, and the prostate is vascularized by several small branches along the latero-prostatic course of the aPA, which then gives the penile vascularization. As soon as the connections with the internal pudendal artery are of a certain size (we can consider that the visibility of a true course in angiography is a good cut-off) there is a significant risk of non-target embolization, including with low-flow embolization. These connections must, therefore, be protected prior to embolization.

How to manage a large connection from the prostatic to the internal pudendal artery?

- First case: the central prostatic branches can be supraselectively catheterized. In this case, a very careful embolization can be performed. Most attention must be paid to avoid reflux into the aPA.
- Second case: a supraselective catheterization is impossible. It is then necessary to occlude the accessory pudendal artery in its post-prostatic portion to be able to embolize upstream "by collaterality" of the prostatic branches. Nevertheless, the consequences of the occlusion of the aPA on penile vascularization must be taken into account. A recent study found no difference between a patient who received embolization of penile collateral in terms of erectile function [14]. These are still debated, despite numerous studies on the subject in the context of radical prostate surgeries for prostate

cancer. These anatomical studies classified penile vascularization according to three categories [15] depending on whether the vascularization is performed only by the internal pudendal (type I, 61.9%), by the internal and accessory pudendal (type II, 32.8%), or only via the accessory pudendal arteries (type III, 5.4%). Put another way, this means that when an aPA is founded, it is the only supply to the penile in 14% of the case (type III/(type II + III)). By cross-referencing these data with MacLean [14], who reported around 12% of penile/aPA protection coiling during PAE, we arrived at a number of 1.7% (12% × 14%) of patients who are potentially at risk of protective occlusion of a type III vascularization. We, therefore, recommend before occluding an aPA to ensure that it is not the only artery supplying the penis, in which case the risk of post-occlusion impotence seems real to us. In our experience, the presence of selectively non-catheterizable prostatic branches in the context of type III penile vascularization in young subjects wishing to preserve their sexual activity is the only situation contraindicating embolization.

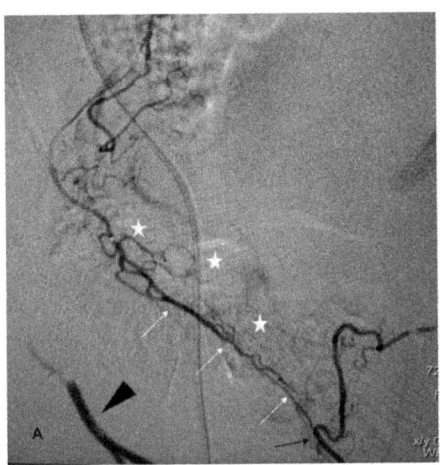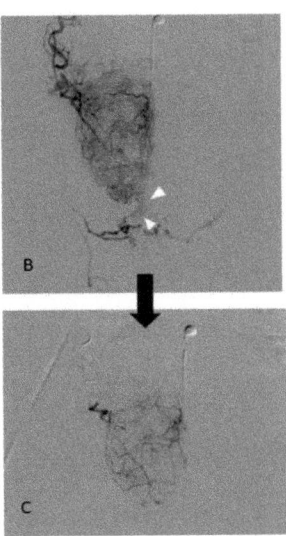

Figure 6. Different patterns of a shunt between prostatic and penile arteries. Image (**A**): an accessory pudendal artery arising from the peripheral prostatic artery (white arrow) with a direct connection to the internal pudendal artery (black arrow) which is retrogradely opacified (black arrowhead). Prostate vascularization (white stars) arises from small branches along the aPA. In this case, embolization should not be performed without protection of the anastomosis [14]. Image (**B**): an intra-prostatic capsular shunt (arrowhead) with a high injection rate (0.7 cc/s). Unlike image A, there is no real individualizable branch between prostatic and penile territory. Image (**C**): at a lower injection rate (0.3 cc/s), the shunt is no longer present. Embolization can be performed safely.

Ultimately, the study of the prostate and penile anatomy and the possible interconnections between these two systems seems to be an essential time in the preoperative analysis.

From our point of view, this is an additional argument in favor of the use of preoperative CT. Indeed, when the CT scan is carried out according to an adequate protocol, connections of significant size can be detected easily, and give the operator the possibility to anticipate at-risk situations and adapt the procedure to the anatomy.

3. Perspective, Evolution, and Discussion about PAE

3.1. PAE Safety and Complications

The safety of PAE procedures from the prospective study is presented in Table 1, including four randomized clinical trials (RCT) of PAE vs. TURP, 1 RCT of PAE vs. an open adenomectomy, one RCT of PAE vs. a sham procedure, and one prospective cohort on PAE only. The results show an excellent safety profile with an absence of grade 4 and 5 adverse events, and grade 3 adverse events in only one study, affecting 4.3% of the total patients treated with PAE. Grade I adverse events range from 7.5 to 67.3% of patients and grade II from 1 to 47.8%. The significant variability between studies is probably explained by the fact that some studies have included the symptoms of post-embolization syndrome in the complications whereas others did not. These data confirm that PAE is a safe procedure, with a few side effects except the post-embolization syndrome.

Table 1. Adverse events after PAE from seven prospective studies [16–22].

Study	Pisco, 2019 [19]	Insauti, 2020 [18]	Abt, 2018 [16]	Carnevale, 2015 [17]	Russo, 2015 [21]	Ray, 2018 [20]	Salem, 2018 [22]
Patient Number	n = 78	n = 23	n = 48	n = 15	n = 80	n = 199	n = 45
Design	RCT, PAE vs. Sham	RCT, PAE vs. TURP	RCT, PAE vs. TURP	RCT, PAE vs. TURP	RCT, PAE vs. prostatectomy	Registry-based study	Prospective, PAE only
Total adverse event, n (%)	25 (32.0)	15 (65.2)	36 (75)	4 (46.7)	7 (8.7)	136 (68.3)	26 (57.8)
Clavien Dindo grade							
grade I	21 (26.9)	4 (17.3)	54%		6 (7.5)	134 (67.3)	24 (53.3)
grade II	3 (3.8)	11 (47.8)	17%		1 (1.3)	2 (1)	2 (4.4)
grade III	1 (1.3)	0	4.30%		0	0	0
grade IV	0	0			0	0	0
grade V	0	0			0	0	0
Description (number, %)							
Urinary frequency and urgency							3 (6.6)
Burning perineal pain	1 (1.3)	1 (4.3)	15 (31.3)				
Burning urethral pain	3 (3.8)	4 (17.3)					
Dysuria	3 (3.8)				5 (6.3)		13 (28.9)
Ecchymosis	2 (2.6)						
Haematospermia	7 (9.0)			1 (6.7)	1 (1.3)	25 (12.6)	2 (4.4)
Haematuria	5 (6.4)	1 (4.3)	4 (8.3)	2 (13.3)		37 (18.6)	6 (13.3)
Inguinal haematoma	4 (5.1)					4 (2)	
Penile ulcer						2 (1)	
Artery dissection						4 (2.0)	
Acute urinary retention		5 (21.7)	1 (2.1)				2 (4.4)
Radiodermitis		1 (4.3)					
Erectile dysfunction		1 (4.3)					
Change in ejaculation volume		1 (4.3)		2 (13.3)		48 (24.1)	
Incontinence						2 (1)	
Prostate fragment expelled	1 (1.3)						
Rectorrhagia/rectal ischemia	2 (2.6)	1 (4.3)		1 (6.7)			
Urinary tract infection	1 (1.3)		10 (20.1)		1 (1.3)	14 (7.0)	
Other			6 (12.5)	1 (6.7)			

3.2. PAE Limitations

Results of the RCT conducted by Abt demonstrated no difference in IPSS score improvement between PAE and TURP. Nevertheless, TURP seems to achieve better results in terms of debimetric results [23]. To date, no large prospective study with a long follow-up has been published to compare these two technics. PAE should have a higher recurrence rate, as a recent publication reported a reintervention rate of 58% at 10 years [24], whereas TURP seems to have a reintervention rate of around 20% [3].

3.3. Embolization Agent

Historically, EAP was performed with particles. Recently some studies have been published with the use of alternative embolic agents such as n-butyl-cyanoacrylate, ethylene vinyl alcohol copolymer, and alcohol [25,26]. A recent study [27] showed a decrease in fluoroscopy time and radiation dose with the use of glue, without a difference in terms of IPSS score.

3.4. Particle Size

The size of the ideal particles to be used remains subject to discussion. A randomized trial [28] comparing the use of 100–300 vs. 300–500 micron caliber particles did not show a significant difference between the two groups. Nevertheless, various studies have shown a more extensive prostatic necrosis on post-operative MRI, the greatest decrease in prostatic volume and PSA level was when the size of the particles decrease [28,29]. It would make sense that a more aggressive embolization would allow greater prostatic necrosis and, therefore, a greater clinical benefit, in particular on the risk of recurrence in the medium/long term. However, this remains to be proven, and the aggressiveness of the embolization must be weighed against the undoubtedly increased risk of nontarget embolization, as the small particles cross the small shunts more easily. Our team tends to favor aggressive embolization (a particle caliber from 50 to 300 microns) when supraselective angiography of the prostatic artery does not show that any collateral potentiality is at risk of nontarget embolization, but these remain out of the guidelines which recommend to use 300–500 micron particles [4].

3.5. Peripheral vs. Central Prostate

The prostate adenoma develops mainly at the expense of the transition zone. Considering both the fact that the adenoma is vascularized almost exclusively by the central branch of the prostatic artery and that, on the contrary, the majority of extra-prostatic anastomoses arise from the peripheral artery (78% of cases [30]), the idea of an aggressive embolization of the central artery (particles of calibers less than 150 microns or embolization with a liquid agent) could be attractive, thus supplementing it with micro-particles of a higher caliber for the continuation of the embolization. Once again, studies would be needed to find out if such an attitude offers better results, and current guidelines do not recommend it.

In conclusion, PAE is a technically and intellectually challenging intervention. A precise knowledge of both theoretical and angiographic anatomy is essential in order to embolize the entire adenoma while avoiding nontarget embolization. The learning curve is arguably one of the longest of all vascular radiology procedures, but performed by a trained operator, both technical and clinical success rates are excellent, with a low risk of major complication.

Author Contributions: Conceptualization, B.M. and A.H.; methodology, B.M. and M.D.P.; software, O.V. and J.L.S.; validation, G.A., M.D.P. and A.H. Resources, M.D.P., A.H. and G.A.; writing—original draft preparation, B.M.; writing—review and editing, A.H., M.D.P. and G.A.; supervision, A.H.; project administration, O.V. and J.L.S.; funding acquisition, no funding. All authors have read and agreed to the published version of the manuscript.

Funding: This research received no external funding.

Institutional Review Board Statement: Not applicable.

Informed Consent Statement: Informed consent was obtained from all subjects involved in the study.

Data Availability Statement: Not applicable.

Conflicts of Interest: The authors declare no conflict of interest.

References

1. Berry, S.J.; Coffey, D.S.; Walsh, P.C.; Ewing, L.L. The Development of Human Benign Prostatic Hyperplasia with Age. *J. Urol.* **1984**, *132*, 474–479. [CrossRef] [PubMed]
2. Ahyai, S.A.; Gilling, P.; Kaplan, S.A.; Kuntz, R.M.; Madersbacher, S.; Montorsi, F.; Speakman, M.J.; Stief, C.G. Meta-analysis of Functional Outcomes and Complications Following Transurethral Procedures for Lower Urinary Tract Symptoms Resulting from Benign Prostatic Enlargement. *Eur. Urol.* **2010**, *58*, 384–397. [CrossRef] [PubMed]
3. Reich, O.; Gratzke, C.; Bachmann, A.; Seitz, M.; Schlenker, B.; Hermanek, P.; Lack, N.; Stief, C.G. Urology Section of the Bavarian Working Group for Quality Assurance† Morbidity, Mortality and Early Outcome of Transurethral Resection of the Prostate: A Prospective Multicenter Evaluation of 10,654 Patients. *J. Urol.* **2008**, *180*, 246–249. [CrossRef] [PubMed]
4. Cornelis, F.H.; Bilhim, T.; Hacking, N.; Sapoval, M.; Tapping, C.R.; Carnevale, F.C. CIRSE Standards of Practice on Prostatic Artery Embolisation. *Cardiovasc. Intervent. Radiol.* **2020**, *43*, 176–185. [CrossRef] [PubMed]
5. Malde, S.; Umbach, R.; Wheeler, J.R.; Lytvyn, L.; Cornu, J.-N.; Gacci, M.; Gratzke, C.; Herrmann, T.R.W.; Mamoulakis, C.; Rieken, M.; et al. A Systematic Review of Patients' Values, Preferences, and Expectations for the Diagnosis and Treatment of Male Lower Urinary Tract Symptoms. *Eur. Urol.* **2021**, *79*, 796–809. [CrossRef]
6. de Assis, A.M.; Moreira, A.M.; de Paula Rodrigues, V.C.; Harward, S.H.; Antunes, A.A.; Srougi, M.; Carnevale, F.C. Pelvic Arterial Anatomy Relevant to Prostatic Artery Embolisation and Proposal for Angiographic Classification. *Cardiovasc. Intervent. Radiol.* **2015**, *38*, 855–861. [CrossRef]
7. Bilhim, T.; Pisco, J.; Pinheiro, L.C.; Rio Tinto, H.; Fernandes, L.; Pereira, J.A. The Role of Accessory Obturator Arteries in Prostatic Arterial Embolization. *J. Vasc. Interv. Radiol.* **2014**, *25*, 875–879. [CrossRef]
8. du Pisanie, J.; Abumoussa, A.; Donovan, K.; Stewart, J.; Bagla, S.; Isaacson, A. Predictors of Prostatic Artery Embolization Technical Outcomes: Patient and Procedural Factors. *J. Vasc. Interv. Radiol.* **2019**, *30*, 233–240. [CrossRef]
9. Bagla, S.; Isaacson, A.J. Tips and Tricks for Difficult Prostatic Artery Embolization. *Semin. Interv. Radiol.* **2016**, *33*, 236–239. [CrossRef]
10. Bhatia, S.; Harward, S.H.; Sinha, V.K.; Narayanan, G. Prostate Artery Embolization via Transradial or Transulnar versus Transfemoral Arterial Access: Technical Results. *J. Vasc. Interv. Radiol.* **2017**, *28*, 898–905. [CrossRef]
11. Dudeck, O. Safety and Efficacy of Target Vessel Catheterization with the New Steerable Microcatheter Direxion Compared with a Standard Microcatheter: A Prospective, Preclinical Trial. *Cardiovasc. Intervent. Radiol.* **2014**, *37*, 1041–1046. [CrossRef]
12. Picel, A.C.; Hsieh, T.-C.; Shapiro, R.M.; Vezeridis, A.M.; Isaacson, A.J. Prostatic Artery Embolization for Benign Prostatic Hyperplasia: Patient Evaluation, Anatomy, and Technique for Successful Treatment. *RadioGraphics* **2019**, *39*, 1526–1548. [CrossRef]
13. Bilhim, T.; Pisco, J.M.; Rio Tinto, H.; Fernandes, L.; Pinheiro, L.C.; Furtado, A.; Casal, D.; Duarte, M.; Pereira, J.; Oliveira, A.G.; et al. Prostatic Arterial Supply: Anatomic and Imaging Findings Relevant for Selective Arterial Embolization. *J. Vasc. Interv. Radiol.* **2012**, *23*, 1403–1415. [CrossRef]
14. Maclean, D.; Vigneswaran, G.; Maher, B.; Hadi, M.; Harding, J.; Harris, M.; Bryant, T.; Hacking, N.; Modi, S. The effect of protective coil embolization of penile anastomoses during prostatic artery embolization on erectile function: A propensity-matched analysis. *J. Vasc. Interv. Radiol.* **2022**, *33*, S1051044322012787. [CrossRef]
15. Henry, B.M.; Pękala, P.A.; Vikse, J.; Sanna, B.; Skinningsrud, B.; Saganiak, K.; Walocha, J.A.; Tomaszewski, K.A. Variations in the Arterial Blood Supply to the Penis and the Accessory Pudendal Artery: A Meta-Analysis and Review of Implications in Radical Prostatectomy. *J. Urol.* **2017**, *198*, 345–353. [CrossRef]
16. Abt, D.; Hechelhammer, L.; Müllhaupt, G.; Markart, S.; Güsewell, S.; Kessler, T.M.; Schmid, H.-P.; Engeler, D.S.; Mordasini, L. Comparison of prostatic artery embolisation (PAE) versus transurethral resection of the prostate (TURP) for benign prostatic hyperplasia: Randomised, open label, non-inferiority trial. *BMJ* **2018**, *361*, k2338. [CrossRef]
17. Carnevale, F.C.; Iscaife, A.; Yoshinaga, E.M.; Moreira, A.M.; Antunes, A.A.; Srougi, M. Transurethral Resection of the Prostate (TURP) Versus Original and PErFecTED Prostate Artery Embolization (PAE) Due to Benign Prostatic Hyperplasia (BPH): Preliminary Results of a Single Center, Prospective, Urodynamic-Controlled Analysis. *Cardiovasc. Intervent. Radiol.* **2016**, *39*, 44–52. [CrossRef]
18. Insausti, I.; Sáez de Ocáriz, A.; Galbete, A.; Capdevila, F.; Solchaga, S.; Giral, P.; Bilhim, T.; Isaacson, A.; Urtasun, F.; Napal, S. Randomized Comparison of Prostatic Artery Embolization versus Transurethral Resection of the Prostate for Treatment of Benign Prostatic Hyperplasia. *J. Vasc. Interv. Radiol.* **2020**, *31*, 882–890. [CrossRef]
19. Pisco, J.M.; Bilhim, T.; Costa, N.V.; Torres, D.; Pisco, J.; Pinheiro, L.C.; Oliveira, A.G. Randomised Clinical Trial of Prostatic Artery Embolisation Versus a Sham Procedure for Benign Prostatic Hyperplasia. *Eur. Urol.* **2020**, *77*, 354–362. [CrossRef]
20. Ray, A.F.; Powell, J.; Speakman, M.J.; Longford, N.T.; DasGupta, R.; Bryant, T.; Modi, S.; Dyer, J.; Harris, M.; Carolan-Rees, G.; et al. Efficacy and safety of prostate artery embolization for benign prostatic hyperplasia: An observational study and propensity-matched comparison with transurethral resection of the prostate (the UK-ROPE study). *BJU Int.* **2018**, *122*, 270–282. [CrossRef]
21. Russo, G.I.; Kurbatov, D.; Sansalone, S.; Lepetukhin, A.; Dubsky, S.; Sitkin, I.; Salamone, C.; Fiorino, L.; Rozhivanov, R.; Cimino, S.; et al. Prostatic Arterial Embolization vs Open Prostatectomy: A 1-Year Matched-pair Analysis of Functional Outcomes and Morbidities. *Urology* **2015**, *86*, 343–348. [CrossRef] [PubMed]
22. Salem, R.; Hairston, J.; Hohlastos, E.; Riaz, A.; Kallini, J.; Gabr, A.; Ali, R.; Jenkins, K.; Karp, J.; Desai, K.; et al. Prostate Artery Embolization for Lower Urinary Tract Symptoms Secondary to Benign Prostatic Hyperplasia: Results From a Prospective FDA-Approved Investigational Device Exemption Study. *Urology* **2018**, *120*, 205–210. [CrossRef] [PubMed]

23. Knight, G.M.; Talwar, A.; Salem, R.; Mouli, S. Systematic Review and Meta-analysis Comparing Prostatic Artery Embolization to Gold-Standard Transurethral Resection of the Prostate for Benign Prostatic Hyperplasia. *Cardiovasc. Intervent. Radiol.* **2021**, *44*, 183–193. [CrossRef] [PubMed]
24. Bilhim, T.; Costa, N.V.; Torres, D.; Pinheiro, L.C.; Spaepen, E. Long-Term Outcome of Prostatic Artery Embolization for Patients with Benign Prostatic Hyperplasia: Single-Centre Retrospective Study in 1072 Patients Over a 10-Year Period. *Cardiovasc. Intervent. Radiol.* **2022**, *45*, 1324–1336. [CrossRef] [PubMed]
25. Moulin, B.; Hakime, A.; Kuoch, V. Percutaneous Prostatic Artery Embolization with Absolute Alcohol: A Case Report. *J. Vasc. Interv. Radiol.* **2022**, *33*, 1008–1010. [CrossRef] [PubMed]
26. Chau, Y.; Rambaud-Collet, C.; Durand, M.; Léna, P.; Raffaelli, C.; Brunner, P.; Quintens, H.; Sédat, J. Prostatic Artery Embolization with Ethylene Vinyl Alcohol Copolymer: A 3-Patient Series. *J. Vasc. Interv. Radiol.* **2018**, *29*, 1333–1336. [CrossRef]
27. Salet, E.; Crombé, A.; Grenier, N.; Marcelin, C.; Lebras, Y.; Jambon, E.; Coussy, A.; Cornelis, F.H.; Petitpierre, F. Prostatic Artery Embolization for Benign Prostatic Obstruction: Single-Centre Retrospective Study Comparing Microspheres Versus n-Butyl Cyanoacrylate. *Cardiovasc. Intervent. Radiol.* **2022**, *45*, 814–823. [CrossRef]
28. Torres, D.; Costa, N.V.; Pisco, J.; Pinheiro, L.C.; Oliveira, A.G.; Bilhim, T. Prostatic Artery Embolization for Benign Prostatic Hyperplasia: Prospective Randomized Trial of 100–300 µm versus 300–500 µm versus 100- to 300-µm + 300- to 500-µm Embospheres. *J. Vasc. Interv. Radiol.* **2019**, *30*, 638–644. [CrossRef]
29. Wang, M.Q.; Zhang, J.L.; Xin, H.N.; Yuan, K.; Yan, J.; Wang, Y.; Zhang, G.D.; Fu, J.X. Comparison of Clinical Outcomes of Prostatic Artery Embolization with 50-µm Plus 100-µm Polyvinyl Alcohol (PVA) Particles versus 100-µm PVA Particles Alone: A Prospective Randomized Trial. *J. Vasc. Interv. Radiol.* **2018**, *29*, 1694–1702. [CrossRef]
30. Anract, J.; Amouyal, G.; Peyromaure, M.; Zerbib, M.; Sapoval, M.; Barry Delongchamps, N. Study of the intra-prostatic arterial anatomy and implications for arterial embolization of benign prostatic hyperplasia. *Prog. Urol.* **2019**, *29*, 263–269. [CrossRef]

Disclaimer/Publisher's Note: The statements, opinions and data contained in all publications are solely those of the individual author(s) and contributor(s) and not of MDPI and/or the editor(s). MDPI and/or the editor(s) disclaim responsibility for any injury to people or property resulting from any ideas, methods, instructions or products referred to in the content.

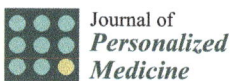

Article

Preventive Proximal Splenic Artery Embolization for High-Grade AAST-OIS Adult Spleen Trauma without Vascular Anomaly on the Initial CT Scan: Technical Aspect, Safety, and Efficacy—An Ancillary Study

Skander Sammoud [1,*], Julien Ghelfi [2,3], Sandrine Barbois [4], Jean-Paul Beregi [1], Catherine Arvieux [5] and Julien Frandon [1]

1. Department of Radiology, Nîmes Carémeau University Hospital, 30900 Nimes, France
2. Institute for Advanced Biosciences, Inserm U 1209, CNRS UMR 5309, Université Grenoble Alpes, 38000 Grenoble, France
3. Department of Radiology, Grenoble-Alpes University Hospital, 38000 Grenoble, France
4. Department of Digestive Surgery, University Hospital Grenoble Alpes, 38043 Grenoble, France
5. Department of Digestive and Emergency Surgery, Grenoble Alpes University Hospital, 38043 Grenoble, France
* Correspondence: skander.sammoud@tutanota.com

Citation: Sammoud, S.; Ghelfi, J.; Barbois, S.; Beregi, J.-P.; Arvieux, C.; Frandon, J. Preventive Proximal Splenic Artery Embolization for High-Grade AAST-OIS Adult Spleen Trauma without Vascular Anomaly on the Initial CT Scan: Technical Aspect, Safety, and Efficacy—An Ancillary Study. J. Pers. Med. 2023, 13, 889. https://doi.org/10.3390/jpm13060889

Academic Editor: Nariman Nezami

Received: 3 April 2023
Revised: 18 May 2023
Accepted: 18 May 2023
Published: 24 May 2023

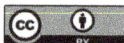

Copyright: © 2023 by the authors. Licensee MDPI, Basel, Switzerland. This article is an open access article distributed under the terms and conditions of the Creative Commons Attribution (CC BY) license (https://creativecommons.org/licenses/by/4.0/).

Abstract: The spleen is the most commonly injured organ in blunt abdominal trauma. Its management depends on hemodynamic stability. According to the American Association for the Surgery of Trauma-Organ Injury Scale (AAST-OIS ≥ 3), stable patients with high-grade splenic injuries may benefit from preventive proximal splenic artery embolization (PPSAE). This ancillary study, using the SPLASH multicenter randomized prospective cohort, evaluated the feasibility, safety, and efficacy of PPSAE in patients with high-grade blunt splenic trauma without vascular anomaly on the initial CT scan. All patients included were over 18 years old, had high-grade splenic trauma (≥AAST-OIS 3 + hemoperitoneum) without vascular anomaly on the initial CT scan, received PPSAE, and had a CT scan at one month. Technical aspects, efficacy, and one-month splenic salvage were studied. Fifty-seven patients were reviewed. Technical efficacy was 94% with only four proximal embolization failures due to distal coil migration. Six patients (10.5%) underwent combined embolization (distal + proximal) due to active bleeding or focal arterial anomaly discovered during embolization. The mean procedure time was 56.5 min (SD = 38.1 min). Embolization was performed with an Amplatzer™ vascular plug in 28 patients (49.1%), a Penumbra occlusion device in 18 patients (31.6%), and microcoils in 11 patients (19.3%). There were two hematomas (3.5%) at the puncture site without clinical consequences. There were no rescue splenectomies. Two patients were re-embolized, one on Day 6 for an active leak and one on Day 30 for a secondary aneurysm. Primary clinical efficacy was, therefore, 96%. There were no splenic abscesses or pancreatic necroses. The splenic salvage rate on Day 30 was 94%, while only three patients (5.2%) had less than 50% vascularized splenic parenchyma. PPSAE is a rapid, efficient, and safe procedure that can prevent splenectomy in high-grade spleen trauma (AAST-OIS) ≥ 3 with high splenic salvage rates.

Keywords: spleen; trauma; embolization; proximal; preventive

1. Introduction

The spleen is the organ most often damaged by blunt abdominal trauma, with an estimated 40,000 splenic traumas occurring each year in the United States, mainly affecting a young population and potentially resulting in life-threatening bleeding [1,2]. However, this organ plays a vital role regarding red blood cells and the immunity system. Splenectomy is avoided whenever possible in cases of splenic damage to prevent the onset of overwhelming post-splenectomy sepsis, a complication caused by encapsulated bacteria, which may be lethal [3]. Trauma protocols are subject to variations depending on the institution. Hemodynamically unstable patients undergo hemostatic splenectomy. Stable patients with high-grade splenic trauma and vascular anomalies on the CT scan are prone to embolization, whereas stable patients with high-grade splenic trauma and no vascular anomalies on CT represent a high-risk subgroup for whom, currently, there is no consensus on their treatment [4–7]. Schematically, with high-grade splenic trauma, proximal embolization is performed to decrease the perfusion pressure within the spleen, thus preventing secondary ruptures. In contrast, distal embolization is reserved for focal parenchymal injuries [8]. A randomized multicenter clinical trial, SPLASH [9], showed that proximal preventive splenic artery embolization (PPSAE) in patients with high-grade spleen trauma without vascular abnormality on the initial CT reduced complications related to splenic trauma and secondary vascular anomalies requiring embolization, and improved rescue splenectomy rates. PPSAE is a promising therapeutic option that every interventional radiologist should learn. However, PPSAE is still considered a high-risk embolization with the risk of distal migration of the material into the splenic hilum with extensive ischemia of the spleen or ischemic complication of the pancreas with coverage of the pancreatic arteries. Others prefer not to perform PPSAE in the absence of a vascular anomaly on the initial CT because they are afraid of blocking access to the splenic artery in case a secondary vascular anomaly develops during follow-up, requiring distal embolization.

This ancillary study on the sub-population of embolized patients of the SPLASH study aimed to specifically explore the feasibility, safety, and efficacy of PPSAE in patients with high-grade blunt splenic trauma without vascular anomaly on the initial CT scan and to give a technical insight.

2. Materials and Methods

2.1. Study Design

This ancillary study focused on the technical aspects of PPSAE using data from the SPLASH prospective randomized multicenter clinical trial [9] to assess the feasibility, safety, and efficacy of PPSAE in patients with recent (<48 h) high-grade blunt splenic trauma according to the American Association for the Surgery of Trauma-Organ Injury Scale (AAST-OIS ≥ 3) (Table 1) without active bleeding, who have been hemodynamically stabilized according to the French Society of Anesthesia & Intensive Care Medicine criteria [10]. SPLASH was conducted in sixteen Level 1 trauma centers in France from 6 February 2014 to 1 September 2017. This prospective study was approved by the ethical committee under the number: 2013-A00409-36. Each participating institution provided an institutional review board approval for the study protocol, and all patients or their legal representatives had provided written informed consent before participation.

Table 1. AAST-OIS spleen injury scale.

Grade	Imaging Findings
I	Subcapsular hematoma < 10% surface area Parenchymal laceration < 1 cm depth capsular tear
II	Subcapsular hematoma 10–50% surface area; intraparenchymal hematoma < 5 cm Parenchymal laceration 1–3 cm
III	Subcapsular hematoma > 50% surface area; ruptured subcapsular or intraparenchymal hematoma ≥ 5 cm Parenchymal laceration > 3 cm depth
IV	Any injury in the presence of a splenic vascular injury or active bleeding confined within the splenic capsule Parenchymal laceration involving segmental or hilar vessels producing > 25% devascularization
V	Any injury in the presence of a splenic vascular injury with active bleeding extended beyond the spleen into the peritoneum Shattered spleen

This ancillary study followed the STROBE checklist guidelines. Only patients attributed to the embolization group who received PPSAE and had a one-month follow-up CT scan and a consultation on Day 30 were included.

2.2. Patients

Male and female patients (>18 years old) with high-grade blunt splenic trauma ($\geq$AAST-OIS 3) admitted through the emergency department, shock treatment unit, intensive care unit, or surgery department were enrolled in this study. Each patient completed a baseline evaluation before enrolment, including a medical history interview and physical examination (age, sex, and AAST score). In the standard procedure, a whole-body multidetector CT scan with contrast injection was performed on all hemodynamically stable patients with abdominal injuries upon admission. The CT protocol included the thorax, abdomen, and pelvis during the arterial phase and the abdomen and pelvis during the portal venous phase. Depending on the CT findings, delayed acquisition was left to the on-call radiologist's discretion. An initial injection of 1–2 cc/kg of iodine contrast was given, followed by 15 to 20 cc of normal saline at 3 cc/s. Inclusion criteria were AAST-OIS 3 with substantial hemoperitoneum (peri splenic associated with pelvic effusion), AAST-OIS 4, or AAST-OIS 5 with residual vascularized parenchyma > 25%. Hemodynamically unstable patients (AAST-OIS 5) with a shattered spleen, stable but requiring immediate spleen or other abdominal organ embolization based on CT findings, were excluded. The New Injury Severity Score (NISS) was used to give an overall score for the anatomical lesions of each patient with multiple traumas. Each organ involved is scored according to the OIS from 1 (mild) to 5 (total destruction or devascularization of the organ), according to the American Association for the Surgery of Trauma criteria. The NISS is calculated from the AAST-OIS of the three most serious lesions as follows: NISS = $a^2 + b^2 + c^2$ (e.g., a patient with a minor kidney injury rated OIS = 2, a spleen fracture rated OIS = 4, and minor hepatic injury rated OIS = 2 will have a NISS of 4 + 16 + 4 = 24).

2.3. Procedures

Interventional radiologists with varying levels of experience (3 years to 20 years) performed all endovascular procedures in dedicated angio suites. A technical manual was prepared beforehand to describe the anatomy of the celiac trunk and splenic artery, correct micro/catheter tip position for imaging and embolization, and angiographic images of each artery before and after embolization. All operators had viewed this manual before the trial began.

PPSAE procedures were performed under local anesthesia or sedation, depending on the institution. Percutaneous arterial access was obtained preferably via common femoral artery access or via radial artery access for cases with unfavorable anatomy. Ultrasound guidance was recommended. In most cases, an angiographic Cobra 2 catheter was used to select the celiac trunk (CeT) and a Sim 1 catheter where the CeT was compressed by the median arcuate ligament [1]. The CeT was selected using a multipurpose angiographic catheter when radial access was performed. Digital subtraction angiography (DSA) was performed from the splenic artery, with an automatic injection of 16 mL of contrast medium at a 4–5 mL/s injection rate, to study the anatomy, prepare for embolization, and identify a potential parenchymal splenic vascular injury (arteriovenous fistula, pseudoaneurysm, vessel truncation, or rarely contrast extravasation). In cases of focal vascular anomaly, a primary distal embolization was performed; a microcatheter was advanced to the injured vessel and, once in position, mircocoils, fragments of gelatin sponge, or liquid agent were used. Proximal embolization was then performed at the truncal splenic artery downstream from the dorsal pancreatic artery and upstream of the great pancreatic artery, i.e., the left lateral aspect of the spine (Figure 1). The choice of embolization equipment was left to the operator's discretion and included: (1) The AMPLATZER™ Vascular Plug (AVP) (Abbott Medical, Abbott Park, IL, USA), a self-expanding device made of nitinol, which comes in varying sizes; (2) The Penumbra occlusion device (POD®) (Penumbra Inc., Alameda, CA,

USA), a detachable metallic coil with a specific anchor system, delivered through a standard 2.8 F microcatheter (Progreat; Terumo, Japan), available in several sizes depending on the diameter of the splenic artery; (3) Other regular coils. The embolization equipment was 20–50% bigger than the diameter of the splenic artery measured on procedural imaging acquired during angiography.

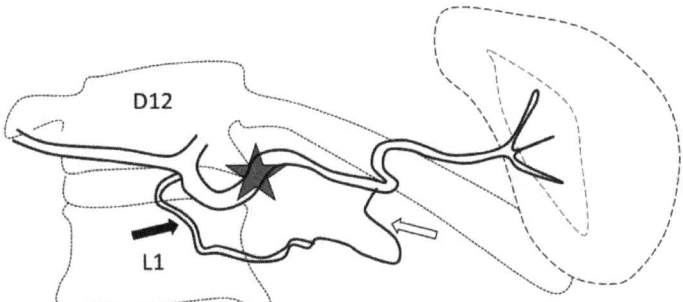

Figure 1. Optimal site of preventive proximal splenic artery embolization. The optimal site of embolization (star) is downstream from the dorsal pancreatic artery (arrow) and upstream of the great pancreatic artery (blank arrow). Classically, at the left edge of the spine.

2.4. Technical Assessment

Technical success was defined as the adequate deployment of the embolization equipment, resulting in complete flow stasis in the splenic artery downstream from the occlusion site. Subsequent collateral circulation develops at a variable time after the endovascular occlusion. The procedure time and quantity of iodine contrast medium were also documented.

2.5. Safety and Efficacy Assessments

Safety evaluation was based on adverse events according to the classification of the Society of Interventional Radiology (SIR) [11]. Day 5 and Day 30 post-intervention visits were conducted by senior radiologists to evaluate the efficacy of the treatment. Primary efficacy was defined as the absence of death or complementary intervention during the first month, including rescue splenectomy, vascular spleen anomalies, urgent embolization or re-embolization, and hemorrhagic complications. There was also a focus on pancreatic complications secondary to dorsal pancreatic artery occlusion. The percentage of residual spleen parenchyma was evaluated one month after the follow-up CT scan by two consenting expert radiologists.

2.6. Statistics

The statistical analysis was performed using Biostatgv. Qualitative variables were described in numbers and proportions, and quantitative variables were represented as median values and standard deviations (SDs). The χ^2 test was used to compare categorical variables. A nonparametric Fisher's exact test was used if these were not validated. The continuous values were compared using the Student t-test (parametric variables) or the Wilcoxon–Mann–Whitney test (nonparametric variables). Results were deemed statistically significant at $p < 0.05$.

3. Results

3.1. Patients

A total of 71 patients from sixteen Level 1 trauma centers in France were enrolled in the study from 6 February 2014 to 1 September 2017. The surgical team refused one patient, three patients were excluded due to non-inclusion criteria, one patient withdrew consent, one refused PPSAE treatment, and eight were lost to follow-up or had no CT on Day 30. Finally, 57 patients were reviewed (Figure 2). The leading traumatic cause was a traffic accident (n = 35/57, 61.4%), followed by sports (n = 14/57, 24.5%), work (n = 3/57, 5.2%), and domestic accidents (n = 2/57, 3.5%). Most patients had AAST-OIS 3 (n = 33/57, 57.9%) or AAST-OIS 4 (n = 23/57, 40.3%) spleen injury; however, AAST-OIS 5 lesions were less common (n = 1/57, 1.8%) (Table 2). All patients underwent PPSAE. Thirty-seven patients (n = 37/57, 64.9%) were polytrauma patients with a mean NISS of 19.6 (SD = +/−8.1).

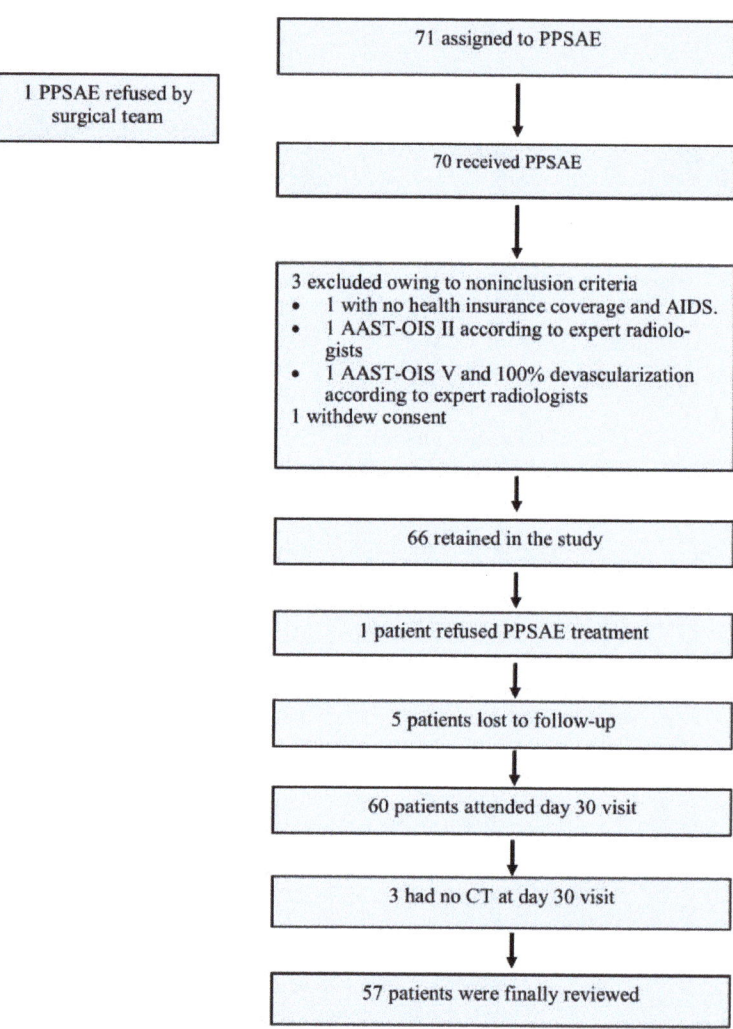

Figure 2. Flowchart.

Table 2. Patient characteristics.

Characteristics	Patients
Sex	
Male	47/57 (82.4%)
Female	10/57 (17.6%)
Age	31 (SD = +/−7.5 years)
Circumstances of injury	
Traffic	35/57 (61.5%)
Domestic	2/57 (3.5%)
Sport	14/57 (24.6%)
Work	3/57 (5.2%)
Other	3/57 (5.2%)
AAST-OIS grade	
3	33/57 (57.9%)
4	23/57 (40.3%)
5	1/57 (1.8%)
NISS	19.6 (SD = +/−8.1)

3.2. Technical Results

Fifty-three patients had femoral access and only four patients had radial access. Six patients (10.5%) had combined embolization (proximal + distal) due to focal vascular anomalies identified on the DSA but not visible on the initial CT. Embolic agents for distal embolization included gelatin sponge, microcoils, and Onyx®. PPSAE was performed with an Amplatzer™ vascular plug (AVP) in 29 patients (50.9%), a Penumbra occlusion device (POD®) in 18 patients (31.6%), and coils in 10 of the 57 patients (17.5%) (Figure 3).

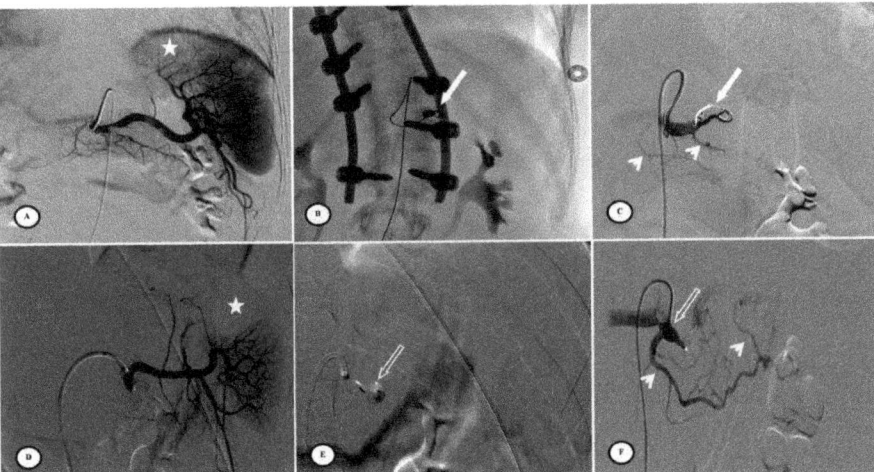

Figure 3. Preventive proximal splenic artery embolization materials. (**A**) Upper pole splenic trauma without focal vascular anomaly (star). (**B**) Penumbra occlusion device (arrow) deployment through a microcatheter along the left lateral aspect of the spine; note that the patient had osteosynthesis material. (**C**) Final control shows complete flow stasis in the splenic artery downstream from the embolic material (arrow) and the development of collateral circulation (arrowheads). (**D**) Another upper pole splenic trauma without focal vascular anomaly (star). (**E**) Amplatzer vascular plug deployment (blank arrow) directly through the Cobra 2 4F catheter. (**F**) Final control displays the development of a collateral pathway through the dorsal pancreatic artery and the great pancreatic artery (arrowheads).

Technical success was achieved in 54 of the 57 patients (94.7%) with complete splenic artery stasis and the development of collateral circulation. Inadvertent distal coil migration occurred in four patients in the other coils group ($n = 4/10$, 40%; $p < 0.01$). There were no procedural complications with AVP or POD. The mean procedure time for all techniques was 56.5 min (SD = 38.1 min) with no significant difference between groups. The mean quantity of iodine contrast injected was 70.0 mL (SD = 42.0 mL), with less contrast injected in the AVP group ($p < 0.01$) (Table 3).

Table 3. Comparison of technical and clinical parameters according to embolization equipment.

	AVP ($n = 29$)	POD ($n = 18$)	Microcoils ($n = 10$)	p
OIS-AAST grade				
Grade 3	18	11	4	0.48
Grade 4	10	7	6	0.40
Grade 5	1	0	0	1
Technical success (%)	100	100	60	<0.01
Clinical efficacy (%)	96.6	94.4	100	1
Procedure time (min, mean +/− SD)	52.3 (41.4)	61.4 (39.3)	67 (68.7)	0.2
Contrast (mL, mean +/−SD)	57 (25.8)	83.2 (56.4)	88.3 (57.8)	<0.01
Spleen parenchyma J30 (%, mean+/−SD)	90.5 (11.1)	82.8 (17.9)	82.9 (10.3)	<0.01

3.3. Safety, Efficacy, and One-Month Splenic Salvage

According to the SIR classification, no procedure-related Grade 3 or higher adverse events (AEs) existed. Mild AEs included puncture site hematoma ($n = 2/57$, 3.5%) and puncture site pain ($n = 5/57$, 8.7%). Primary efficacy was achieved in 97% of cases but two patients were re-embolized; one for active bleeding on Day 6 (Figure 4) and the other for an arteriovenous fistula on Day 30 (Figure 5). No deaths, rescue splenectomies, or hemorrhagic, infectious, or thromboembolic complications occurred. Secondary efficacy was high, with no cases of necrotic pancreatitis and a high splenic salvage rate (94.7%), as only three cases of < 50% vascularized spleen parenchyma were observed at the consultation on Day 30. The average percentage of vascularized spleens at one month was 86.7% (SD = 14.2%), with more vascularized parenchyma in the AVP group ($p < 0.01$).

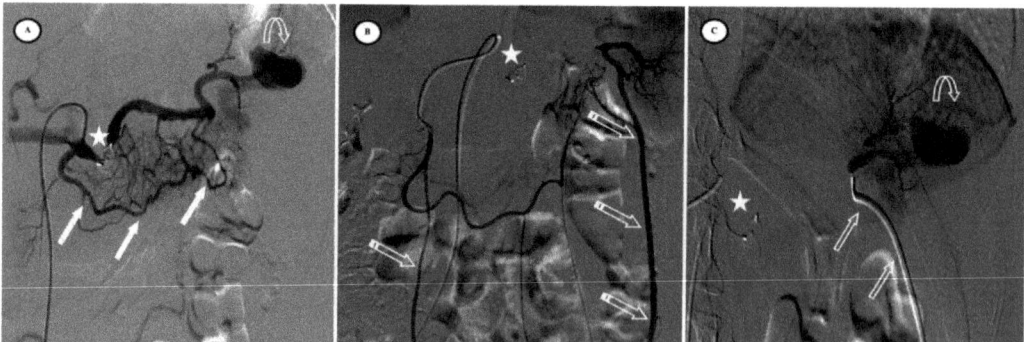

Figure 4. Secondary pseudoaneurysm formation 6 days after preventive proximal splenic artery embolization (PPSAE). (**A**) shows PPSAE with a vascular plug (star) and the development of collateral circulation (arrows) alongside pseudoaneurysm formation (curved arrow). (**B**) displays the dominant collateral circulation via the gastroepiploic artery (striped arrows). (**C**) Microcatheter selection of the gastroepiploic artery for distal embolization (blank arrows).

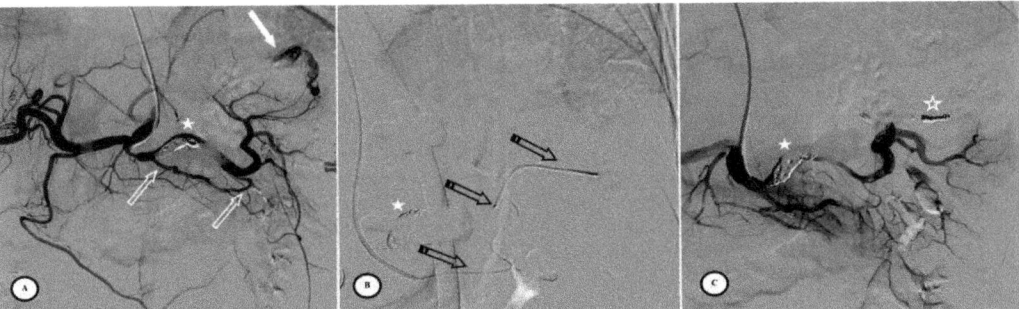

Figure 5. Secondary arteriovenous (AV) fistula development 30 days after preventive proximal splenic artery embolization (PPSAE). (**A**) shows PPSAE using Penumbra occlusion device (star), the subsequent development of collateral circulation mainly through the dorsal pancreatic artery and the great pancreatic artery (blank arrows), and the secondary AV fistula (arrow). (**B**) illustrates the distal microcatheter selection (striped arrow) through radial access. (**C**) shows microcoil embolization (blank star) with satisfying angiographic results.

4. Discussion

This study demonstrates the safety and efficacy of PPSAE treatment in high-grade blunt splenic trauma without active bleeding detected on the initial CT. Technical success was defined as the correct deposition of embolic material with complete flow stasis downstream with the development of collateral circulation. This was achieved in 94.1% of cases. No patients suffered any major adverse events according to the SIR classification. Based on the absence of complications or reinterventions before 1 month, primary efficacy was achieved in 97% of cases; two patients were re-embolized, one for active bleeding on Day 6, and another for an arteriovenous fistula on Day 30. The splenic salvage rate was as high as 94.7%, with only three patients having less than 50% of vascularized spleen parenchyma on Day 30. No splenectomies were performed. No instances of ischemic pancreatitis were reported.

The current study provided prospective data about PPSAE in patients with high-grade (AAST-OIS $\geq$ 3) splenic injuries, which is lacking in the literature. It illustrates the real-life daily practice conditions of various French teams with varied experience, using different materials, which increases generalizability. PPSAE was very safe with no salvage splenectomy. One recent study concluded that PPSAE reduces the need for splenectomy even in hemodynamically unstable patients [12]. In line with the findings of other studies [11,12], secondary complications, such as splenic abscess/infarction and pancreatitis, feared in splenic embolization, were not observed. PPSAE contributes to splenic preservation, considering its vital role in the immune system since splenectomy is associated with recurrent, potentially fatal, systemic infections [13].

As in previous studies, the spleen rescue rate was 94.7%, with no SIR Grade 3 or higher procedure-related AEs [1,4,14–25]. Less spleen necrosis was significantly found after embolization with AVP. It is reasonable to assume that embolizing the shortest possible splenic artery segment potentially reduces ischemic complications because this approach preserves proximal and distal side branches that can function as collateral pathways [8]. Combined distal and proximal embolization may be performed in instances of focal vascular injury. Distal embolization results in the occlusion of smaller segmental branches, which are end arteries; thus, there is an increase in potential parenchymal wedge infarction or abscess development. Some patients have multiple bleeding sites, which may be missed due to vasospasm caused by trauma. This could lead to rebleeding at sites that were not selectively embolized, which is unlikely after proximal splenic artery embolization. Some authors consider distal splenic artery embolization to be more technically challenging than proximal embolization. This is because the catheter must be navigated throughout the splenic artery, which may be tortuous, and segmental branches must be microcatheterized. Distal splenic embolization can be more time-consuming than proximal splenic embolization and may be counterproductive in potentially life-threatening traumatic settings [26]. After successful distal embolization, PPSAE is recommended because some arterial anomalies may not be seen on the initial angiography and may cause delayed bleeding after the vasospasm has subsided [3]. Collaterals keep blood flowing to the spleen, preventing infarction and abscess formation, maintaining the splenic immune system, and saving an access route if re-embolization is indicated [8,11,12]. There are several collateral pathways to the splenic artery after PPSAE: (1) The dorsal pancreatic artery to the transverse pancreatic artery to the great pancreatic artery pathway, leading to the mid/distal splenic artery. The great pancreatic artery should, therefore, not be embolized distally; (2) The great pancreatic artery to the caudal pancreatic artery for cases of inadvertent embolization distal to the great pancreatic artery; (3) The right gastroepiploic artery to the left gastroepiploic, leading to the distal splenic artery/inferior polar branch; (4) The left gastric artery to short gastric arteries (region of the fundus), leading to branches of the splenic artery (10–12). As a general rule, coils should be sized to be 20–30% larger, and plugs should be sized 30–50% larger than the target vessel [27]. Following the current Advisory Committee on Immunization Practices recommendations, we defined the threshold of the vascularized spleen to be 50% under which the patient is considered asplenic on the Day 30 consultation [9,28]. We also insist that complications are relevant to the procedure but also to the severity of trauma, i.e., with a high AAST-OIS score [29].

The mean procedure time was 57 min, whatever the equipment used, thus making this technique a fast, reliable option for intensive care doctors, as it remains within the golden hour field of damage control radiology. Studies have suggested that AVP has a shorter procedural time than POD or coils, but the difference is not always statistically significant [30–32]. Similarly, the use of AVP results in shorter fluoroscopy than other techniques [30,32]. The mean quantity of contrast medium injected was 71 mL, i.e., around 1 mL/kg, per FDA prescribing information [33]. Less iodine was injected using AVP in favor of procedures requiring less iterative control. The AVP procedures were, therefore, faster, with less iodine injection, and less fluoroscopy time. Thus, meeting the criteria of damage control radiology, equivalent to damage control surgery, leads us to recommend using AVP when anatomically possible.

Regarding procedural complications, coil migration with conventional microcoils was the most notable complication occurring in 40% of cases. This is probably related to the flexible nature of these coils, which are not really anchored in the splenic artery's wall. Initially well-positioned, they will be mobilized by the high-flow splenic artery. Thus, we recommend using either AVP or POD devices, which are more rigid, better anchored in the artery wall and, therefore, less mobilizable by the flow. Indeed, technical success was 100% with these two devices. If an endovascular reintervention is needed, the AVP results in a shorter occluded segment, theoretically sparing the collateral pathways through the dorsal and great pancreatic arteries [34].

Following splenic artery embolization, clinical and radiological assessments are essential during post-intervention visits. According to the SPLASH study, a contrast-enhanced CT scan should be carried out on Day 5 and Day 30 following the intervention [9]. Apart from severe splenic infarction, possible side effects include ischemic pancreatitis or other nontarget embolization. None of these possible complications were reported in this ancillary study. The patient should, nevertheless, be regularly monitored for the emergence of pseudoaneurysms or secondary splenic rupture [34].

PPSAE is a promising preventive and therapeutic option for high-grade spleen trauma and is deemed safe and efficient when the proper technique is used. AVP is advantageous due to a lower degree of iodine contrast agent use and a higher splenic salvage rate. However, using AVP may be a challenge in cases of catheter instability or when the median arcuate ligament compresses the CeT; thus, we recommend using rigid microcoils, such as

POD, through a microcatheter. We discourage using softer microcoils due to the high risk of distal migration.

Our study has certain limitations. First, it was not designed to analyze differences between embolization equipment. There were no restrictions and the choice of the material was left to the operator's discretion. This is why we have different types of materials used and heterogeneous groups. Second, we did not include radiation exposure parameters. Unfortunately, this information was not available to all centers and was not part of the prospectively collected data. Third, we did not include microeconomic data.

5. Conclusions

To conclude, PPSAE for high-grade splenic trauma without vascular anomaly on initial CT, using AVP or POD, resulted in excellent splenic salvage. It was safe and quick, without major complications, and did not prevent secondary embolization of the splenic artery downstream of the material due to the high vascular collaterality. Thus, PPSAE seems to be a solid therapeutic option for managing high-grade (AAST-OIS $\geq$ 3) splenic trauma, providing high feasibility, safety, and efficacy rates.

Author Contributions: Conceptualization: J.-P.B.; methodology: J.F.; software: J.G.; validation: C.A. and S.B.; writing—preparation of the original draft, review and editing: S.S. All authors have read and agreed to the published version of the manuscript.

Funding: This research received no external funding.

Institutional Review Board Statement: The study was conducted in accordance with the Declaration of Helsinki, and approved by the Institutional Review Board of CHU de Grenoble (Réf CCP 13-CHUG-21, accepted 21 June 2013).

Informed Consent Statement: Informed consent was obtained from all subjects involved in the study.

Data Availability Statement: Data is unavailable due to privacy and ethical restrictions.

Acknowledgments: We wish to thank Teresa Sawyers, Medical Writer at the BESPIM, Nîmes University Hospital, France, for her help with the final version of this article.

Conflicts of Interest: The authors declare no conflict of interest.

References

1. Requarth, J.A.; D'Agostino, R.B.; Miller, P.R. Nonoperative management of adult blunt splenic injury with and without splenic artery embolotherapy: A meta-analysis. *J. Trauma* **2011**, *71*, 898–903, discussion 903. [CrossRef] [PubMed]
2. Zarzaur, B.L.; Croce, M.A.; Fabian, T.C. Variation in the Use of Urgent Splenectomy After Blunt Splenic Injury in Adults. *J. Trauma Acute Care Surg.* **2011**, *71*, 1333. [CrossRef] [PubMed]
3. Quencer, K.B.; Smith, T.A. Review of proximal splenic artery embolization in blunt abdominal trauma. *CVIR Endovasc.* **2019**, *2*, 11. [CrossRef] [PubMed]
4. Banerjee, A.; Duane, T.M.; Wilson, S.P.; Haney, S.; O'Neill, P.J.; Evans, H.L.; Como, J.J.; Claridge, J.A. Trauma center variation in splenic artery embolization and spleen salvage: A multicenter analysis. *J. Trauma Acute Care Surg.* **2013**, *75*, 69–74, discussion 74–75. [CrossRef]
5. Stassen, N.A.; Bhullar, I.; Cheng, J.D.; Crandall, M.L.; Friese, R.S.; Guillamondegui, O.D.; Jawa, R.S.; Maung, A.A.; Rohs, T.J., Jr.; Sangosanya, A.; et al. Selective nonoperative management of blunt splenic injury: An Eastern Association for the Surgery of Trauma practice management guideline. *J. Trauma Acute Care Surg.* **2012**, *73* (Suppl. S4), S294–S300. [CrossRef]
6. Patil, M.S.; Goodin, S.Z.; Findeiss, L.K. Update: Splenic Artery Embolization in Blunt Abdominal Trauma. *Semin Intervent. Radiol.* **2020**, *37*, 97–102. [CrossRef]
7. Padia, S.A.; Ingraham, C.R.; Moriarty, J.M.; Wilkins, L.R.; Bream, P.R.; Tam, A.L.; Patel, S.; McIntyre, L.; Wolinsky, P.R.; Hanks, S.E. Society of Interventional Radiology Position Statement on Endovascular Intervention for Trauma. *J. Vasc. Interv. Radiol.* **2020**, *31*, 363–369.e2. [CrossRef]
8. Xu, S.S.; Eng, K.; Accorsi, F.; Cool, D.W.; Wiseman, D.; Mujoomdar, A.; Cardarelli-Leite, L. Proximal splenic artery embolization using a vascular plug in grade IV or V splenic trauma—A single centre 11-year experience. *CVIR Endovasc.* **2023**, *6*, 1. [CrossRef]
9. Arvieux, C.; Frandon, J.; Tidadini, F.; Monnin-Bares, V.; Foote, A.; Dubuisson, V.; Lermite, E.; David, J.-S.; Douane, F.; Tresallet, C.; et al. Effect of Prophylactic Embolization on Patients With Blunt Trauma at High Risk of Splenectomy: A Randomized Clinical Trial. *JAMA Surg.* **2020**, *155*, 1102–1111. [CrossRef]

10. Duranteau, J.; Asehnoune, K.; Pierre, S.; Ozier, Y.; Leone, M.; Lefrant, J.Y. Recommandations sur la réanimation du choc hémorragique. *Anesth. Réanim.* **2015**, *1*, 62–74. [CrossRef]
11. Khalilzadeh, O.; Baerlocher, M.O.; Shyn, P.B.; Connolly, B.L.; Devane, A.M.; Morris, C.S.; Cohen, A.M.; Midia, M.; Thornton, R.H.; Gross, K.; et al. Proposal of a New Adverse Event Classification by the Society of Interventional Radiology Standards of Practice Committee. *J. Vasc. Interv. Radiol.* **2017**, *28*, 1432–1437.e3. [CrossRef]
12. Zoppo, C.; Valero, D.A.; Murugan, V.A.; Pavidapha, A.; Flahive, J.; Newbury, A.; Fallon, E.; Harman, A. Splenic Artery Embolization for Unstable Patients with Splenic Injury: A Retrospective Cohort Study. *J. Vasc. Interv. Radiol.* **2023**, *34*, 86–93. [CrossRef]
13. Demetriades, D.; Scalea, T.M.; Degiannis, E.; Barmparas, G.; Konstantinidis, A.; Massahis, J.; Inaba, K. Blunt splenic trauma: Splenectomy increases early infectious complications: A prospective multicenter study. *J. Trauma Acute Care Surg.* **2012**, *72*, 229. [CrossRef]
14. Schnüriger, B.; Inaba, K.; Konstantinidis, A.; Lustenberger, T.; Chan, L.S.; Demetriades, D. Outcomes of proximal versus distal splenic artery embolization after trauma: A systematic review and meta-analysis. *J. Trauma* **2011**, *70*, 252–260. [CrossRef]
15. Bhangu, A.; Nepogodiev, D.; Lal, N.; Bowley, D.M. Meta-analysis of predictive factors and outcomes for failure of non-operative management of blunt splenic trauma. *Injury* **2012**, *43*, 1337–1346. [CrossRef]
16. Sclafani, S.J.; Shaftan, G.W.; Scalea, T.M.; Patterson, L.A.; Kohl, L.; Kantor, A.; Herskowitz, M.M.; Michael, M.; Hoffer, E.K.; Henry, S.; et al. Nonoperative salvage of computed tomography-diagnosed splenic injuries: Utilization of angiography for triage and embolization for hemostasis. *J. Trauma* **1995**, *39*, 818–825, discussion 826–827. [CrossRef]
17. Haan, J.M.; Bochicchio, G.V.; Kramer, N.; Scalea, T.M. Nonoperative management of blunt splenic injury: A 5-year experience. *J. Trauma* **2005**, *58*, 492–498. [CrossRef]
18. Haan, J.M.; Biffl, W.; Knudson, M.M.; Davis, K.A.; Oka, T.; Majercik, S.; Dicker, R.; Marder, S.; Scalea, T.M. Splenic embolization revisited: A multicenter review. *J. Trauma* **2004**, *56*, 542–547. [CrossRef]
19. Rong, J.J.; Liu, D.; Liang, M.; Wang, Q.H.; Sun, J.Y.; Zhang, Q.Y.; Peng, C.-F.; Xuan, F.-Q.; Zhao, L.-J.; Tian, X.-X.; et al. The impacts of different embolization techniques on splenic artery embolization for blunt splenic injury: A systematic review and meta-analysis. *Mil. Med. Res.* **2017**, *4*, 17. [CrossRef]
20. Dent, D.; Alsabrook, G.; Erickson, B.A.; Myers, J.; Wholey, M.; Stewart, R.; Root, H.; Ferral, H.; Postoak, D.; Napier, D.; et al. Blunt splenic injuries: High nonoperative management rate can be achieved with selective embolization. *J. Trauma* **2004**, *56*, 1063–1067. [CrossRef]
21. Bessoud, B.; Denys, A.; Calmes, J.M.; Madoff, D.; Qanadli, S.; Schnyder, P.; Doenz, F. Nonoperative management of traumatic splenic injuries: Is there a role for proximal splenic artery embolization? *AJR Am. J. Roentgenol.* **2006**, *186*, 779–785. [CrossRef] [PubMed]
22. Rajani, R.R.; Claridge, J.A.; Yowler, C.J.; Patrick, P.; Wiant, A.; Summers, J.I.; McDonald, A.A.; Como, J.J.; Malangoni, M.A. Improved outcome of adult blunt splenic injury: A cohort analysis. *Surgery* **2006**, *140*, 625–631, discussion 631–632. [CrossRef] [PubMed]
23. Miller, P.R.; Chang, M.C.; Hoth, J.J.; Mowery, N.T.; Hildreth, A.N.; Martin, R.S.; Holmes, J.H.; Meredith, W.J.; Requarth, J.A. Prospective trial of angiography and embolization for all grade III to V blunt splenic injuries: Nonoperative management success rate is significantly improved. *J. Am. Coll. Surg.* **2014**, *218*, 644–648. [CrossRef] [PubMed]
24. Albrecht, R.M.; Schermer, C.R.; Morris, A. Nonoperative management of blunt splenic injuries: Factors influencing success in age >55 years. *Am. Surg.* **2002**, *68*, 227–230, discussion 230–231. [CrossRef]
25. McIntyre, L.K.; Schiff, M.; Jurkovich, G.J. Failure of nonoperative management of splenic injuries: Causes and consequences. *Arch Surg.* **2005**, *140*, 563–568, discussion 568–569. [CrossRef]
26. Splenic Artery Embolization: Proximal or Distal? Endovascular Today. Bryn Mawr Communications. Available online: https://evtoday.com/articles/2018-apr/splenic-artery-embolization-proximal-or-distal (accessed on 11 April 2023).
27. Vaidya, S.; Tozer, K.R.; Chen, J. An Overview of Embolic Agents. *Semin Intervent. Radiol.* **2008**, *25*, 204–215. [CrossRef]
28. Crooker, K.G.; Howard, J.M.; Alvarado, A.R.; McDonald, T.J.; Berry, S.D.; Green, J.L.; Winfield, R.D. Splenic Embolization After Trauma: An Opportunity to Improve Best Immunization Practices. *J. Surg. Res.* **2018**, *232*, 293–297. [CrossRef]
29. Frandon, J.; Rodiere, M.; Arvieux, C.; Vendrell, A.; Boussat, B.; Sengel, C.; Broux, C.; Bricault, I.; Ferretti, G.; Thony, F. Blunt splenic injury: Are early adverse events related to trauma, nonoperative management, or surgery? *Diagn. Interv. Radiol.* **2015**, *21*, 327–333. [CrossRef]
30. Gunn, A.J.; Raborn, J.R.; Griffin, R.; Stephens, S.W.; Richman, J.; Jansen, J.O. A pilot randomized controlled trial of endovascular coils and vascular plugs for proximal splenic artery embolization in high-grade splenic trauma. *Abdom. Radiol.* **2021**, *46*, 2823–2832. [CrossRef]
31. Jambon, E.; Hocquelet, A.; Petitpierre, F.; Le Bras, Y.; Marcelin, C.; Dubuisson, V.; Grenier, N.; Cornelis, F. Proximal embolization of splenic artery in acute trauma: Comparison between Penumbra occlusion device versus coils or Amplatzer vascular plug. *Diagn. Interv. Imaging* **2018**, *99*, 801–808. [CrossRef]
32. Johnson, P.; Wong, K.; Chen, Z.; Bercu, Z.L.; Newsome, J.; West, D.L.; Dariushnia, S.; Findeiss, L.K.; Kokabi, N. Meta-analysis of Intraprocedural Comparative Effectiveness of Vascular Plugs vs. Coils in Proximal Splenic Artery Embolization and Associated Patient Radiation Exposure. *Curr. Probl. Diagn. Radiol.* **2021**, *50*, 623–628. [CrossRef]

33. FDA. OMNIPAQUE-Iohexol Injection, Solution. FDA Report. Available online: https://fda.report/DailyMed/ba2fb00e-ba4c-48d4-81ad-93371a63a902 (accessed on 21 December 2022).
34. Boscà-Ramon, A.; Ratnam, L.; Cavenagh, T.; Chun, J.Y.; Morgan, R.; Gonsalves, M.; Das, R.; Ameli-Renani, S.; Pavlidis, V.; Hawthorn, B.; et al. Impact of site of occlusion in proximal splenic artery embolisation for blunt splenic trauma. *CVIR Endovasc.* **2022**, *5*, 43. [CrossRef]

Disclaimer/Publisher's Note: The statements, opinions and data contained in all publications are solely those of the individual author(s) and contributor(s) and not of MDPI and/or the editor(s). MDPI and/or the editor(s) disclaim responsibility for any injury to people or property resulting from any ideas, methods, instructions or products referred to in the content.

MDPI AG
Grosspeteranlage 5
4052 Basel
Switzerland
Tel.: +41 61 683 77 34

Journal of Personalized Medicine Editorial Office
E-mail: jpm@mdpi.com
www.mdpi.com/journal/jpm

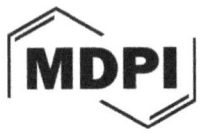

Disclaimer/Publisher's Note: The statements, opinions and data contained in all publications are solely those of the individual author(s) and contributor(s) and not of MDPI and/or the editor(s). MDPI and/or the editor(s) disclaim responsibility for any injury to people or property resulting from any ideas, methods, instructions or products referred to in the content.

www.ingramcontent.com/pod-product-compliance
Lightning Source LLC
LaVergne TN
LVHW070735100526
838202LV00013B/1238